A Manifesto for Menta

Peter Kinderman

A Manifesto for Mental Health

Why We Need a Revolution in Mental Health Care

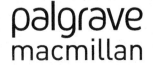

Peter Kinderman
Department of Psychological Sciences
University of Liverpool
Liverpool, UK

ISBN 978-3-030-24385-2   ISBN 978-3-030-24386-9   (eBook)
https://doi.org/10.1007/978-3-030-24386-9

Cover credit: MirageC/gettyimages

This Palgrave Macmillan imprint is published by the registered company Springer Nature Switzerland AG
The registered company address is: Gewerbestrasse 11, 6330 Cham, Switzerland

Contents

1

Introduction

We are changing—and improving—the ways in which we plan and deliver mental health services. But if we are to continue to improve, we need to change the way we think about mental health. Instead of a 'disease model', which assumes that emotional distress is merely a symptom of biological illness, we would all benefit if we were to embrace and implement a social and psychological approach to mental health and wellbeing that recognises our essential and shared humanity.

I am an optimist. Our mental health services are far from perfect. But if we elect the right kinds of politicians and implement the right kinds of policies, change is possible.

In 1967, Martin Luther King said that: '*...there are some things in our society, some things in our world, to which we... must always be maladjusted if we are to be people of good will.... There comes a time when one must take a stand that is neither safe, nor politic, nor popular. But one must take it because it is right*'.[1] When we look at our current approach to mental health care, we still have a lot about which we should be 'maladjusted', and there is a lot about which we must take a stand. As I was making final preparations for the publication of this book, a doctoral student was interviewing people on mental health wards in the

© The Author(s) 2019
P. Kinderman, *A Manifesto for Mental Health*,
https://doi.org/10.1007/978-3-030-24386-9_1

North–West of the UK about their views on the protection of their human rights. One participant reported that she didn't feel safe on her psychiatric ward (a damning comment in itself). She reported how she had woken up the night before to see one of the other residents with her hands around another woman's neck. *'It's a risk...'*, she said, *'... but, I've learned to cope. I smear Vaseline on my neck; it means their hands can't get a grip'*. What an indictment. In the fifth largest economy in the world, and in a nation that prides itself on its values, a woman in our mental health care system has to use Vaseline to protect herself from assault.

Many of the horrors of previous generations' attempts to offer 'care' are thankfully behind us. My generation have not had to run the risk of lobotomy or insulin coma therapy. The people I love have not been forced to weigh up the possible risk and benefits of having an ice pick hammered into their brains through the thin bone just above the orbit of the eye, and then wiggled from side to side to destroy the delicate nerve tissue in the frontal lobes of the brain. We are lucky. Around 66,000 people were subjected to lobotomies before the Soviet Union banned the practice (which had won its inventor a Nobel Prize in 1949) in 1950 on moral grounds and the use of lobotomy declined worldwide.

But we have absolutely no reasons to rest on our laurels. As I was preparing this book, some of my colleagues were preparing for a twenty-first-century version of lobotomy. At the 2018 Annual Conference of the UK's Royal College of Psychiatrists, delegates promoted the benefits of localised destruction of brain tissue. The claim (in the words of one colleague via a personal email) is that *'...precise lesioning... interrupts the neural circuits that drive obsessional thoughts...'* There is something chilling, incidentally, in the use of the words 'precise lesioning'. The now notorious 'ice pick' lobotomy technique used in the past was euphemistically called the 'precision method'. I don't doubt the motivations of my colleagues looking to help people with serious and even life-threatening problems. But I do doubt the wisdom of approaching things from such a reductionist biomedical perspective.

A short time ago, I accompanied a friend to a stressful appointment with her family doctor. My friend wanted to discuss an 'advance directive', a quasi-legal summary of her wishes as to how she expected to be cared for if she became unable to make decisions for herself. Because of aversive experiences with mental health care in the past, my friend made it clear that, under no circumstances whatsoever would she accept psychiatric care. And she knew that the law, in the form of the Mental Health Act, was insufficient to protect her. Rather than ensuring that her needs are met, my friend feared that the Mental Health Act gives unprecedented powers to mental health professionals, without any immediate need to seek judicial approval, to detain and medicate any person whom they believe to be 'ill', despite—or, more properly, against—the wishes of that person.

Care rather than Containment

In the UK, we spend around 10% of our (substantial) national wealth on health care, a figure which has risen steadily over the years (although substantially dependent on which politicians we elect).[2] In general, we spend that investment efficiently, because we have a nationalised healthcare system, the National Health Service (NHS). And we spend a relatively high proportion of that healthcare budget on mental health, around 12% in the UK, compared to only 5.5% as the European average. That's all good, but we have a long way to go.

I am not in any sense undermining the efforts of my hard-working colleagues, but the care that people receive, both in community and residential care settings, is inadequate. In 2011, the charity and pressure-group *Rethink Mental Illness* established the independent *Schizophrenia Commission* and in 2012 published the report '*Schizophrenia—The Abandoned Illness*'.[3] The Commission recognised that there will always be a need for some form of residential care for people in acute distress. It seems clear that there will always be individuals within even the most advanced and democratic societies whose problems leave them desperate, at risk of harm from neglect or self-harm, or very occasionally so distressed and angry that they pose a risk to others. Among some excellent recommendations (which echo many of my own views, e.g., in calling for greater access to psychological therapies, a right to a second opinion on medication, greater reliance on the skills of pharmacists and general practitioners, etc.), the Commission called for 'a radical overhaul of poor acute care units'. The Commission's chair, Professor Sir Robin Murray, concluded: '... *the message that comes through loud and clear is that people are being badly let down by the system in every area of their lives'*.

Recently, in the UK, there has been extensive media coverage (appropriately) of the challenges faced by clinicians needing crisis care for children. Our front-line colleagues have found it so difficult to find residential care that children have been placed in residential care only in settings so far from their homes that their parents were practically unable to visit; journalists reported cases where children in serious distress could only be found suitable accommodation 200 miles from home, and a 400 mile round trip, even if parents could afford and had access to transport, takes the whole day.[4] In a remarkable outburst, Sir Justice James Munby, President of the English High Court's family division, ruled that a (normally private) judgement should be made public. The case concerned a girl who had made 'determined' attempts to kill herself since being detained, and desperately needed a safe, therapeutic, place to live. For legal reasons, the place in which she was resident was no longer suitable, but the staff caring for her reported that they had simply been unable to find a suitable alternative. Sir James Mumby used his power as a judge to warn of 'blood on our hands' and to order (because judges make 'orders') that the news should not only be made public but also sent to senior government ministers to expose the 'outrage' over the 'lack of proper provision for X – and, one fears, too many like her'. The upshot, through the combined influences of a high court judge, the media and government ministers, was that (fortunately) a suitable place was then swiftly found.[5]

We're faced with an unenviable choice. When in acute distress (and perhaps when we're finding it difficult to make decisions for ourselves), we are faced with a choice between neglect on the one hand and, on the other, residential units plagued by stress, boredom, a lack of purposeful activity, a lack of staff–patient interaction, and inadequate physical environments. Pressure for 'beds' means that people are often discharged before their problems are resolved or without proper care having been planned for after their discharge. Because there is an emphasis on the treatment of so-called mental illnesses, the idea that the root causes of our problems (violence from parents or spouses, sexual abuse, poverty, unemployment, etc.) would be addressed is a faint hope in any case. On these residential units, there are often unacceptable levels of violence against both staff and members of the public who use mental health services, sexual harassment and theft, with drug and alcohol problems common.

We need to make residential mental health units 'places of safety'. Recently,[6] media in the UK were alerted to a powerful report by one of those regulatory bodies mentioned earlier, the Care Quality Commission. They concluded that sexual harassment, assaults and rapes are 'commonplace' on mental health units in the UK. These crimes were (it was reported) mainly committed by patients. For perfectly under-standable reasons, many people in receipt of mental health care are sexually disinhibited. Many others have had deeply troubling experiences of sexual abuse, experiences which can clearly put us at risk of further, later, exploitation. We must, therefore, ensure that mental health care is genuinely safe and therapeutic. As the care regulator reported, these risks are well-known and predictable, and, and this is the point, the services placed people at risk by having too few members of staff available to provide a safe environment. This is wholly unacceptable. When we are distressed, we need an 'asylum', a place of safety and calm, where we can resolve tension and stress and overcome trauma... not be exposed to abuse and assault.

As I suggested earlier, respectable commentators have suggested that the UK has one of the better mental healthcare systems (at least in 2006)[7] and so we should; we're wealthy enough to afford it. Rather unfortunately, that suggests that people in other countries have much worse provision still. In the USA, for example, and reflecting the social inequity in that wealthy society, there are very high levels of investment for the rich, but also neglect for poor and socially disadvantaged people. It's widely estimated that until very recently, with the very welcome development of 'Obamacare', which aimed to make healthcare insurance mandatory, universal and automatic, some 40% of citizens had no healthcare insurance. Despite 'Obamacare', and because of policies by Donald Trump that have dismantled the progress made by Obama, we're still living with that legacy, meaning that only about half of all people with mental health problems receive any form of planned care. For the rest, there's a mixed picture, from various forms of charitable services through to state mental institutions with poor reputations. In the developing world, the picture is again complex. It seems likely that for people who avoid formal psychiatric care, the prognosis is if anything at least as good as in the industrialised world.[8] Formal, institutional, care in much of the developing world is concerning, with disturbing stories of physical restraint, chemical sedation and very poor standards of care.

I have no desire to criticise the hard work of my colleagues, but standards of care in many mental healthcare clinics are disgraceful. I occasionally receive unsolicited letters documenting people's experiences. One recent letter reported: '… *Rather than engaging with the patients on the ward, the staff instead shepherded them around like sheep with bullying commands, threats of "jabs" (injections), and removal to an acute ward elsewhere in the hospital, if they did not co-operate. The staff also stressed medication rather than engagement as a way of controlling the patients. And the staff closeted themselves in the ward office, instead of being out and about on the corridors and in the vestibule where they should have been. The staff wrote daily reports on each patient on the hospital's Intranet system; these reports were depended upon by the consultant psychiatrists for their diagnoses and medication prescriptions, but were patently fabricated and false, because the staff had never engaged or observed properly the patient they were writing about in their reports. The psychiatrists themselves were rarely seen on the ward, and only consulted with their patients once a week*'.

Sadly, many of the stories that emerge from psychiatric hospitals imply that physical force and restraint are used when we either wish to leave environments that we experience as untherapeutic and harmful (perhaps because they are harmful and untherapeutic) or when we decline to take medication that we believe is doing more harm than good (quite possibly because… that's precisely true).[9] Sadly, the stories that emerge seem to have much more to do with punitive practices than anything therapeutic. Early in 2018, the UK government released figures on the use of tasers (electrical stun-guns) by police officers.[10] These revealed that tasers had been used inside mental health units 58 times in a six-month period.

It's true that our low mood, risk of suicide, confusion or disturbed behaviour sometimes puts us at extreme risk or, in very unusual cases, renders us a risk to others. Some form of mental health legislation may well be needed, as I acknowledged when I contributed to the drafting of both the Mental Health Act 2007 and the Mental Capacity Act 2005 on behalf of the British Psychological Society. It is important to offer a robust legislative framework for us if our difficulties put us at significant personal risk, or if we pose a risk to others. But this is a social and psychological problem, not a medical one. Diagnosis and even severity of an 'illness' do not relate to risk and dangerousness. Decisions do need to be made about the necessary care of people with serious problems who are at risk. And, after the fact, decisions need to be made about how to deal with people who have committed crimes. In both cases, current practice in a 'disease model' driven system is flawed. A more coherent and fair approach would be to agree to take decisions on behalf of other people if they are unable to make decisions for themselves, regardless of whether they have a diagnosis… and to make judicial decisions in the criminal justice field on the same basis. This doesn't mean 'letting them off'; it means making appropriate decisions on rational bases.

We are all in the process of escaping an unfortunate history of coercion, with many mental health treatments rooted in moral judgements and punitive approaches.[11] We need to invest appropriately in mental health care. We need to maintain Britain's enviable record in this respect. But we also need to ensure that our investment is leading to high-quality care and ensuring greater wellbeing.

Morality

A psychological perspective on mental health would also be a more positive, optimistic, empathic moral perspective, too. It's often argued that the idea of 'mental illness' protects us from moral judgements. If we aren't seen as 'ill', the argument goes, we'll be seen as lazy or weak. That argument sounds good, but it fails to follow through on its promises. Moral judgements are additional to illness labels, not alternatives. We can see this particularly clearly when it comes to sexuality. In 1952, the

World War II code-breaker Alan Turing took his own life after being prosecuted for an indecency offence; he had been the victim of a theft by his lover and when he reported it to the police, his sexuality was both criminalised and pathologised. Obliged to take Stilboestrol (oestrogen) in an attempt to alter his hormone balance, Turing killed himself with a bite from a cyanide-coated apple. With homosexuality at the time both a mental illness (hence the 'treatment') and a crime, it seems a stretch to argue that illness labels protect us. Homosexuality may no longer be a crime in the UK (we achieved something approaching parity with the passage of the Marriage [Same Sex Couples] Act 2013) and was removed from the American list of mental illnesses in 1973 and from the World Health Organization classification system in 1992. Nevertheless, in 2018, we found it necessary to campaign for political support[12] to end the practice of 'conversion therapy'; the term for therapy that assumes certain sexual orientations and gender identities is inferior to others and seeks to change or suppress them on that basis. The point here is that, instead of protecting us from moral judgements, the illness narrative or 'disease-model' thinking actively uses the idea of physiological pathology to support pejorative moral attitudes.

Of course, the Brain is Important

We all have complex psychological mechanisms that determine how we make sense of the world; how we understand ourselves, other people, relationships, plan for the future, predict people's behaviour and confidently anticipate the outcome of events. Just as language use requires a functioning brain, but the functioning of the brain fails to dictate which dialect is learned, so we need a functioning brain to make emotional sense of the world, but the ways in which we each develop our own framework of understanding is far from biologically predetermined.

Our mental health reflects the way we make sense of the world, our thoughts about ourselves, other people, the world and the future. These 'cognitive schemas' have many of the characteristics of cultural beliefs, and as such any differences between people seem more likely to be learned than biologically determined. Of course, such schemas are emotional and have consequences for our mood and our behaviour, even our physiological status. But that is true for cultural issues too, as anyone attending a rock concert, a religious ceremony, a marriage, a court case or an employment tribunal could testify. Moreover, our past experiences affect how we experience and interpret things that happen in the present. Everybody interprets and reacts to new events and challenges in the light of previous experience.

The human brain makes and 'prunes' around a million synapses a second. It does this in support of learning. Our synaptic networks are fundamental to our emotions, thoughts, beliefs and desires. But it is also a network shaped by and responsive to events. This shaping of associative networks can be extremely elegant. The 'interacting cognitive subsystems' model[13] allows us to map how we learn, from pre-cognitive 'machine learning' (deciphering lines and edges in our visual landscape, for instance, or plotting the patterns of contingent reinforcement that lie behind conditioning of behaviour) through to the derivation of abstract meaning and concepts such as love, belief, trust, truth and justice.

Our brains enable us to learn about the world, rather than dictating our behaviours. This learning must use biological mechanisms, but that does not imply that the learning process can be meaningfully reduced to the level of biology. There are many possible analogies, but one that springs to mind is the steering wheel of a car. The steering wheel is a vital, necessary, logically indispensable (without the invention of alternative technology) element in determining the trajectory of a car. But the steering wheel doesn't determine the direction of travel. The steering wheel enables the car to be driven, but it doesn't drive the car.

Our brains rely on biochemical processes ultimately dependent on gene expression, common to all of us, interacting with our very different experiences. One example of this comes from recent research into inflammatory processes, psychotic experiences and loneliness. We know that a variety of social disadvantages are related to mental health problems. Interestingly, lonely people (and, in fact, lonely macaque monkeys) have inflamed brains; the lonelier we are, the more inflammation researchers have found. This is important. Inflammatory processes interfere with the formation and pruning of synapses, presumed to be part of the process of learning. That illustrates at least one route by which social disadvantage (in this case loneliness) may influence biological systems to affect learning. And, equally interestingly, loneliness has an impact on our genes. That seems a slightly counter-intuitive idea; we're used to thinking of genes as 'blueprints'. Which, in a way, they are. But genes code for proteins. And the biological production of proteins is not constant; it responds to environmental challenges. So, when a person (or a macaque monkey) experiences a particular challenge, whether that's drought or loneliness, genes are 'switched on'; chemical signals lead to increases in the genetic production of particular proteins. In the case of loneliness, genes involved in our inflammatory response are 'switched on' when an individual is socially isolated. That's fascinating in itself, but it's important to point out that these are not genetic differences between people. We all have these genes. They're just 'switched on' when we're lonely.

Most mental health problems are associated with a very large number of different genes, each of which seems to contribute something, but none of which is the complete explanation. And these genes seem to be non-specific, conveying a tiny (but significant) additional risk of a broad spectrum of mental health problems (and other consequences, including benefits). Where gene variants contribute additively (when the gene variants all add, independent of each other, a little extra risk), then a normal distribution of the consequent problems is the most likely outcome. Where genes interact with each other (when, e.g., the presence of one particular gene variant has a more significant effect when a second gene variant is also present), then the more likely distribution of the consequent problems is exponential (where most of us experience relatively little effect, with only a very few more significantly affected). In other words, very many genes seem to play a role in a broad range of mental health problems (referred to as polygenic load or polygenic risk), and these genetic risk factors can add and interact in a range of different complex ways. But perhaps most importantly, differences between people in the expression of these genes may not depend too much on whether or not people were born with different genetic variants. What seems much more important is how our genes give us the fantastic capacity of our brains to learn and respond to the environment. And the environment still presents us all with huge challenges to our mental health and wellbeing.

Making Sense of Things

We don't merely react passively to life events. Learning is core to the human experience, and for humans, this learning is abstract, complex and cognitive. We construct mental models of the world as a consequence of our experiences, through our relationships and by learning from others, through the conscious and unconscious development of meaning. Life events impact on our mental health through their effects on our psychological mechanisms. Economic recessions hurt us, but they do so through the psychological responses to the threat of unemployment, job insecurity and poverty, which includes a range of concepts about meaning and purpose in life, our relationships, the expectations of other people (including the expectations set out for us by our politicians) and even what we understand that it means to be a working man or working woman and our obligations to provide for our families.

One of the supreme accomplishments of the human brain is the capacity for abstract thought. We have an enormous potential for learning. Uniquely among all the animals, we made a huge evolutionary leap by developing the ability to extract abstract, meaningful or 'implicational', representations of the world and then manipulate these abstractions. We can predict the future and understand the rules behind schedules of reinforcement. We learn to understand problems in order to solve them, not merely act in hope of reward. And we model our behaviour on other people; we learn the rules of social behaviour. What we believe about ourselves, our abilities, strengths and weaknesses, what we hope—or fear—for the future and our beliefs about the nature of the world, especially the social world, is crucial to our mental health. If we believe someone close to us is untrustworthy, or even dangerous, it really does matter. It obviously matters if we believe that there is no hope, no future and no point in carrying on living. It is ridiculous to assume that, unless a doctor has diagnosed an 'illness', all we can do is condemn people for their weakness.

What we believe, how we think about the world, how we have learned to think about the world, is profoundly important. It has real causal power. If you believe that your life has no meaning, that the future is bleak, then there are profound consequences. It is important to recognise that these beliefs do not arise merely as some form of symptom of an illness. There are reasons why people learn to view the world in the ways they do; we learn. But it's also important to recognise the fundamental importance of these psychological issues.

Only Us: Labels are for Objects, not People

A terrible murder was committed in 1860 at Road Hill House in the village of Road in Wiltshire, which shocked Victorian society. The murder became the real-life inspiration for crime thrillers by authors like Wilkie Collins and was detailed by Kate Summerscale in 'The Suspicions of Mr Whicher'.[14] Because the house was locked up securely for the night, there was the inescapable conclusion that one member of the extended family (parents, siblings, step-children, servants, etc.) must have been responsible for the fatal knife-wounds on the body of a four-year-old boy. The mystery itself was never fully solved, and we don't know for sure who killed the child. But what shocked the Victorians was the idea that an apparently normal middle-class family might be harbouring a murderous secret. Moreover, that secret lay on the cusp between evil, madness, and sanity. As the newspaper-reading classes speculated, *The Times* newspaper published a rather remarkable editorial on Saturday 22 July 1854:

> Nothing can be more slightly defined than the line of demarcation between sanity and insanity. Physicians and lawyers have vexed themselves with attempts at definitions in a case where definition is impossible. There has never yet been given to the world anything in the shape of a formula upon this subject which may not be torn to shreds in five minutes by any ordinary logician. Make the definition too narrow, it becomes

meaningless; make it too wide, the whole human race are involved in the drag-net. In strictness, we are all mad as often as we give way to passion, to prejudice, to vice to vanity; but if all the passionate, prejudiced, vicious, and vain people in this world are to be locked up as lunatics, who is to keep the keys to the asylum?[15]

This speaks to a truth recognised at least implicitly for over 100 years; that we cannot reliably and validly dissect categorical diagnoses in the field of mental health. As long ago as 1854, this editorial concluded that we are unable to agree, reliably and validly, on the presence or absence of madness, the 'line of demarcation between sanity and insanity'. Moreover, in this editorial is the observation that such problems lie on continua. Nobody doubts that we are discussing very real problems. Nobody is suggesting that the issues are either fanciful or trivial. In 1854, a child was murdered. That may be an extremely rare event, but it highlights the serious issues at stake.

A short while ago, in response to significant criticism of psychiatric diagnosis, Alex Langford, a young psychiatrist, published a blog[16] entitled 'Categorically Ill', in which he argued that rejecting a psychiatric diagnosis: '...*mean looking all your friends and family who've had a mental illness in the eye and telling them that their diagnoses were nonsense and they weren't really ill, they shouldn't have seen their doctor for that, they shouldn't have been allowed health insurance or sick leave or medication or treatment for that, that they were just sad, obsessed, stressed or weak...*'. There are many errors in this argument. But central to this way of thinking is the idea that only the concept of psychiatric illness protects us from stigmatising people, ignoring them or castigating them as morally weak or worse. This approach seems to assume that only 'illnesses' are real.

In truth, the benefits of this way of thinking are, like the false dualistic argument, moral rather than scientific. One member of the public put it nicely on Twitter in reply to a thread discussing the benefits of psychiatric diagnosis: '*Amen! If I don't have a diagnosis then I'm not unwell, just weak and imagining things*'. This is the same point as Alex Langford, but from the recipient's position. My position isn't, however, to accept this false dichotomy. I simply don't accept that the only alternative to pathologizing psychiatric diagnosis is either to refuse people *'health insurance or sick leave or medication or treatment'* (as Langford has argued), or that we are *'just sad, obsessed, stressed or weak…'*. Yes, I would agree that sometimes we are sad or stressed, and of course many of us are severely affected by obsessional thoughts, but that alone points out how there is a perfectly logical alternative to diagnosis: simply describe our experiences. The alternative to diagnosis is not *'weakness'* or *'just imagining things'*. Quite apart from the fact that there is absolutely no reason to assume that being given a traditionally pathologizing, stigmatising, psychiatric label that, for many people, acts as a simple synonym for *'lazy, weak and obsessional'*, will act as any protection, the logical alternative isn't a binary choice. I and my colleagues who reject diagnostic labels simply don't regard those of us who are depressed as *'weak'* and *'lazy'*; we regard them as… depressed. Some of us are troubled by obsessional, intrusive, thoughts and they aren't *'weak'* or *'lazy'*, either. They aren't *'ill'*, but they are not *'weak'* or *'lazy'*, either. They are perfectly ordinary (or extraordinary, if you like) people who are experiencing distressing but understandable psychological phenomena. *'Weak'* and *'lazy'* are moral judgements. *'Major depressive disorder'* is a diagnostic label. 'Depression' is an understandable psychological phenomenon. I would suggest: *'Amen! I'm not unwell, I'm not just weak and imagining things. I'm depressed'*.

The traditional diagnostic system runs the risk of pathologising nearly all aspects of our lives, with the inevitable danger that we are 'treated' for what's normal. In the case of children, this risk is very real. We now have the worrying situation that, in the USA in 2014, over 80,000 prescriptions were issued for antidepressants to be taken by children aged 2 and younger, with a truly alarming 20,000 prescriptions for antipsychotic medication for this age group.[17] In the UK, nearly a million prescriptions for Ritalin and related drugs for 'attention deficit hyperactivity disorder' ('ADHD') were dispensed last year, more than double the number of a decade ago.[18] In the USA, the numbers are even higher.

The criteria for such diagnoses are deeply worrying as well as scientifically perplexing. It is important to recognise that children and adults occasionally have very serious problems. Criticism of the diagnostic approach does not mean 'domesticating' people's problems or pretending they don't exist. Quite the opposite, we must acknowledge the deep reality of the difficulties that adults and children face. But that recognition is undermined in the attempt to fit these problems into a disease model.

In the case of 'ADHD', applying a diagnostic framework to the normal variations of childhood behaviour, including even serious problems, has attractions, but ultimately leads to paradoxes and difficulties. When our children are distressed, failing to thrive or presenting challenges to parents, peers or teachers, we need to understand them, and we need to offer realistic and effective help. But I have very serious concerns over the use of psychiatric diagnoses such as 'ADHD' or 'Attention Deficit Hyperactivity Disorder', concerns widely shared by other mental health professionals. Most children (indeed, most people) often fail to '*give close attention to details*' or make '*careless mistakes in schoolwork, at work, or with other activities*'. Most of us often have '*trouble holding attention on tasks or play activities*' and have '*trouble organizing tasks and activities*'. Almost everybody '*avoids, dislikes, or is reluctant to do tasks that require mental effort over a long period of time (such as schoolwork or homework)*', and often '*loses things necessary for tasks and activities (e.g. school materials, pencils, books, tools, wallets, keys, paperwork, eyeglasses, mobile telephones)*'. It's unnecessary to continue; these are examples of distractibility, impulsivity and 'hyperactivity' that have huge overlap with everyday life. It is absolutely true to say that, in order to receive the formal diagnosis of 'ADHD' as a recognised 'disorder', these experiences '*show a persistent pattern of inattention and/or hyperactivity-impulsivity that interferes with functioning or development*' and that they are '*inappropriate for developmental level*'. That's important. Some children experience real difficulties and there are children for whom these kinds of problems are real threats to their wellbeing. But these very real problems aren't abnormal, aren't quintessentially different from normal experiences and aren't pathological. Quite the reverse. These are very real problems… but they are normal problems. As the commentator Phil Hickey points out: '*Has there ever been a small child who didn't fail to give close attention to details or didn't make careless mistakes? Isn't this almost a defining feature of early childhood?… Remember, we're talking about children below the age of seven. Not many five/six year-olds are great organizers*'.[19]

Most psychological phenomena lie on continua like this. Generally, scientific analyses of the distribution of psychological problems have failed to find clear distinctions between the supposedly diagnosable 'illnesses', with authors sharing the conclusions of researchers such as Godfrey Pearlson and Judith Ford that there is '*no point of symptomatic rarity between schizophrenia, psychotic bipolar disorder, and schizoaffective disorder*' and '*the boundaries between clinical entities defined by phenomenology appear to be distributed on a continuum and to lack sharp demarcations*'.[20]

These are not simple, straight-line, relationships. Psychologists understand a wide range of mental health problems through understanding vicious cycles and feedback loops. When something bad happens, maybe somebody passes on a piece of bad news, we tend to feel a little low. The way that human memories work means that, when our mood drops, we are more likely to think about more negative things. It does not follow that, because there is a continuum of experiences, that the one extreme is somehow no longer being differentiated from the other. Indeed, many important physical health problems exist on continua, too. Many of us, these days, are overweight. Some people could do with losing a few pounds, but some people are in serious and acute danger. In these areas, very few people argue that the presence of a continuum implies that we aren't taking these issues seriously.

When it comes to psychological wellbeing, however, the battle to retain the concept of diagnosis seems particularly significant. This may be because there is perceived to be more of a need for spurious certainty in the complex and fluid arena of human emotions. Robert Kendell and Assen Jablensky[21] inadvertently pointed out this paradox when they wrote that: '*most diagnostic concepts have not been shown to be valid in this sense*'... but ... '*possess high utility by virtue of the information about outcome, treatment response, and aetiology that they convey. They are therefore invaluable working concepts for clinicians*'. This is a fascinating quote. Despite the lack of scientific validity, the notion of categorical diagnosis in mental health seems irresistibly attractive. These labels are invaluable 'for clinicians'. It could be argued that, although psychiatric diagnoses fail to differentiate natural entities, they serve functions for traditional psychiatry by emphasising the supposed biological nature of the problems.

Psychiatric language tends to form diagnoses by adding the word 'disorder' to otherwise normal and understood psychological phenomena. The differentiation of a problematic 'disorders' from normal experiences is usually achieved through the use of phrases such as: '...*that cause social or occupational dysfunction*' or '...*are inappropriate for developmental level*' (the latter used in the case of children's problems). These kinds of phrases are circular; a problem is a 'disorder' when it causes problems. They also reflect the idea that such problems lie on continua. Otherwise, why would such criteria be needed?

Using these criteria, a very wide range of normal psychological issues become 'disorders'. We all experience social anxiety from time to time and to different levels of intensity. Converting 'social anxiety' into 'social anxiety disorder' sends many messages, but few of them good. On the positive side of the equation, it might let people know that their problems are recognised (in both senses of the word), understood, validated, explained (and explicable) and have some relief. But often, unfortunately, most people find that diagnosis offers only a spurious promise of such benefits. And such benefits can be achieved without the consequent problems. When we turn 'social anxiety' into 'social anxiety disorder' we offer spurious certainty, we suggest that the problems are pathological, different and the product of pathology. These linguistic games occur throughout psychiatry. We turn 'depression' into 'major depressive disorder', the experience of intrusive thoughts and compulsive behaviours into 'obsessive-compulsive disorder', distress after a traumatic, stressful, event into 'PTSD'.

Most interestingly, we don't seem to feel the need to pathologise otherwise normal experiences in other areas of medicine. We don't diagnose 'fracture disorder' when we suffer broken bones, and we don't have 'tuberculosis disorder'. Perhaps most pertinently, we don't seem to need to add these labels of disorder even when the person's problems lie on continua. Like many people in the West, I have relatively high cholesterol levels. There are various tests, including blood tests, and clinical algorithms that help clinicians decide whether or not prescription is justified. These take into account the fact that levels of cholesterol vary continuously across the general population, but also that high levels of cholesterol are likely to be associated with sharply increased risks of cardiovascular disease. And yet the word hypercholesterolemia isn't followed by the word 'disorder'; I don't have 'hypercholesterolemia disorder', I have high cholesterol levels, and I have been advised to take a statin.

When we reject the diagnostic approach, there is greater prospect for both humane and rational approaches to care. The wonderful Only Us Campaign disputes the idea of 'them' and 'us' and instead proposes that: *'there's a continuum, a scale along which we all slide back and forth during our lives, sometimes happy, occasionally depressed or very anxious; mostly well balanced but with moody moments; usually in touch with reality, but at times detached or even psychotic. When we separate ourselves and imagine humanity divided into two different groups, we hurt those labelled as sick, ill, even mad. We allow stigma, prejudice and exclusion to ruin potentially good and creative lives. But we also hurt ourselves, because we stress ourselves out with false smiles and the suppression of our own vulnerabilities. There is no them and us, THERE'S ONLY US'.*[22]

A New Ethos

The pressure for a new ethos, although often resisted by people in powerful professional roles, has surprisingly influential support.

In 2012, the World Health Organization argued that the way that we care for people with mental health problems is a hidden human rights emergency. The United Nations' international human rights treaty, the *'Convention on the Rights of Persons with Disabilities'*, was issued in 2006, and its implementation is monitored by a body of independent experts appointed by the Human Rights Council known as Special Rapporteurs. In June 2017, Special Rapporteur Dainius Pūras, a practising psychiatrist from Lithuania, issued a report on the right of everyone to the enjoyment of the highest attainable standard of physical and mental health.[23]

The report is soundly based on psychological science, but is also groundbreaking in its honesty. It's worth quoting at length; *'For decades, mental health services have been governed by a reductionist biomedical paradigm that has contributed to the exclusion, neglect, coercion and abuse of people with intellectual, cognitive and psychosocial disabilities, persons with autism and those who deviate from prevailing cultural, social and political norms.... ..... We have been sold a myth that the best solutions for addressing mental health challenges are medications and other biomedical interventions.... Public policies continue to neglect the importance of the preconditions of poor mental health, such as violence, disempowerment, social exclusion and isolation and the breakdown of communities, systemic socioeconomic disadvantage and harmful conditions at work and in schools... Reductive biomedical approaches to treatment that do not adequately address contexts and relationships can no longer be considered compliant with the right to health'.*

The report pulls no punches in condemning neglect of '*the preconditions of poor mental health, such as violence, disempowerment, social exclusion and isolation and the breakdown of communities, systemic socioeconomic disadvantage and harmful conditions at work and in schools...... There exists an almost universal commitment to pay for hospitals, beds and medications instead of building a society in which everyone can thrive...*' It has a stern warning about the dangers of permitting the unrestricted export of a Western, psychiatric, disease-model approach to mental health, one which stresses technical diagnosis, biological explanations and a reliance on pharmacological interventions; '*An effective tool used to elevate global mental health is the use of alarming statistics to indicate the scale and economic burden of "mental disorders".....(t)he current "burden of disease" approach firmly roots the global mental health crisis within a biomedical model, too narrow to be proactive and responsive in addressing mental health issues at the national and global level. The focus on treating individual conditions inevitably leads to.... narrow, ineffective and potentially harmful outcomes... (and) paves the way for further medicalization of global mental health, distracting policymakers from addressing the main risk and protective factors affecting mental health for everyone... The scaling-up of care must not involve the scaling-up of inappropriate care'.*

Drawing on a range of examples and resources, including the British Psychological Society's report '*Understanding psychosis*' (which I helped write), Dr. Pūras's report emphasises the need for a 'paradigm shift' towards offering culturally appropriate psychosocial interventions as the first-line; working in partnership with members of the public who use mental health services and carers; respecting diversity; and taking steps to eliminate coercive treatment and forced confinement. We need all of this to be backed up by a firm commitment to social policy that addresses the root causes, such as poverty, discrimination, abuse and structural inequalities, of poor mental health across whole populations. Among the report's recommendations are that '*The urgent need for a shift in approach should prioritize policy innovation at the population level, targeting social determinants and abandon the predominant medical model that seeks to cure individuals by targeting "disorders". The crisis in mental health should be managed not as a crisis of individual conditions, but as a crisis of social obstacles which hinders individual rights. Mental health policies should address the "power imbalance" rather than "chemical imbalance"*'.

Many of our shared responses to this challenge are uncontroversial; increased funding, calls for greater compassion and understanding, calls to reduce or eliminate stigma, a focus on effective care… but there are also some clear differences between professionals as to the right way forwards.

There are very many good reasons to argue for greater investment in mental health services. The question is whether we're better off investing in more of the same or whether we might gain more if we were to do things differently. We urgently need substantial improvement in our mental health care system. The Organisation for Economic Co-operation and Development estimated in 2018[24] that the direct costs of mental health problems to the UK economy are around £94 billion per year (4% of gross domestic product). Worldwide, the annual costs of mental health problems have been estimated at $2.5 trillion. The personal costs are even higher. In the UK, around 6000 people take their own lives each year, and (partly as a result of advances in the treatment of infection) the most common cause of death in women in the first year after childbirth is now suicide. Every 40 seconds someone kills themselves somewhere in the world. That's nearly a million deaths by suicide each year.

We need, therefore, to invest. But we shouldn't simply double investment into an imperfect system. Reinforcing failure is no solution. Despite the expertise and dedication of NHS staff, our current mental

health services (in the words of the 'Schizophrenia Commission') are: '…
badly letting people down in every area of their lives'. One in five (20%)
of the adult population in the UK takes a psychiatric drug on any given
day, and the numbers are rising. Both the number of adults taking antidepressants and the number of children prescribed stimulants have doubled over the past decade. While many people report benefits of such
medication, many also report serious adverse effects, both immediately
and on discontinuation. In the UK, now, we have a million people on
incapacity benefit, and prescriptions are highest in areas with greater
socio-economic deprivation. The relationship between economic deprivation, distress and the identification of various mental health problems
and state welfare benefits is complex, but in the UK and worldwide,
we can see that, as more people are prescribed antidepressant medication (e.g.) the number of people receiving welfare payments increases[25];
increased use of psychiatric medication is associated with increased (not
decreased) disability rates. This does not necessarily mean that the drugs
are actually causing the problems (although many colleagues believe
that the research indicates that the medication quite literally does more
harm than good). It might just mean that, as we experience very real
challenges in our everyday lives, we suffer.

Excessive long-term use of psychiatric drugs is causing significant
harm, and there is little evidence that these harms are outweighed by
any tangible benefits. Indeed, while outcomes in most areas of physical medicine have improved dramatically over the past few decades, the
outcomes in mental health care are not getting better.[26] In a rather dramatic comment, the former Director of the US National Institute of
Mental Health, Thomas Insel, recently acknowledged that the biomedical framework (which he promoted) and $20 billion dollars in research
funding failed to 'move the needle' in improving people's lives.[27] While
generating thousands of research papers we have not seen clinically useful 'biomarkers' or robust theoretical models, and while we have seen
millions of people prescribed medication and other physical treatments,
we have also seen increased mortality rates and worsening outcomes.[28]

Our services are fragmented, under-resourced and do not deliver
what people want. Mental health care requires adequate funding, but
we would do well to avoid the 'more of the same approach', which

would merely see increasing funding for services with poor outcomes. Current mental health services fail to invest sufficiently in alternative yet more effective provision, including psychological therapies, psychosocial care as well as support in the community (rather than costly long-term hospitalisation). Cost-effective psychosocial options are under-resourced, difficult to access and poorly integrated with other health and social care services. Instead, we should prioritise investment in effective alternatives that will improve outcomes (including psychological therapies, psychosocial support and early intervention and primary prevention) and shift funding from ill-coordinated and fragmented biomedical services to integrated and whole-person care.

Providing these services properly will entail significant change. Many of these issues are currently largely ignored, and most are ill-coordinated. Apologists for the present systems will argue that all these services are currently part of the care offered to clients. The experiences of those who have passed through the system would tend to suggest otherwise. We don't need more hand-wringing self-justification. We need change.

Notes

1. Martin Luther King's speech can be read here: https://www.apa.org/monitor/features/king-challenge and was published as: Martin Luther King, "The role of the behavioral scientist in the civil rights movement," *Journal of Social Issues* 24, no. 1 (1968): 1–12.
2. See, for example, this article in *The Guardian* newspaper: http://www.guardian.co.uk/news/datablog/2012/may/02/uk-healthcare-spending-gdp.
3. The report of the '*Schizophrenia Commission*'; '*Schizophrenia: The Abandoned Illness*' can found here: http://www.schizophreniacommission.org.uk/the-report/.
4. More detail can be found in this article in *the Daily Telegraph* newspaper: https://www.telegraph.co.uk/news/2017/05/09/seven-ten-children-severe-mental-health-problems-sent-hospitals/.
5. Details of Judge Mumby's ruling can be found here: https://www.independent.co.uk/news/uk/home-news/girl-x-suicidal-teenage-

judge-warning-sir-justice-munby-nhs-finds-safe-bed-blood-on-hands-secure-a7878351.html.

6. Details of the level and frequency of abuse in mental health care settings can be found here: https://www.theguardian.com/society/2018/sep/11/nhs-care-regulator-says-sexual-incidents-commonplace-in-mental-health-units.

7. This newspaper article from 2006 discusses the relative quality of UK mental health care... it may be out of date by now, after several years of right-wing government: http://www.guardian.co.uk/society/2006/oct/25/mentalhealth.socialcare.

8. Assen Jablensky, Norman Sartorius, Gunilla Ernberg, Martha Anker, Ailsa Korten, John E. Cooper, Robert Day, and Aksel Bertelsen, "Schizophrenia: Manifestations, incidence and course in different cultures: A World Health Organization ten-country study," *Psychological Medicine Monograph Supplement* 20 (1992): 1–97. This paper and its implications are discussed in greater length in James Davies' excellent book "Cracked": James Davies, *Cracked: Why psychiatry is doing more harm than good* (London: Icon Books, 2013).

9. Discussion as to whether psychiatric care does more harm than good occurs in many places (including this book). One journalistic account from the BBC can be found here: https://www.bbc.co.uk/news/uk-england-41914555.

10. Details of the use of tasers (and other forms of force) in mental health care settings can be found here: https://www.bbc.co.uk/news/uk-42820284.

11. For more information on the history of psychiatry, try reading: Roy Porter, *Madness: A brief history* (Oxford: Oxford University Press, 2002); or Edward Shorter, *A history of psychiatry: From the era of the asylum to the age of Prozac* (New York: Wiley, 1997).

12. Discussion of 'conversion therapy' in the context of LGBTQ+ rights can be found here: https://www.independent.co.uk/news/uk/politics/gay-conversion-therapy-uk-theresa-may-lgbt-equality-plan-a8427406.html.

13. The interacting cognitive subsystems model is a very technical, complicated, psychological theory of how our thoughts work. But although it's complicated, it's also brilliant. Probably the easiest to read paper is: Philip J. Barnard and John D. Teasdale, "Interacting cognitive subsystems: A systemic approach to cognitive-affective interaction and change," *Cognition & Emotion* 5, no. 1 (1991): 1–39. http://www.tandfonline.com/doi/abs/10.1080/02699939108411021.

14. Kate Summerscale, *The suspicions of Mr. Whicher, or, The murder at Road Hill House* (London: Bloomsbury, 2008).
15. *The Times* is, remarkably, searchable online from as early as 1785 (although you need an account: www.thetimes.co.uk/archive). The Editorial quoted is for Saturday, 22 July 1854, p. 8.
16. Alex Langford's blog can be found here: https://psychiatrysho.wordpress.com/2014/02/12/categorically-ill-my-argument-in-favour-of-the-diagnosis-of-mental-illnesses/.
17. Details of US Ritalin prescription can be found here: http://www.nytimes.com/2015/12/11/us/psychiatric-drugs-are-being-prescribed-to-infants.html.
18. Details of UK prescription trends can be found here: http://www.theguardian.com/society/2015/aug/15/ritalin-prescriptions-double-decade-adhd-mental-health.
19. Phil Hickey's excellent blog can be found here: http://behaviorismandmentalhealth.com/2015/12/08/allen-frances-still-trying-to-excuse-psychiatrys-and-his-own-role-in-the-adhd-epidemic/.
20. Godfrey D. Pearlson and Judith M. Ford, "Distinguishing between schizophrenia and other psychotic disorders," *Schizophrenia Bulletin* 40, no. 3 (2014): 501–503. http://schizophreniabulletin.oxfordjournals.org/content/early/2014/03/1/schbul.sbu055.full.
21. Robert Kendell and Assen Jablensky, "Distinguishing between the validity and utility of psychiatric diagnoses," *American Journal of Psychiatry* 160, no. 1 (2003): 4–12. http://ajp.psychiatryonline.org/doi/10.1176/appi.ajp.160.1.4.
22. The wonderful 'OnlyUs' campaign is to be found here: https://twitter.com/onlyuscampaign.
23. Dainius Pūras, *Special Rapporteur on the right of everyone to the enjoyment of the highest attainable standard of physical and mental health* (United Nations, 2017). http://ap.ohchr.org/documents/dpage_e.aspx?si=A/HRC/35/21.
24. Coverage of the economic costs of mental health problems can be found here: https://www.theguardian.com/society/2018/nov/22/mental-illness-costs-uk-94bn-a-year-oecd-report-says-employment-economy-productivity.
25. Robert Whitaker, *Anatomy of an epidemic: Magic bullets, psychiatric drugs, and the astonishing rise of mental illness in America* (Random House, 2010).

26. For detailed discussion of all these issues, see Richard P. Bentall, *Doctoring the mind: Why psychiatric treatments fail* (London: Penguin, 2009); James Le Fanu, *The rise & fall of modern medicine* (London: Abacus, 1999); and James D. Hegarty, Ross J. Baldessarini, Mauricio Tohen, Christine Waternaux, and Godehard Oepen, "One hundred years of schizophrenia: A meta-analysis of the outcome literature," *American Journal of Psychiatry* 151, no. 10 (1994): 1409–1416.

27. An interview including Tom Insel's "$20bn" comment can be found here: https://www.psychologytoday.com/gb/blog/theory-knowledge/201705/twenty-billion-fails-move-the-needle-mental-illness

28. Sukanta Saha, David Chant, and John McGrath, "A systematic review of mortality in schizophrenia: Is the differential mortality gap worsening over time?" *Archives of General Psychiatry* 64, no. 10 (2007): 1123–1131.

2

Events and Consequences

Our mental health is profoundly affected by the events that happen in our lives, including through the impact that they have on our brains. There is very clear evidence that life events, especially social adversity, shape how we make sense of the world... and hence affect our thoughts, emotions and behaviour. But it's often our interpretation of events that affects us more than the events themselves and that this can explain why events that affect one person may not upset another.

We are immersed in societies that form, support and mould us. The World Health Organization entitled its 2003 report on the social determinants of health 'The Solid Facts'.[1] In that report, Richard Wilkinson and Michael Marmot pointed out the fundamental impact that social, political and environmental factors have on our general health. For mental health, that impact is much greater.

John Read, Richard Bentall and colleagues[2] recently conducted an extensive review of the effects of childhood trauma (including, but not limited to, abuse) on our mental health. It's obvious... distressing events distress us. You don't have to be a genius to realise that we're affected by the things that happen to us. There is overwhelming evidence that adverse childhood events; abuse, poverty, poor housing, unemployment

© The Author(s) 2019
P. Kinderman, *A Manifesto for Mental Health,*
https://doi.org/10.1007/978-3-030-24386-9_2

and social disadvantage of all kinds contribute to mental health problems.

Research conducted at the University of Liverpool by Ben Barr, David Taylor-Robinson, Alex Scott-Samuel, Martin McKee and David Stuckler[3] illustrates how the recent economic recession impacted on suicide rates, a rather dramatic (and sad) example of how social factors impact on our mental health. More recently, Ben has expanded on this research, showing how 'work capability assessments'—a scheme whereby people receiving benefits as a consequence of health problems, whether physical or mental, are assessed to consider whether or not such benefits are justified—impact on mental health and suicide rates.[4]

Not long ago, public health colleagues in Liverpool analysed the impact of the economic recession on suicide rates. They concluded that around a thousand people had taken their own lives as a result of the recent financial crisis and recessions; the economic mismanagement of our banks really is a matter of life and death. To be precise, it's a sad fact that around 6000 people take their lives every year. The statistics are relatively stable. What my colleagues found was that the numbers spiked immediately after the 2008 economic crash. While we can't be absolutely sure that the economic crisis <u>caused</u> the deaths, the UK's Royal College of Psychiatrists tweeted in 2017 that: '*The selling of sub prime mortgages by big banks caused a reverse in the downward trend of suicide in the UK … credit crunch caused 700 suicides per year and set trend for increase over following years*',[5] citing the detailed work of Professor Louis Appleby, tracking the socio-economic (and other) causes of suicide.

Inequalities, both economic and social, are important. In their book, *The Spirit Level*, Richard Wilkinson and Kate Pickett argued that the wellbeing of a nation's citizens is much more closely linked to economic equality than to average economic performance, once a nation has achieved a certain basic level of economic performance.[6] Wilkinson and Pickett compared the 'G20' nations (that is, the 20 most economically successful, industrialised nations) and found that the greater the difference between the rich and poor, the worse a nation performs on a series of measures such as physical health, obesity, substance misuse, education, crime and violence and (of course) mental health.

Wilful Ignorance

Research into both social and biological causes of mental health problems has revealed that the more abuse and deprivation suffered by individuals, the more likely they are to experience psychological or mental health problems. This 'dose–response' effect is hardly surprising. What is surprising is the way that many mental health professionals respond. Despite the evidence, it is not unknown for quite senior scientists simply to deny that social factors play any role in the origin of, for example, 'schizophrenia'. Or, as the evidence mounts, its importance is minimised or sidelined. People sometimes seem to go to extreme lengths to fit inconvenient facts into their existing world view. For example, one scientist commented on a recent paper discussing the emotional impact of childhood abuse with the suggestion that: *'the possibility cannot be ruled out that a child destined to develop schizophrenia may show characteristics in childhood that increase the risk of abuse'*.[7]

The tendency of many influential figures in mental health to emphasise biological and genetic factors and minimise or ignore social and psychological aspects was reflected in a discussion about the genetics of 'attention deficit hyperactivity disorder' or 'ADHD'. A study had revealed that 16% of children who had been given a diagnosis of 'ADHD' had a particular genetic variant, in comparison with only 8% of children without the diagnosis. This was a statistically significant difference, and the researcher had claimed that, therefore, *'now we can say with confidence that ADHD is a genetic disease'*.[8] But, as Ben Goldacre pointed out in his column *'bad science'*, 84% of children with a diagnosis of so-called 'ADHD' did not possess the particular genetic variant at the heart of the research.[9] Some of my colleagues seemed to be genuinely shocked and confused by the criticism of the statement. They tried to argue that the researcher had really meant nothing more than that there was a genetic element to 'ADHD' and wasn't trying to say that environmental factors were unimportant. My view was then, and remains now, that when a doctor states *'with confidence'* that a particular problem is *'a genetic disease'*, then members of the public would assume that the problems are genetically determined. If the researcher had meant merely that her research had found a genetic element, explaining relatively little in a problem that was largely social and psychological in nature, given that 84% of children receiving the (highly controversial) diagnosis possessed no such variant, then she should have said that. Researchers need to be very careful about how they report their work.

If we are to provide for one another the kind of humane care that we deserve, we need genuinely to understand—scientifically, rationally, empathically—the reasons for our distress and difficulties. That means acknowledging the enormous weight of evidence showing that people are distressed as a result of the events and circumstances of our lives and the ways in which we have learned to appraise and respond to them. A profound change is required, both in the way we think about 'mental health' and in how we help people in distress.

Spectra and Continua

It's worth remembering that our current ways of thinking about 'mental health' are relatively new. It was only as recently as the nineteenth century that the ideas that auditory hallucinations represented a different form of experience from 'normal' perceptions and that we need to distinguish 'false' beliefs or 'delusions' from any other belief that a person might have were developed. Until then, it appears terms 'delusion' and 'hallucination' were frequently used more or less interchangeably.[10]

Many of my colleagues from a more traditional, medical, perspective would argue that this represents progress. They would argue that the recognition of different, in their terms 'abnormal', modes of thought is a rational step forwards. But conceptual models of mental health change, and our understanding of psychotic experiences changes over time. We are taught to think of phenomena such as hearing voices and unusual beliefs as both quintessentially biological in nature and categorically different from 'normal' experiences. But the most complicated and serious mental health problems such as hallucinations, unusual beliefs and even the complex patterns of communication difficulty rather insultingly termed 'thought disorder' lie on continua.

Paul Bebbington and colleagues[11] looked at the experience of paranoia. They examined the number of people who endorsed a variety of questions about paranoia, from a vague sense unease through to an unshakeable belief that there is an active plot to harm you. Unsurprisingly, more members of the public reported generalised mistrust of others than endorsed the more extreme questions about active plots to kill them. Importantly, psychotic phenomena (in this case, paranoia): '...*appear to form a continuum with normal experience and beliefs*...' with a '... *lack of a clear distinction from normal experiences and processes*'.

Paul Bebbington and colleagues went on to point out another conclusion from their research that '*persecutory ideas build on more common cognitions of mistrust, interpersonal sensitivity and ideas of reference*'. Although the discovery of these continua is a threat to a simple disease model of mental health, this pattern of experiences is exactly what one would expect if these were the statistical consequences of more or less common, and more or less problematic, normal experiences. Most of us are relatively trusting of our friends, families and neighbours. Only a few of us have developed the kind of mistrust that ruins lives and leads to tragedies. When that happens, it can be dramatic and life-changing. But Paul and colleagues' research strongly suggests that those most serious instances represent the far end of a bell curve and not a quintessentially different experience.

A similar pattern of continua and spectra, rather than categorical distinctions, seems to apply to other phenomena commonly described as symptoms of serious mental illness. The definition of a 'delusion' is itself contentious. The current definition of 'delusions' in DSM-5 is: '*fixed beliefs that are not amenable to change in light of conflicting evidence*'. The problem with this as a definition is that, as DSM-5 itself acknowledges, '...*the distinction between a delusion and a strongly held idea is sometimes difficult to make*...'. This reflects the fact that 'delusional' beliefs are merely beliefs, and therefore the attempt at clarity is merely one of distinguishing two different belief systems. Moreover, as we know from everyday life, many of our family and friends maintain a bewildering variety of beliefs with absolute conviction despite what appears to everyone else to be clear evidence of their falsehood. For example, political beliefs are seemingly held 'with absolute conviction despite what appears to everyone else to be clear evidence of their falsehood'. Friends honestly believe that capitalism has been responsible for improvements in the wellbeing of our citizens, that 'trickle-down' economics works, that financial and social inequity is good for societies and that 'owners', but not workers, deserve a disproportionately large share in the profits of a shared enterprise, despite putting in a disproportionately low level of labour. These beliefs exist despite all the evidence to the contrary.

Research reveals not a discrete and categorical distinction between 'well' and 'ill', but instead a set of continua in respect to our more troubling experiences. An opinion poll[12] suggested that three quarters (73%) of Americans believe in some form of supernatural power ... and that doesn't include religion! So; 41% of people believed in extra-sensory perception, 37% in haunted houses, 25% in astrology, etc. Only 27% of respondents rejected all of the beliefs listed, and this level of belief in frankly bizarre ideas is consistent over time. This simple survey does not assess the degree of 'delusional conviction' associated with these beliefs, and it doesn't differentiate between beliefs that are unusual or idiosyncratic and beliefs that are equally illogical but are widely shared across society. Equally, it doesn't refer to the consequences of such belief systems on our lives. But it is consistent with the idea of multiple continua across many dimensions.

Auditory hallucinations are often seen as quintessential 'symptoms of mental illness' and a marker of the difference between 'well' and 'ill'. But, again,[13] hallucinations of various kinds are common. In a European sample, 39% of people reported experiencing hallucinations. These were unevenly distributed. Only 2.4% of people reported hallucinations more than once a week (although that is much more common than the incidence of so-called 'schizophrenia'), 6% monthly and 20% less frequently than once a month. Again, these experiences occurred for a wide variety of reasons. Many people reported hallucinations while dropping off to sleep (named 'hypnagogic hallucinations' and reported by 25% of the sample) or immediately on waking ('hypnopompic hallucinations'; 7%). Unsurprisingly, people who had received a diagnosis of a 'psychotic disorder' were around six times more likely to report hallucinations, but taking 'street' or recreational drugs made it around ten times more likely that someone would report these experiences. People experience visual and auditory hallucinations for a huge variety of reasons and not simply as a result of 'categorical illnesses'.

A final quintessential 'psychotic' phenomenon is so-called thought disorder. This (highly insulting) term refers to a pattern of disorganised thinking or, at least, as far as we can assess a person's thinking through their disorganised speech. In brutal terms, it refers to speech characterised by; derailment (a sequence of unrelated or apparently unconnected ideas), poverty of speech (very little speech, few details, monosyllabic answers), tangentiality (where the conversation wanders without focus), illogicality, perseveration (repetition) and thought blocking (when a conversation suddenly stops, with people reporting that the ideas simply empty from the mind). This is usually thought of as a core 'symptom' of 'schizophrenia', but it's also widely observed in times of extreme stress. The picture is understandably complex, but we know that people who have experienced childhood abuse, and abuse in adulthood, are more likely to report 'thought disorder'.[14] We also know that, for those of us who are experiencing mental health problems, when we are talking about emotionally charged issues, quite understandably, we exhibit significantly more evidence of complex and confused thinking.[15]

At the risk of revealing my political sympathies, there's a rather wonderful example of thought disorder in the public domain from a well-known politician. I need to stress that in no sense does this imply the presence of any mental health problems (and certainly not a 25th Amendment issue). Quite the reverse; it's an example of how phenomena like 'thought disorder' occur in everyday life. On 21st July 2015, the then Republican presidential contender, Donald Trump, addressed supporters in Bluffton, South Carolina.[16] His speech has no inherent worth, but it illustrates how 'thought disorder' crops up all the time when we make off-the-cuff and emotionally charged statements.

> Look, having nuclear—my uncle was a great professor and scientist and engineer, Dr. John Trump at MIT; good genes, very good genes, OK, very smart, the Wharton School of Finance, very good, very smart—you know, if you're a conservative Republican, if I were a liberal, if, like, OK, if I ran as a liberal Democrat, they would say I'm one of the smartest

people anywhere in the world—it's true!—but when you're a conservative Republican they try—oh, do they do a number—that's why I always start off: Went to Wharton, was a good student, went there, went there, did this, built a fortune—you know I have to give my like credentials all the time, because we're a little disadvantaged—but you look at the nuclear deal, the thing that really bothers me—it would have been so easy, and it's not as important as these lives are (nuclear is powerful; my uncle explained that to me many, many years ago, the power and that was 35 years ago; he would explain the power of what's going to happen and he was right—who would have thought?), but when you look at what's going on with the four prisoners—now it used to be three, now it's four—but when it was three and even now, I would have said it's all in the messenger; fellas, and it is fellas because, you know, they don't, they haven't figured that the women are smarter right now than the men, so, you know, it's gonna take them about another 150 years—but the Persians are great negotiators, the Iranians are great negotiators, so, and they, they just killed, they just killed us.

The clear evidence of continua undermines the idea of a categorical distinction between 'well' and 'ill'. But the argument here isn't merely one of continua; there are many medical conditions that lie on continua. We understand that lipid levels vary, but we identify 'hypercholesterolemia'; we understand that our body weight varies, but we also understand the meaning of 'obese'. Our bone density ('osteoporosis') and memory functioning vary in complex but continuous ways, especially as we age, not as discrete, 'on/off' entities. But it's not just an issue of continua and, therefore, the establishment of the statistical 'normality' of these experiences. There's also overwhelming evidence that these continua of experience are related to what happens to us in our lives and reflect the complex variety of our social circumstances, the things that happen to us and the ways in which we make sense of them and respond.

Cowardice, Sickness and Empathy

The First World War poet, Wilfred Owen, asked: '*Who are these? Why sit they here in twilight? These are men whose minds the Dead have ravished... Pawing us who dealt them war and madness*'.[17] Owen was well aware of the impact of war on our mental health. After serving on the front line, he was evacuated in 1917 to Craiglockhart Military Hospital in Scotland suffering from 'shell shock'.

We've known about the psychological impact of combat for thousands of years. The Greek historian Herodotus describes an episode in the battle of Marathon in 490 BCE. The warrior Epizelus reported that in the middle of the battle, a heavily armed man stepped past him and killed the man next to him, at which point he: '... *was deprived of sight though wounded in no part of his body, not struck from a distance; and that he continued to be blind from that time for the remainder of his life*'.[18] My friend and colleague, Professor Jamie Hacker Hughes, together with Dr. Walid Abdul-Hamid, discovered references to such psychological trauma following warfare from 1300 BCE. In documents from the Assyrian Dynasty in Mesopotamia, there are accounts of soldiers being visited by '*ghosts they faced in battle*', traumatised flashbacks to hand-to-hand combat.[19]

During the First World War, the impact of 'shell shock' on the officer class led to a partial re-thinking about how mental ill-health should be understood. It was generally accepted among the establishment that the officers, as selected and admired members of the upper classes, and trained and educated since youth, were ideal examples of manhood. Faced with the realities of war, a disturbingly large number of young men succumbed to 'shell-shock', 'combat fatigue' or what those of us who like attaching diagnostic labels to problems would now call 'PTSD' or 'post traumatic stress disorder'. Many were the junior officers, who were expected to lead from the front. Some were shot for cowardice (although, inevitably, those victims tended to be from lower down the social hierarchies). Then, as now, the dominant explanation for mental health problems was biological. The most common view, reaching its peak in the eugenics movement, was that psychological weakness was biological and constitutional in origin. But this was incompatible with the young men of the officer class succumbing to psychological problems. In response to the overwhelming horror of the trenches, mental illness could no longer be thought only as the consequence of constitutional weakness. It was tragically obvious that stress could unbalance the mind.

Commonplace Trauma

Psychological problems are common after all kinds of traumatic events. Around 25% of refugees and survivors of conflict, as well as combatants, report high rates of depression and those problems (hypervigilance, anxiety, memory problems, traumatic recollections of events and avoidance) that attract the label of 'PTSD'. Many women sadly report that childbirth is traumatic. There is a tendency to want to believe that the birth of a child will be a uniquely happy and positive experience, but for many women, it's a painful, terrifying, experience of lack of control. Some women secretly fear for the future, some secretly regret the birth of their child, and some are physically damaged by the delivery. Not surprisingly, then, many women report traumatic flashback memories of the experience.

It is shocking that one woman in ten in the UK has been raped, but only 20% of those women report their assault to the police. Most of the women who are attacked know their assailants, and an even greater proportion of women—around 50%—have experienced domestic violence from a spouse, partner or family member. This violence has major long-term consequences for women's physical and psychological health.[20]

Shamefully, we also damage too many of our children, and we can see the effects on their psychological health. About one child in every ten is sexually abused in the UK, and about one child in four is physically abused. It's almost redundant to point out that psychologists and psychiatrists have found that abuse is very common in people with mental health problems. Such events affect us grievously. It's easy to see how abuse leads to depression and relationship difficulties. It's often tempting to assume that other types of mental health difficulties are attributable to biological causes or the innate constitution of the individual. But abuse and other childhood experiences are very common precursors of later serious mental health issues. Between 50 and 80% of people experiencing psychotic phenomena report having survived childhood sexual abuse. Moreover, around 80% of the reports of childhood sexual abuse are corroborated by other sources (such as social worker or police investigations), and people who report psychotic experiences don't appear to be more likely to make incorrect allegations than anybody else. Filippo

Varese and colleagues at the University of Liverpool[21] have demonstrated a clear link between traumatic childhood experiences (poverty, abuse, etc.) and later psychotic experiences. This is important because many people tend to think that serious problems such as hallucinations and delusional beliefs are quintessentially biological in origin, and this paper suggests an important social dimension. Filippo and colleagues' conclusions (as reported in the abstract of their paper) were: '... *These findings indicate that childhood adversity is strongly associated with increased risk for psychosis...*'.

Much of this evidence has been summarised by Paul Bebbington and colleagues.[22] People who have survived childhood sexual abuse appear to be about 15 times more likely to experience psychotic problems. This is a stunningly powerful statistic. We all know the risks associated with smoking cigarettes. Smoking increases our risk of developing lung cancer such that smokers are somewhere between 10 and 25 times more likely to develop lung cancer than non-smokers. We are comfortable with saying 'smoking causes cancer'; it's on the packets of cigarettes. The evidence is equally consistent with stating that 'abuse causes psychosis'.

These kinds of traumatic events are dramatic, but we also need to think about the psychological consequences of, for instance, bullying at school and at work. It doesn't take a lot of imagination to think of the impact on the psychological health of a child who, every day, has to walk to school knowing not only that she will be taunted and possibly assaulted, told she is inadequate and ugly, but also knowing that the teachers will see all this but ignore it. And we don't only experience trauma or abuse as children. We also suffer from traumatic events in adulthood. We are bullied, abused, assaulted, robbed and raped. Workers (especially women) are abused and assaulted. We are insulted and humiliated. Even the everyday choices of capitalism will affect our mental health. Do we smile at the customer who's humiliating us or lose our job? Do we accept hours of work that mean it's impossible to care for our children properly? Do we accept a job that involves more commuting, or longer hours, in return for higher wages? And should we have to put up with verbal abuse? The emotional and psychological consequences of balancing these unpleasant choices and conflicting goals can be distressing and affect our wellbeing and mental health.

'Prevention is better than Cure'

The founding Charter of the World Health Organization describes health as '*a state of complete physical, mental and social well-being and not merely the absence of disease or infirmity*'.[23] Medical practitioners have always done more than merely treat the illness. Doctors in a variety of specialisms (general practitioners, obstetricians, paediatricians) contribute to the care of, for example, pregnant women. Pregnancy can sometimes have potentially serious medical complications. But pregnancy, itself, is not an illness. To be blunt, the physiology of the female body is doing exactly what it has evolved to do. Of course, there are things that can go wrong. But a normal pregnancy is a normal part of human life. The analogous error would be to assume that our mental health problems are evidence of pathology. The training and ethos of the medical profession, and the pharmaceutical industry, understandably promote the idea of illnesses and their treatment. Many people may also find this approach appealing; for example, they may feel that it offers a way of explaining problems without blame. But it is misleading and unnecessary, not least because the science simply fails to support a biomedical explanatory model of mental health.[24]

I am lucky to work with public health specialists in Liverpool, and Liverpool's history includes the legacy of Dr. William Duncan. Like most doctors in Victorian Britain, Duncan came from a privileged background. After qualifying as a doctor in 1829 and working as a general practitioner (family doctor) in a working-class area of Liverpool, he became interested in the links between the health and the living conditions of his poor patients. He was shocked by the poverty he found and in the clear link between housing conditions and the risk of diseases such as cholera, smallpox and typhus. Dr. Duncan started a lifelong campaign for improved living conditions and, together with Liverpool's Borough Engineer, James Newlands and Thomas Fresh, the wonderfully titled 'Inspector of Nuisances', tried to address the problems. This led to Duncan's appointment as Liverpool's first Medical Officer of Health, and to the passing of Liverpool's Sanitary Act in 1846, acknowledged as a breakthrough in public health.[25]

Public health specialists protect us against risks such as diabetes and coronary heart disease, often as a result of obesity, poor diet or not enough exercise. Many doctors provide vital medical interventions to treat these illnesses, but public health physicians and family doctors aim to prevent illness and promote health. This is a recognised and integral part of medicine: the General Medical Council and the medical Royal Colleges (the Royal College of General Practitioners, the Royal College of Physicians, etc.) all stress the importance of the promotion of health as well as the treatment of illness. At the University of Liverpool, my colleague Professor Dame Margaret Whitehead is responsible for leading a World Health Organization Collaborating Centre for Policy Research into the Social Determinants of Health, exploring, in particular, how social and economic inequalities contribute to poor health outcomes in disadvantaged communities.

The point is that, in physical medicine at least as much as in the fields of psychiatry and psychology, doctors embrace the concept of health and wellbeing and the connection between our health and our physical and social circumstances. In 2001, the World Health Organization defined mental health as: '*a state of well-being in which the individual realizes his or her own abilities, can cope with the normal stresses of life, can work productively and fruitfully, and is able to make a contribution to his or her community*'.[26] The European Commission takes a step further, describing mental health as: '*a resource which enables them to realise their intellectual and emotional potential and to find and fulfil their roles in social, school and working life. For societies, good mental health of citizens contributes to prosperity, solidarity and social justice*'.[27] The European Commission also notes that: '*the mental condition of people is determined by a multiplicity of factors including biological (e.g., genetics, gender), individual (e.g., personal experiences), family and social (e.g., social support) and economic and environmental (e.g., social status and living conditions)*'. As well as echoing points I made earlier, this approach links concepts of mental health to much wider aspects of wellbeing, which is becoming a key element of government policy. It's almost certainly what we want from our health professionals, and it is just about possible to reconcile a traditional approach to psychiatry with these aspirational ideas. Psychiatry is increasingly embracing the promotion of positive psychological wellbeing rather than merely treating illnesses when they are diagnosed, and the present UK government's strategy for mental health, launched in 2011,[28] reflects this focus on wellbeing and prevention.

In October 2018, the British Medical Association published a report entitled: *'Tackling the Causes: promoting public mental health and investing in prevention'*,[29] which addressed the increasing demands on the workload of GPs specifically to address mental health problems. From the perspective of the BMA, this reflects a worry that demands for traditional mental health care is increasing faster than resources are being made available. In large part, this is simply because our politicians fail to provide the kind of sustainable long-term funding for our healthcare systems. But, as people are more aware of their mental health needs and as they are—thankfully—less reticent in talking about these issues, there is a duty to provide the right kinds of response. That does not mean more diagnosis and more drugs; it means addressing the root causes. These include trauma, but also more insidious pressures on our mental health, including the ongoing psychological pressures of poverty, loneliness, boredom and neglect.

Deprivation

We all have to manage stressful events in our lives. We are all affected by the normal and inevitable cycles of birth, childhood, adolescence, success and failure in examination, employment, marriage, moving house, divorce, disease and death. Even if positive, such as marriage and childbirth, these major life events are often stressful. And everyday 'hassles', or ongoing lower-level stress, can also affect our mental health; overwork, poor housing, financial difficulties, transport problems, relationship problems, etc. And all these pressures are worse if we're poor.

In 2018, the British Medical Association called for a major focus on public mental health, with a (long) list of important elements. These are genuinely wonderful, but also ambitious and political, reducing poverty (especially its effects on parents and their children), reducing unemployment and supporting the mental health of unemployed people, providing parenting programmes to targeted families, putting mental health at the centre of the schools' curriculum and providing early help to distressed pupils at school, mental health support forums and anti-bullying campaigns: putting social media to use for the greater good, maintaining a life course approach (from infancy and childhood, through the workplace and including older adults), examining the effects of public health cuts on social determinants of mental health and wellbeing, promoting exercise in its own right (which the BMA estimates would reduce depression by a third) and promoting 'social prescribing'. They point out, however, that we spend very little on public mental health; only 1.6% of the total spent on public health and that, itself, is pitifully low.[30]

These issues affect children most severely. We know that adverse childhood experiences, both at home (e.g. domestic violence, substance misuse by parents, abuse of various kinds) and at school (e.g. academic pressures and bullying), impact on our mental health, and we know that these problems are more acute in areas of greater social deprivation. Children from low-income families are more likely to act in anti-social ways and benefit less from education. Poverty is strongly associated with neglect of children, and this has predictable impacts on mental health, academic achievement and crime. Accidental and 'non-accidental' injuries in children are more common in poorer families and in areas of socio-economic deprivation. In the words of the World Health Organization: '...*mental disorders occur in persons of all genders, ages, and backgrounds. No group is immune to mental disorders, but the risk is higher among the poor, homeless, the unemployed, persons with low education...*'.[31]

It would be ridiculous to suggest that these kinds of stressful events or circumstances would affect us without affecting the functioning of the brain. It's perhaps also worth pointing out that these stresses may affect the functioning of the child's developing brain. Stress during childhood may affect what is called the 'hypothalamic-pituitary-adrenal (HPA) axis'. This is a neural system that responds to external threats, including by controlling the release of cortisol, the so-called stress hormone.

At the same time, there's more to this than merely an interaction of sociology and biology. We make sense of the world around us. We make sense of the world using our brain, and our brain is a physical organ of the body. But we are not just the product of our genes and brains, nor are our moods and behaviours completely dictated by the circumstances of our social environment and the events that happen to us. We are not passive sponges of these external influences, because human beings, perhaps uniquely, make sense of the world.

Political Failure

Political decisions, too, impact on our mental health. In the UK, we use a process known as 'work capability assessments' to assess whether or not a person is eligible for welfare benefits. If a person is 'ill'—or, rather, in the regime of our regrettably right-wing government, sufficiently ill—then they are no longer expected to look for work and receive a higher rate of financial support. But the assessments themselves are major stressors. A senior civil servant in the Department of Work and Pensions, whom I know well on a personal level, was not long ago subjected to significant pressure from political leaders and senior managers. His error was to acknowledge in an internal memo, now leaked on the Internet and reported in national media, that the assessment process may trigger suicidal responses in applicants for benefits.

I have personal experience of this. One applicant for state benefits is a close relative of mine. He was in receipt of the 'Employment and Support Allowance' paid to people unable to work. As is common, he was subjected to a 'work capability assessment', a short medical test carried out by a private contractor. There is considerable suspicion that the policies and working practices of these contractors extend and develop the political decisions to make the application process for benefits particularly difficult and challenging. Indeed, a recent report by a (different) United Nations Special Rapporteur on extreme poverty and human rights, Philip Alston,[32] was very critical of the political mentality behind 'austerity policies', cuts in public services and reforms. He commented that: '*British compassion for those who are suffering has been replaced by a punitive, mean-spirited and callous approach …*', whereby policies were in place to '*…make the system as unwelcoming as possible, that people who need benefits should be reminded constantly that they are lucky to get anything, that nothing will be made easy*'. Claimants know that. They know that the process is designed to put them off, to limit the financial support available and to question and challenge their applications and that 'sanctions' (use quasi-judicial cuts in benefits akin to fines) are used to threaten and punish deviations from the rules.

For my relative, the anxiety associated with the possibility of losing his only form of financial support, and personal conflict over revealing his most private and intimate mental health issues to a barely trained stranger, meant that he had difficulty sleeping. As a consequence, his mental health deteriorated significantly.

In the summer of 2018, the Trussell Trust,[33] a UK anti-poverty charity, which operates a network of over 420 food banks, reported that it was preparing emergency food packs for children during the school summer holidays. Many children in the UK receive free school meals during term time if their parents receive state benefits. But, during the holiday periods (and the summer holidays are the longest), these free meals are no longer available because the children aren't in school. Consequently, according to the Trussell Trust, there is an extra financial pressure of around £30 and £40 a week on poor families and so children suffer. Food banks and 'emergency packs' are needed. In fact, the number of these three-day emergency food packs supplied by the charity has been rising steadily, from 913,000 in 2013 to 1.3 million in 2018.

For the children involved, the impact on their mental health is profound. Physically, these children may even be slightly malnourished; there's evidence of children's academic performance being affected by tiredness and at least anecdotal comments by teachers that some of the kids in their classes are handicapped by missing out on decent breakfasts. But as a psychologist, I'm interested in psychological impact. Put yourself in the shoes of the children. Kids relying on free school meals, children attending food banks, watching their parents arguing with officials from the privatised, outsourced, private companies charged with implementing the policies the UN Special Rapporteur so overtly criticised—these children will realise that they are growing up in a deprived family. They grow up comparing themselves against their peers in this respect, knowing that their parents are poor and that they can't provide for everything they need. In other words, it's a continual grinding social pressure on their mental health. At one level, were we actually to think differently, we might alleviate some of these pressures, as well as using our position as the fifth richest economy in the world to provide decent social services, for example by giving ALL children free school meals. That would nourish them, but also minimise perceived differences. Although this might involve a modest financial investment (a French proposal to provide free breakfasts croissants, of course, for 100,000 disadvantaged children was estimated to cost €6m euro a year[34]), this is fairly insignificant relative to the cost of the impact on our children's mental health.

We need a wholesale revision of the way we think about psychological distress. We could start by acknowledging that such distress is a normal, not abnormal, part of human life. We humans respond to distressing circumstances by becoming distressed. Any system for identifying, describing and responding to distress would most effectively, most accurately and most humanely use language and processes that reflect this position.

Notes

1. Richard G. Wilkinson and Michael Marmot, eds., *Social determinants of health: The solid facts* (World Health Organization, 2003).
2. John Read and Richard P. Bentall, "Negative childhood experiences and mental health: Theoretical, clinical and primary prevention implications," *The British Journal of Psychiatry* 200, no. 2 (2012): 89–91. https://doi.org/10.1192/bjp.bp.111.096727. See also: Filippo Varese, Feikje Smeets, Marjan Drukker, Ritsaert Lieverse, Tineke Lataster, Wolfgang Viechtbauer, John Read, Jim Van Os, and Richard P. Bentall, "Childhood adversities increase the risk of psychosis: A meta-analysis of patient-control, prospective-and cross-sectional cohort studies," *Schizophrenia Bulletin* 38, no. 4 (2012): 661–671. https://doi.org/10.1093/schbul/sbs050.

3. Ben Barr, David Taylor-Robinson, Alex Scott-Samuel, Martin Mckee, and David Stuckler, "Suicides associated with the 2008–10 economic recession in England: Time trend analysis," *British Medical Journal* 345 (2012): e5142. http://www.bmj.com/content/345/bmj.e5142.

4. Ben Barr, David Taylor-Robinson, David Stuckler, Rachel Loopstra, Aaron Reeves, and Margaret Whitehead, "'First, do no harm': Are disability assessments associated with adverse trends in mental health? A longitudinal ecological study," *Journal of Epidemiology and Community Health* 70, no. 4 (2016): 339–345. http://dx.doi.org/10.1136/jech-2015-206209.

5. The tweet by the Royal College of Psychiatrists, quoting Professor Appleby, can be found here: https://twitter.com/rcpsych/status/938480947279941632.

6. Richard G. Wilkinson and Kate Pickett, *The spirit level: Why more equal societies almost always do better* (London: Allen Lane, 2009). ISBN 9780241954294. The associated website also provides some useful information—www.equalitytrust.org.uk.

7. Lucia Sideli, Alice Mule, Daniele La Barbera, and Robin M. Murray, "Do child abuse and maltreatment increase risk of schizophrenia?" *Psychiatry Investigation* 9, no. 2 (2012): 87.

8. Nigel M. Williams, Irina Zaharieva, Andrew Martin, Kate Langley, Kiran Mantripragada, Ragnheidur Fossdal, Hreinn Stefansson, et al., "Rare chromosomal deletions and duplications in attention-deficit hyperactivity disorder: A genome-wide analysis," *The Lancet* 376, no. 9750 (2010): 1401–1408.

9. Ben Goldacre's website (discussing this issue) can be found here: http://www.badscience.net/2010/10/pride-and-prejudice/.

10. Åsa Jansson, "Voice-hearing in 19th-century psychiatry," *The Lancet* 392, no. 10158 (2018): 1618–1619. https://www.thelancet.com/journals/lancet/article/PIIS0140-6736(18)32604-7/fulltext.

11. Paul E. Bebbington, Orla McBride, Craig Steel, Elizabeth Kuipers, Mirjana Radovanovič, Traolach Brugha, Rachel Jenkins, Howard I. Meltzer, and Daniel Freeman, "The structure of paranoia in the general population," *The British Journal of Psychiatry* 202, no. 6 (2013): 419–427. https://doi.org/10.1192/bjp.bp.112.119032.

12. The survey is reported here: http://news.gallup.com/poll/16915/three-four-americans-believe-paranormal.aspx.

13. Maurice M. Ohayon, "Prevalence of hallucinations and their pathological associations in the general population," *Psychiatry Research* 97, no. 2–3 (2000): 153–164. https://www.ncbi.nlm.nih.gov/pubmed/11166087.

14. John Read, Kirsty Agar, Nick Argyle, and Volkmar Aderhold, "Sexual and physical abuse during childhood and adulthood as predictors of hallucinations, delusions and thought disorder," *Psychology and Psychotherapy: Theory, Research and Practice* 76, no. 1 (2003): 1–22. https://onlinelibrary.wiley.com/doi/abs/10.1348/14760830260569210_.

15. Sara Tai, Gillian Haddock, and Richard P. Bentall, "The effects of emotional salience on thought disorder in patients with bipolar affective disorder," *Psychological Medicine* 34, no. 5 (2004): 803–809. https://www.cambridge.org/core/journals/psychological-medicine/article/effects-of-emotional-salience-on-thought-disorder-in-patients-with-bipolar-affective-disorder/7E271280A82DDE7B5651050C96718C3D.

16. Donald Trump's chaotic speech can be found here: https://www.c-span.org/video/?327258-1/donald-trump-remarks-sun-city-south-carolina.

17. Wilfred Owen's poems can be found online at the Project Gutenberg website: http://www.gutenberg.org/files/1034/1034-h/1034-h.htm. Project Gutenberg offers free online access to 38,000 books that are out of copyright, and is an excellent reference tool.

18. Herodotus's histories can be read online here: https://archive.org/details/herodotusnewlite00hero/page/398.

19. Walid Khalid, Abdul-Hamid, and Jamie Hacker Hughes, "Nothing new under the sun: Post-traumatic stress disorders in the ancient world," *Early Science and Medicine* 19, no. 6 (2014): 549–557. Doi: https://doi.org/10.1163/15733823-00196p02.

20. https://www.ons.gov.uk/peoplepopulationandcommunity/crimeandjustice/bulletins/domesticabuseinenglandandwales/yearendingmarch2017.

21. Filippo, Varese, Feikje Smeets, Marjan Drukker, Ritsaert Lieverse, Tineke Lataster, Wolfgang Viechtbauer, John Read, Jim Van Os, and Richard P. Bentall, "Childhood adversities increase the risk of psychosis: A meta-analysis of patient-control, prospective- and cross-sectional cohort studies," *Schizophrenia Bulletin* 38, no. 4 (2012): 661–671. https://www.ncbi.nlm.nih.gov/pmc/articles/PMC3406538/.

22. Paul Bebbington, Sarah Jonas, Elizabeth Kuipers, Michael King, Claudia Cooper, Traolach Brugha, Howard Meltzer, Sally McManus, and Rachel Jenkins, "Childhood sexual abuse and psychosis: Data from a cross-sectional national psychiatric survey in England," *The British Journal of Psychiatry* 199, no. 1 (2011): 29–37.

23. World Health Organization, "Constitution of the World Health Organization, 1946," *Bulletin of the World Health Organization* 80, no.

12 (2002): 983. http://www.who.int/governance/eb/who_constitution_ en.pdf.

24. To hear more about this argument, listen to my interview on Australia's ABC radio: https://www.abc.net.au/radionational/programs/ allinthemind/does-mental-illness-exist/9130774.

25. Stephen Halliday, "Duncan of Liverpool: Britain's first medical officer," *Journal of Medical Biography* 11, no. 3 (2003): 142–149. There is also a Duncan Society hosted by the University of Liverpool: http://www.liv. ac.uk/ssp/duncansociety/index.htm.

26. World Health Organization, *Strengthening mental health promotion* (Geneva: World Health Organization, 2001).

27. European Commission, *Promoting the mental health of the population: Towards a strategy on mental health for the European Union* (Brussels: European Commission, 2005).

28. Department of Health, *No health without mental health: A cross-government mental health outcomes strategy for people of all ages* (London: Department of Health, 2011). http://www.dh.gov.uk/en/ Publicationsandstatistics/Publications/PublicationsPolicyAndGuidance/ DH_123766.

29. The BMA report on public mental health can be found here: https:// www.bma.org.uk/collective-voice/policy-and-research/public-and-pop-ulation-health/mental-health/promoting-mental-health-and-prevention.

30. British Medical Association, *Tackling the causes: Promoting public mental health and investing in prevention* (London: British Medical Association, 2018).

31. Richard G. Wilkinson and Michael Marmot, eds., *Social determinants of health: The solid facts* (World Health Organization, 2003).

32. Philip Alston's highly critical report on poverty in the UK can be found here: https://www.theguardian.com/society/2018/nov/16/key-points-un-envoy-philip-alston-report-poverty-britain-uk.

33. Details of the Trussell Trust's work can be found here: https:// www.trusselltrust.org/2018/08/03/call-donations-charity-re-veals-rise-food-children-behind-increased-foodbank-need-holidays/.

34. The French proposal is reported here: https://www.thelocal.fr/20190423/ france-to-launch-free-school-breakfasts-in-fight-against-poverty.

3

We are not the Slaves of our Brains

It is a simple fact of life that all of our thoughts, behaviours and emotions emanate from the biological activity of our brains. But this does not imply that mental health problems therefore need to be regarded as brain diseases. Our brains have evolved to allow us to process information about the world and make sense of our environment. These neurological mechanisms underpin all psychological processes, whether that involves depression, anxiety, falling in love, writing poetry or going to war. It is vital to understand the involvement of neurotransmitters, of synapses and neurones in human behaviour, but it is misleading to suggest that only mental health problems have biological elements. The biology of human thought and human emotion is universal. When things happen to us, there are biological consequences (our brains change, physically, for example, when we're lonely), but those consequences are true for all of us, not just those of us labelled as 'ill'. We all differ in our basic biological makeup, but the science is clear: biological differences between people seem to explain very little of the differences between us in terms of our mental health.

Biological accounts of mental health rest on the idea that our behaviour, thoughts and emotions are products of our brains and are best explained in terms of biological mechanisms, ultimately determined by the expression of our genes. The neurotransmitter dopamine (which

© The Author(s) 2019
P. Kinderman, *A Manifesto for Mental Health*,
https://doi.org/10.1007/978-3-030-24386-9_3

has been linked to many street drugs and to psychosis) seems to have a role in making events seem more personally significant and salient and has been linked to a range of mental health problems, including psychotic experiences such as hallucinations and persecutory delusions. Serotonin (another neurotransmitter) has been linked to mechanisms of reward and social status and therefore to depression and low self-esteem. The power of medical science and its success (in areas other than mental health) means that biological explanations for a whole swathe of psychological phenomena, including our mental health, are seductively popular and commonplace in the media; on TV, the radio, in newspapers.

Biological accounts of psychological phenomena describe the physiological processes underpinning the psychology very well. But descriptions and explanations are not always the same things; we can describe the internal workings of a train, and we can describe the processes of purchasing a ticket, and how the barriers to the platform work, and how the train timetables are constructed, but that doesn't in any sense explain why I was on the 06:15 from Manchester to London. Detailed mechanistic descriptions are not necessarily sufficient explanations, especially of behaviours that have moral implications. Biological explanations are not, in themselves, very good at explaining complex behaviours, and they are particularly poor at explaining differences between people, which is usually what we're interested in. At one level, it's obviously true that our behaviour is the product of the functioning of our brains. Every action and every thought we ever have involves the brain. But since every thought necessarily involves the brain, this merely tells us that we think with our brains (which, to be honest, we already knew). This kind of explanation doesn't add much to our understanding. When confident people think about performing in public, their brains are involved in doing the thinking, but that is also true for anxious people; their brains are also, and equally, involved in doing the thinking. Trying to explain complex human behaviours in neurological terms alone is the equivalent of explaining the origins of the First World War in terms of the mechanisms of high explosives. A simple biological model is 'true' on one level, but loses explanatory power when over-extended.

A more elegant version of biological explanation focusses on individual differences, and more specifically on whether the obvious differences in behaviour, personality and attitudes are best explained by biological differences between people, or by differences in some other domain: in the different things that happen to us, in the different ways that we have learned to respond, or in the different experiences that may have contributed to that learning. Biological approaches explain differences in psychological response to trauma in terms of differences in biological functioning. That has some appeal. In stressful situations, such as natural disasters, some people may experience very significant mental health problems whereas others are strikingly resilient. This may well be seen as indicating inherent, even biological differences.

We might, for example, suggest that some people are likely to experience a significantly greater 'spike' in levels of the 'stress hormone', cortisol, in these circumstances. When it comes to depression, it has been suggested that biological processes involving the neurotransmitter serotonin might have a role to play. Serotonin seems to be involved in brain mechanisms that address reward and reinforcement. Therefore, it has been suggested, differences between people—between those of us prone to depression and those more resilient—might reflect biological differences in the serotonin system. These kinds of explanations have implications for treatment. If you can explain behaviour in terms of biological processes, it would make sense to intervene with biological solutions. In the case of mental health problems, this means medication.

It becomes much more complex when we add in the role of psychology. Traumatic life events impact on our mental health. But not everybody exposed to such traumatic events will suffer to the same extent; some people are more resilient than others. Some of that resilience may come from biological differences, but it may also reflect our learning and upbringing. Our likelihood of responding to a stressful life event with rumination and self-blame is, in part, a consequence of our upbringing and the events we've been exposed to in our lives. If, for instance, our childhoods have been characterised by loss or unpredictability or negativity, we're highly likely to approach any new situations (even opportunities) with caution.

There's a well-known experiment involving children and marshmallows. You place a marshmallow in front of a four-year-old child and say something like; *'I'm going to leave the room now for five minutes. You can eat this marshmallow if you want, but if, when I come back, it's still here, I'll give you two!'* Some children can withstand the temptation to eat the marshmallow, but some can't. What's particularly interesting about this experiment is that the differences in kids' performance at the age of four are still detectable many years later; the test seems to be assessing something important. Children who were able to wait for the second marshmallow tend, when adolescents, to be happier, physically healthier (they have lower body-mass indices, presumably because they eat fewer marshmallows) and do better at school. So, it looks as if an ability to delay gratification is likely to reap a range of benefits later in life. In psychological terms, the way that children approach the challenge ('how can I resist this temptation?') is important; some sit and stare, and some try to distract themselves.[1] So, why are we different?

The most common interpretation of the marshmallow test has been that there is an underlying difference, hard-wired even. Some of us are naturally good at this kind of thing, and will do well, and some aren't. This is usually seen as something located in the innate (presumably biological) character of the children. Michael Bourne, writing in the *New York Times* in 2014,[2] suggested that the point of the marshmallow test is that it *'appears to reduce the complex social and psychological question of why some people succeed in life to a simple, if ancient, formulation: Character is destiny'*.

But... but... but... the marshmallow test does seem to have that predictive power, however probably not for the reasons that people assume. The test does tell us something about why some people succeed in life, but it doesn't seem to be the case that 'character is destiny'. It looks very much more as if the social and material circumstances of our childhoods have profound impacts on how we think, and even on how we go about the business of thinking.

Recent replications of the original marshmallow test[3] have shown that there's a strong correlation between the ability to delay gratification from a young age and later achievement across a range of outcomes. And it does seem as if the children who are able to delay gratification are able to do that by employing a range of cognitive techniques. But there are reasons for these differences, and they are reasons that we already (if we're honest with ourselves), know about. Specifically, the children's home environment and family background, including the socio-economic status of their parents, significantly accounts for the variance (the differences) in the children's ability to defer gratification and therefore later achievement.

This makes perfect sense. The ability to defer gratification is an extremely useful (and adaptive) skill. And the marshmallow test picks up on this skill. There are differences between kids in this respect, and those differences really are important. But it may well not be the case that the kids' differences are explicable in terms of 'innate character'. Rather, the children's abilities to defer gratification—to hold out for a second marshmallow—may well have been shaped by their social and economic background. It makes absolute sense. Turn the question around another way. Can we think of social and economic circum-stances that could lead a child to defer gratification, or, put another way, could lead a child to be confident that something good won't be taken away; that rewards in the future can be confidently predicted, that promises will be kept…? Some children will learn that it's wise and sen-sible to take rewards when you can, because they come around only sel-dom. Other children learn that they receive presents all the time. Some children will learn that promises made by adults are rarely kept. Other children learn to trust adults with much greater confidence. Some children, sadly, know what it feels like to be hungry, disappointed, neglected. It seems obvious (at least to me) that children will learn to predict different things in situations like this depending on the environ-ment in which they're grown up. The point of the human brain—its evolutionary advantage—is that it helps us to learn these kinds of les-sons and apply them in life to our advantage.

Psychological mechanisms, like the ability to use strategies to defer gratification, and other mechanisms—the ability to see things from more than one perspective, to stand back from our emotions, the abil-ity to empathise with other people, the way that we make sense of and predict the world around us—are absolutely vital to our mental health, because all are intimately associated with thoughts, behaviour and emotions. We respond to the events in our lives, by appraising and making sense of those events, and our brains are the organs that do this work. The best way to think about the issue of 'cause' in mental health is therefore to ask whether differences between people in terms of our mental health are best explained by differences in the events we experience, differences in the ways in which we appraise and respond to these events, differences in our upbringing and learning, or differences in the neurological functioning of the brain, the organ with which we're doing the appraising and responding.

We cannot understand human life in full if we don't understand the working of the human brain. However, purely biological or mechanistic accounts are incomplete. Although a better understanding of the brain is vitally important, neuroscience, without psychology, can explain very little about why two people are different. We need to understand the psychology of how we make sense of our world if we hope to understand human behaviour and emotions, and therefore mental health problems.

The Science of the Brain

It's not surprising that psychiatrists take a lead from other branches of medicine. This follows naturally from their training and professional identity, but it also conveys huge privilege—in salary, status, power and influence. Although there are challenges both from within the profession and from outsiders, much of mental health care remains dominated (albeit subtly) by a psychiatric 'disease-model' approach. Our mental health care system applies 'diagnoses' to emotional, behavioural and psychological issues. Most psychiatrists diagnose 'mental illnesses' and are trenchant in their defence of the practice. Once illnesses are diagnosed, people's life experiences and their views on the origin of their problems are often unfortunately seen as effectively irrelevant. Adopting a medical perspective, the 'aetiologies' (causes) of those supposed 'illnesses' are investigated. There is lip-service to the idea of a 'bio-psycho-social' approach and to the notion of the importance of social factors, but in practice these ideas are given short shrift.

That said, refreshing clarity is one of the more attractive aspects of a biomedical, disease-model, approach to mental health. In 1998, the Nobel prize-winning neuroscientist, Eric Kandel, published a '*new intellectual framework for psychiatry*'.[4] In it, he argued several points, two being: that '*... all mental processes, even the most complex psychological processes, derive from operations of the brain*', and that '*learning, including learning that results in dysfunctional behavior, produces alterations in gene expression. Thus all of "nurture" is ultimately expressed as "nature"*'.

On the face of it, these two statements are true (although it's unusual to be quite so reductive as to render learning down to the level of gene expression). That is, our behaviour, thoughts and emotions, and therefore learning, all 'derive from processes of the brain'. What this doesn't mean is that the idea of 'illness' or even 'disorder' is an appropriate metaphor, and much less a solid scientific explanatory framework. If 'all mental processes' derive from operations of the brain, there needs to be something else, something specific, that would justify labelling some of those mental processes as symptomatic of 'illness'. Unwise political, or personal judgements, errors of judgement or even offences—the 'high crimes and misdemeanours' that would justify the impeachment of presidents—are just as surely derived from operations of the brain. And, just to be clear, it would be as much of an offence to label these actions as symptomatic of 'sickness' as it is to mislabel psychological issues as pathological.

Nevertheless, this kind of thinking persists. In 2018, Carmine Pariante, a senior psychiatrist in the UK and a widely cited scientific author, argued[5] that '*...we have a body (which includes a brain) that feels changes in functions or sensations or emotions...*' all of which is undisputable. But he continued by labelling these sensations or emotions as 'symptoms', apparently without hesitation. And, presumably because he thought the argument was indisputable, pointed out that, because these experiences can be '*...induced, or modified, by external agents [such as] the chemical product of a pharmaceutical plant*', then there is '*no difference between medicine and psychiatry... Nothing more, nothing less*'.

Both Kandel and Pariante make an interesting logical progression, but one which is both flawed and illustrative. It's clearly true that our thoughts arise in the brain, and indeed that chemicals (and other 'external agents') can change our thinking. It's perhaps worth pointing out that every time (just to pluck a random image from the many millions) we read a poem, we're changing the neurological functioning of our brains. We think with our brains. Every thought is a biological event, that argument is central to Kandel and Pariante's case. Therefore, when we smell a flower, or watch a movie, or stroke a cat, the events in our life are changing the physical structure of the brain. That's true, but trivial. It's true that the physical structure of the brain must be changing as we have those, or any other thoughts, but that isn't relevant to our understanding of the situation; it isn't a useful level of analysis. The logic advanced here leaps from that important but uncontested point to a much more dubious conclusion; that there is 'no difference' between understanding thoughts as products of a biological brain and viewing psychiatry as a branch of medicine. Thus, my colleagues make the transition from identifying particular thoughts or emotions to labelling them as 'symptoms'. That isn't a neutral act. We have a very well-developed notion of what a 'symptom' is. It's something that indicates the presence of a disease. Moving from recognising that all mental events, by definition, occur in the brain, to describing some of them as 'symptoms' involves a whole set of assumptions; of the presence of 'disease' (or at least disorder), of the validity of distinctions between 'normal' and 'abnormal' psychological states, of the likely origin of these experiences, and so on. It seems to be the case that the only available frame of reference is that any thought judged as 'dysfunctional' must be the product of a disorder or illness and be amenable to medical treatment. No alternative conceptual framework appears available.

Differences between people, which undeniably exist, may reflect differences in biological functioning. This leads to the knee-jerk assumption that underpins much media coverage of mental health. But there are very good reasons to believe that, while the neurological functions of our brains enable us to make sense of the world, we are best thought of as learning creatures—responding, uniquely, to the events that occur in our lives. Learning is fundamental to the human condition and underpins our mental health. Our mental health, or more precisely the differences in mental health experiences between individuals are largely the product of social and environmental factors. There are broad, polygenetic, factors associated with a general susceptibility to develop a wide range of mental health problems. In other words, we may inherit a raised risk of any one of a number of different problems as a result of many thousands of specific genetic differences. That is interesting and important. But it's also clear that genetic differences explain relatively little of the risk of developing mental health problems, as opposed to the contribution of social, environmental and learning experiences. We are absolutely dependent on our genes for the development of our brains, but that applies to everyone. Nobody ignores the importance of genetics, but we need to be scientific and precise.

The Brain and Genes

Our scientific understanding of the brain has increased enormously in the past few years, but it's still worth emphasising how little we really know about how the brain supports thinking. While it's important to understand the biological functioning of our brains, we cannot explain the complexities of human behaviour merely by explanations at the level of the brain, neurons and synapses. To understand people fully, and particularly if we try to explain mental health problems from the perspective of neuroscience, we need to understand how the brain responds to the environment and the things that happen to us, and we need to understand how we make sense of these experiences.

Simplistic, deterministic, explanations need to be treated with scepticism. Firstly, there is only very weak evidence for genetic influences on mental health problems, falling a long way short of 'causes'. On a technical level, much of the evidence used to support a simple or direct biological model is, at best, open to scientific challenge. It is true that many problems appear to have high 'heritability'; that is, they tend to 'run in families'. You are more likely to experience a particular problem if one or both of your parents also had the same problems, but that does not necessarily imply that there are biological, genetically inherited characteristics at work. To try to see what I'm getting at here, imagine two slightly odd, but entirely factual, examples. Firstly, people can inherit things other than genes from their parents. Wealthy people tend to have children who turn out themselves to be wealthy, and people living in developed countries tend to have children who also live in those countries. This means that car ownership is highly 'heritable'; car ownership runs in families. There are many sound reasons for this. Not only do rich people leave physical wealth for their children in their wills, our societies are full of mechanisms in which the opportunities available to the parents are also offered to their children. Not everything that is inherited is biological or genetic.

On the other hand, many things that are undoubtedly determined by biological mechanisms do not resemble 'genetic disorders'. Thus, the likelihood of having five fingers (or, to be exact, four fingers and a thumb) on each hand has a statistical 'heritability' close to zero.[6] Polydactyly (having more than the expected number of fingers) is clearly a biological rather than social phenomenon (although the consequences of an extra digit are realised in a social world), but it's not an inherited condition. So, despite the spurious correlation that you may find if you search the Internet for 'heritability' and 'IQ' or 'mental illness', simple biological determinism is difficult to sustain on close scientific examination. That's not to say that genetics don't play a part; our brains are physical organs, and genetic factors will affect the way our brains develop and function. But it's almost certainly the case that many thousands of genetic variants all conspire to offer generally increased or decreased risks of a wide variety of problems (rather than 'a gene for X'). At the same time, a very wide variety of injuries and insults to the body and brain (influenza in pregnancy, birth difficulties, injury, drug use etc.), again, all conspire in very general ways to increase our risk of developing problems.

We can use a variety of scientific techniques to explore genetic influences on mental health and wellbeing. Twin studies have been common in the past, comparing monozygotic (identical) and non-identical twins, and we have studied the biological and adoptive relatives of people who were subsequently given a diagnosis of a mental health problem. More recently, scientists have used a technique called 'genome-wide association study' or 'GWAS', which has the ability very precisely to determine genetic or genomic differences between people with or without a particular disease.

We know that it is more common for us to experience mental health problems if our parents have had similar problems. But this is not necessarily evidence of genetic factors in the common-sense interpretation of the phrase. It is very difficult to disentangle genetic inheritance from environmental factors such as upbringing and social circumstances. The methodology and results of studies relating to genetic factors in 'schizophrenia', for example, are hotly debated in professional journals. In the early days of genetic research, it was common to discuss the idea of a 'gene for schizophrenia'. Now, it is much more common to discuss more general polygenetic 'risk'. There may be many heritable characteristics which each, very slightly, increases the likelihood of someone experiencing mental health problems if they are exposed to particular life events. That, in itself, is much more complex than: '…schizophrenia is a genetic disease…'. It's largely unsurprising to recognise that a very wide variety of genetic factors interact to influence broad psychological traits.

In that context, we need to remember that the genetic parts of this jigsaw are common to a wide range of mental health problems; psychosis (hearing voices or experiencing paranoia), mood swings, social communication and difficulties in concentration. These genetic factors are important, but do not imply inevitability; genetic factors interact with environmental factors; and modern genetic science has also highlighted the role of 'epigenetics': the phenomenon whereby important parts of our genetic mechanisms are 'switched on' or moderated by external or environmental factors. So, for instance, a gene that is responsible for the production of a specific protein may be more or less active, and may produce more or less of that protein, in different environmental conditions. At the cellular level, environmental pressures lead to distinct chemical changes at the level of DNA. The best-known process is 'methylation' in which methyl groups (CH_3) are added to the DNA molecule. This changes the expression of a DNA strand without changing the sequence of base-pairs that constitute the genome itself. The presence of the methyl group, attached to the chemical strand itself, prevents the biological mechanisms within the cell from producing the relevant proteins and hence yielding the biological effects. The environment, by changing the circumstances that influence methylation and other cellular processes, alters our DNA's functionality.

The science of genomics has given us remarkable insights into the biology of these phenomena, insights that also change what we understand to be 'genetic' influences. The findings are both striking and thought-provoking. Genetic factors play a role in all human phenomena, but in different ways. In the most fundamental sense, all human behaviours that require thought—from voting for political parties to falling in love—rely on our brains, and it is obvious that the physical development of our brains depends on our genes. What matters is how those genes affect the development of the organ of thought.

Biological Psychology, is there any other Kind?

In the history of psychiatry, there seem to have been psychiatrists highly sceptical of a simple, reductionist, biomedical, approach to mental health, and large numbers of psychiatrists who swallow it without question. In his 1989 paper entitled '*Biological psychiatry: is there any other kind?*' Samuel Guze argued that, since those kinds of behaviours, emotions and thoughts that constituted the subject matter of psychiatry had their origins in the brain, we necessarily must look to brain science and biological manipulations of the brain to solve these problems.[7] In his slightly more elegant paper in 1998, Eric Kandel argued that changes in biological functioning (as opposed to psychological functioning) are the 'final common pathway' for mental disorder and, indeed, therapy. So, for Kandel, all the important factors that affect our mental health do so by causing changes in biological functioning. For Kandel, that includes therapy. Kandel argues that therapy works by changing the biology of your brain. There is a superficial (although only superficial) attraction to this argument.

On one level, this analysis is obviously true. All thoughts involve brain activity. There is no conceivable way in which they could not. If I sit back, close my eyes and think of someone I love (or, indeed, dislike), my brain activity will change. If I were to lie in an functional Magnetic Resonance Imaging (fMRI) scanner, then we would be able to see direct biological correlates of that change in brain activity in real time. fMRI technology relies on picking up the resonant signals from water molecules in the blood circulating in the brain. More active neurons require a greater blood flow, and hence, we infer brain activity from the changes in regional blood flow.

Any learning must be based on biological changes in the brain at the molecular and synaptic level, because we don't have any other physical mechanism for learning. However, using such an argument as the basis for a biological reductionist model of either mental health or therapy is intellectually vacuous. All learning, all human behaviour, is dependent on the functioning of the brain, but merely invoking 'the brain' doesn't explain very much. A functioning brain is necessary for all human activities. It isn't logical or necessary to assume that any particular differences in thinking or emotions reflect biological differences.

Life events and experiences alter our brain biology. Our brains change, electrically and chemically, in response to stimuli, to events in the environment. That's how brains work. As Eric Kandel argued, all learning must logically be represented in the neural architecture of the brain. If indeed (as Kandel said, and as I agree) all thoughts, feelings and behaviours are ultimately 'derive from processes in the brain', and the brain is a biological organ, then it's totally unsurprising to find physical correlates of our reactions to life experiences. For example, dopaminergic pathways are influenced by, among other things, abuse and chronic victimisation.[8]

It is conceivable that important differences in our emotions, thoughts and behaviours reflect biological differences. But it's equally possible that these differences reflect the way in which near identical brains have learned very different things. I am writing this book on a laptop computer, and all the 20 million or so MacBookAirs (or at least those running macOS 'High Sierra' on a 2.2 GHz processor) are essentially identical. I can be pretty sure, however, that the ideas contained in this book, worded in the way I have chosen, are unique. Moreover, if I were to transfer the word-processing file to a different machine, the ideas stay the same, even if the hardware of the computer changes. I'm not trying to say that mental health issues and brains are identical to word-processing and computers, but it is reasonable to ask whether our more distressing thoughts, emotions or behaviours reflect the phenomenon of learning as opposed to the physical infrastructure for learning.

1.8 Million new Synapses a Second

Our brains are made of a staggering 86 billion neurons. In addition to the neurons, there are perhaps another 85 billion glial cells. Glial cells provide 'life-support' to the neurons. They maintain the temperature, oxygen levels, energy levels of the neurons, clear away dead neurons and provide the insulating myelin sheath that wraps around the neurons. They also seem to magnify or attenuate the signals transmitted by the neurons. The neurons themselves connect with each other through a branching network of thread-like tendrils or 'dendrites'. Where the neurons connect, they form synapses, such that each of the 86 billion neurons will make connections to tens of thousands of other neurons. Although most psychology or biology textbooks illustrate these with drawings that look a little like trees, with branches and twigs joining each other at the tips, the physical reality is more like tiny cotton-wool balls; there are so many connections that the cells are furry rather than branch-like.

The physical rate of growth of the human brain is staggering. Research conducted on young rhesus monkeys suggests that around 40,000 new synapses are created every second, and it's entirely likely that human brains are even more complex. New synapses are created very rapidly early in a child's development, but continue to be made, and broken, throughout life. Some estimates suggest that each of us makes between 1 and 1.8 million new neural connections every second of our lives.[9] These changes occur in response to the stimuli and experiences, the learning, that we are exposed to over our lifetime. And this figure, while staggering, takes no account of any changes in the activity of the 85 billion glial cells, modulating the activity of neurones, no account of any changes in the trillions of neurotransmitter receptors, or the environmentally determined methylation of trillions of DNA base-pairs and the consequent production and release of neurotransmitter molecules, each of which binds to receptor molecules to trigger the 'firing' of neurones. Our brains, in their hugely complex set of shifting, developing, changing, connections, reflect our memories, habits and learning through new physical structures. There isn't really any other way we'd have evolved to do it, but equally it is therefore not in the slightest bit surprising that each person's brain is physically different.

The Brain and the Environment

Interaction between genes and environment is fundamentally important. Without changing the DNA sequence, nature has evolved a chemical process by which our environment interacts with our DNA. That affects a wide range of human behaviours and physical processes. But there are other ways in which we can see complex, subtle, but powerful interactions at work.

If we all smoked 40 cigarettes a day, the prevalence of lung cancer would be enormously high. But not all of us would develop lung cancer. Some of us are genetically more vulnerable than others. In a world in which everybody smokes, these genetic differences would be the only real source of differential risks. The same would be true if nobody smoked; again, any genetic differences would be the principal source of variance. In fact, about 20% of people in the UK smoke cigarettes, and cigarette smoke is carcinogenic. This means that whether or not we expose ourselves to this massive risk factor is more important than our relative genetic vulnerabilities. The same seems to be true in the realm of mental health. Genetic factors are important, but we often ignore the 'elephant in the room'—the environmental causes of distress.

A colleague of mine worked as a professor of psychiatry at the University of Oxford. As such, he was exposed to some highly intelligent, but also quirky, characters. He recalled a conversation with a senior scientist whose story was this. '*I discovered at an early age*', he said, '*that my great-grandfather, my grandfather, and my father had all died from the consequences of excess alcohol. I concluded that they were all alcoholics, and that, since this seemed to be a family trait, that I, too, would be at risk.... so, I decided never to touch a drop*'.

If, then, our colleague had a genetic predisposition to alcohol metabolism, then ... he was nevertheless wise enough to recognise the risk and then do something about it. His decision (which is a psychological issue) changed the trajectory of that biological inheritance. He may have been destined, irredeemably, to possess a certain genome sequence inherited from his parents (if, indeed, his suspicions were accurate), but he was not, in fact, destined to 'be an alcoholic'. His decision, made in the light of the knowledge available to him and his rational faculties, changed his destiny.

Brain research is vitally important as we struggle to understand ourselves better. That applies to mental health and to wider psychology. But we have to be careful how we interpret this kind of research, and in particular not to use biologically reductionist arguments. For instance, there have been several well-developed theoretical models suggesting that the neurotransmitter dopamine plays some kind of role in experiences such as hearing voices (auditory hallucinations) or terrifying fears that we're at risk from a plot to kill us.[10] There could well be a lot of mileage here. Some of the psychological processes involved in both phenomena may well use dopamine as a principal neurotransmitter. Dopamine is associated with various aspects of our reward and motivation systems, and street drugs that boost dopamine functioning (bonding to dopamine receptors in the brain) can lead people to making creative (at lower doses) or bizarre and terrifying (at higher doses) links between apparently unrelated things. That seems, at least to me, to be interesting when trying to make sense of hearing voices when there's nobody there, or becoming terrified of non-existent threats.

Our mental health problems cannot be separated from the events and circumstances of our lives. The function of the brain is to respond to the environment. The underlying, fundamental, purpose of our brain, given that it's a biological system, is to respond to changing environmental conditions or external stimuli by using those biological mechanisms. If I am suddenly confronted with a threat—a snarling dog pokes its head around a corner—I need rapidly to appraise the situation, make decisions and take action. I'll do all that using my brain, and I really don't have any choice other than to use the mechanisms of neural transmission, depolarisation, chemical neurotransmitter receptor affinity, etc. So, when I see the snarling dog, there's a cascade of neurotransmitter and electrochemical activity with all the psychological consequences that follow. But the neurotransmitter and electrochemical mechanisms aren't the cause of the issue (it's the snarling dog) and changes in my brain activity aren't responsible for my actions (it's the dog). It's absolutely important to understand how the brain works, but understanding the mechanisms isn't necessarily the same as understanding the wider picture.

People seem more likely to accept a social or psychological account of relatively common problems such as anxiety or depression. We find it much easier to empathise with the experiences of low mood, fatigue, self-condemnation and fear and to understand the circumstances that give rise to them, simply because they are so much more common, but find it more appropriate to use an 'illness', 'disorder', 'disease' metaphor for problems such as obsessions and compulsions, hearing voices or other psychotic experiences. This may simply be because we have very available explanations for commonplace experiences, but fall back on 'sickness' when we're less familiar with the processes involved.

Many professionals and academics also feel that genetic and biological influences are stronger in the case of psychotic experiences, by which they mean that differences between us in terms of our experiences seem to have more correlation with biological differences or with genetic inheritance in these kinds of phenomena. And that may very well be true. It is highly unlikely to be the case that there are literally no genetic, inherited, factors at play, or that each type of phenomenon is identical in this respect. But psychotic experiences also function as good examples of how biological, psychological and social factors interact ... not to produce an 'illness', but in our complex and sometimes troubling experiences.

The neuroscientist Jim van Os[11] focusses on experiences that lead to a diagnosis of 'schizophrenia', often seen as a quintessential example of a 'mental illness'. His research suggests that psychotic experiences such as hallucinations and delusions can be understood as 'disorders of adaptation to social context'. I have to say that, even here, I would tend not to use the word 'disorder', but for van Os, this means that people have problems as a result of the way they have been forced to adjust to difficult social circumstances. While inherited, genetic, factors are important, environmental factors are also important. van Os points out that psychotic experiences are associated with a range of external, social, stressful events, such as abusive experiences in childhood, growing up in an urban environment, coming from a minority community (including minority ethnic groups, but also people from other minority groups), growing up in socially or economically unequal communities, and the use of cannabis. He concludes that exposure to these environmental threats while the brain (especially the 'social brain') is developing may increase the risk of later psychotic experiences. This implies that psychotic problems might be the consequence of the interaction of sadly common stressful life events with a neurocognitive vulnerability that again might be much more common than the perhaps 1% of people who receive a diagnosis of 'schizophrenia'. The work of Jim van Os (and others) suggests there might be a common pattern of neurocognitive vulnerability to the effects of a wide range of environmental problems, especially at vulnerable ages, affecting maybe 20% of the population. This is important and interesting because it necessarily shifts the attention from a very small number of people (1%) who may be viewed as having 'a specific genetic abnormality', towards a much more common (20% of the population) pattern of vulnerability. Moreover, once we accept that (scientifically more valid) way of thinking, the discussion of genetics moves from a 'cause' of an 'illness' towards a more integrated and useful model. Jim van Os and many other researchers stress that, in their opinion, there is a strong genetic element to the underlying pattern of vulnerability, which appears to relate to perception (and therefore, perhaps, why hallucinations and delusions are associated), motivation, mood and information processing. But there is a strong interaction between genes and environment.

Deliberately Altering Brain Chemistry

The neurotransmitter serotonin is associated with a range of brain processes. This seems to be a characteristic aspect of brain functioning: since there are many more psychological processes than there are neurotransmitters, each neurotransmitter plays more than one role; the pathways responsible for voluntary movement and perception, for example, both involve dopamine. Serotonin, however, has reliably been associated with motivation, mood and perception of social status. As a result, abnormalities in serotonin metabolism have been implicated in depression. Our bodies are efficient in their use of resources. Neurotransmitters are absorbed back into neurons after they have performed their function of transmitting signals across synapses. Many antidepressant drugs, the selective serotonin reuptake inhibitors (SSRIs), block this reuptake of serotonin, increasing the amount of serotonin in the synaptic cleft (the microscopic space between the neurons). This, we presume, tends (in the period immediately after taking the medication) to make it more likely that the neural pathway will become activated; the presence of the additional serotonin means that it's more likely that the threshold for depolarisation will be met.

Serotonin is associated with social status. Dominant male monkeys (the alpha males) have been found to have higher levels of serotonin, but when a dominant male loses his elevated social status, these serotonin levels fall. Most interestingly, when a subordinate male monkey is deliberately given either tryptophan or an antidepressant (both of which will affect serotonin metabolism), they appear to achieve dominant status. In a fascinating but disturbing experiment, researchers allowed monkeys to administer cocaine to themselves. Subordinate macaque monkeys tended to use more cocaine than the dominant monkeys. Cocaine stimulates dopamine and serotonin release. The researchers believe that the subordinate monkeys may be using cocaine to medicate themselves against the consequences of their low social status.[12]

The state we call 'depression' may be a natural response to circumstances that involve failure, lack of reinforcement or reward, low social status, abandonment and loss. This understandable phenomenon (or cluster of phenomena) can also result from physical interference with serotonin production. This makes perfect sense, if we assume that the brain—through neurochemical mechanisms that involve serotonin—is responsible for the information processing relating to the ways in which people see themselves, their world, and their future. Echoing the work of Jim van Os, in this case focussing on depression rather than psychotic experiences, if a person's social circumstances involve prolonged exposure to an environment of failure and loneliness, especially during sensitive developmental periods, there are likely to be long-term implications. A system of neurological processes that use serotonin as a principal neurotransmitter is indeed associated with depression. Serotonin appears to be implicated in the biochemical systems that we use to process information about social status, intimately associated with mood and therefore depression. It does seem to be the case that life events, both immediately and over a longer period of time, can affect both our levels of happiness, our sense of social status and likelihood of receiving a diagnosis of depression. It seems clear, to me, that serotonin is one of the neurotransmitters involved, but I don't think it makes sense to assume that depression is a form of 'illness' any more than it makes sense to say that love (which, at least in my experience, involves a LOT of neurotransmitters) is a disease.

Interactions

When I give lectures about the impact of social factors, a common question follows roughly this format: *'It's clearly terrible that some people are exposed to racism, or poverty, or conflict, or sexual assaults. These kinds of events are unambiguously associated with mental health problems, and it's easy to see why. And, yes, we need to focus on prevention. But... it's simply true to point out that not everybody who is exposed to a stressful event will develop problems. Of course we need to do something about the impact of conflict on civilians, but it's just a fact of life that not every refugee will develop PTSD, not every survivor of childhood sexual abuse will grow up to receive a diagnosis of "emotionally unstable personality disorder", and not every child growing up in poverty will be depressed as an adult'.* So, therefore, the argument goes, we have to look towards vulnerabilities and resilience. *'Surely...'* it is argued *'... the fact that all these people have been exposed to the stressful event and only some of them have developed mental health problems proves that there's some form of vulnerability—presumably genetic—in those who suffer most?'*.

Different people are adversely affected by traumatic events to different extents. And it's reasonable to look to genetics for part of the explanation for that. Several researchers have set out to answer this question in relation to depression. Specifically, they looked at research that explored the impact of both life events and genetic variants on the experience of depression. I mentioned earlier two key pieces of background information, the fact that serotonin is implicated in depression and the role of serotonin reuptake. SSRIs are argued to be effective treatments for depression by inhibiting our ability to re-absorb serotonin for re-use. That leaves serotonin in the inter-cellular gap, presumably therefore increasing the likelihood of triggering depolarisation of serotonergic, motivation-related, neurones. If that's true, the argument goes, then there's a natural, genetic, equivalent. We each have one of two different variants of the 5-HTTLPR gene, the gene that codes for the re-uptake transporter protein. That's a complex protein in the membrane of our neurones which (in a complicated chemical process) physically 'flips' serotonin back inside the neuron and available for re-use. The relevant gene comes in either a 'long' or a 'short' form, and that influences the efficiency of the transporter proteins. If, then, we differ, genetically, in respect to these different genotypes, then it follows that we might be able to see this impact on our vulnerability to mental health problems. We might presume, for instance, that the more 'inefficient' variants of the transporter gene or transporter protein would mirror the effect of a SSRI (the 'inhibition' being similar to the less efficient genetic variant), and yield a person less vulnerable to depression in the face of stressful life events.

A major study in 2003 by Avshalom Caspi and colleagues[13] aimed to investigate why, in the words of the authors: '...*stressful experiences lead to depression in some people but not in others*'. They reported that the 'short/short' example of genetic variance was associated with more depression, and suicidal thinking, following stressful life events ... although it's worth noting that this genetic variant moderated the impact of life events, it didn't offer 100% protection or 100% vulnerability. A similar study in 2005 by Kenneth Kendler and colleagues[14] found a similar pattern; that people with the 'short/short' genetic appeared more likely to become depressed following what the researchers termed 'minor stressors'.

More recently, the neuroscientist Neil Risch and colleagues conducted a meta-analysis (a statistical combination of numerous similar studies) of a large number of previously published research studies examining this kind of interaction between genetics and life events[15] in the context of depression. What Risch and colleagues found is that (unsurprisingly) people who had experienced more life events were slightly, but statistically significantly, more likely to experience depression. However, rather surprisingly, they didn't find that the different genes made any difference at all. In their words: '... *the number of stressful life events was significantly associated with depression... No association was found between 5-HTTLPR genotype and depression in any of the individual studies nor in the weighted average ... and no interaction effect between genotype and stressful life events on depression was observed...'*. Their conclusion: '... *This meta-analysis yielded no evidence that the serotonin transporter genotype alone or in interaction with stressful life events is associated with an elevated risk of depression...'*.

Our genes are important; it would be ridiculous to deny this. And the serotonin transporter gene is fundamentally important in the functioning of the nervous system. There's some intriguing suggestion that the expression of this gene is altered (through epigenetic effects) when we fall in love, which might suggest that reward mechanisms are active there, too.[16] What seems less clear-cut is whether the variants between humans play much of a role. It matters that we all have a serotonin reuptake system, but it might not matter too much whether or not we have either one, or the other, of the common variants.

We do indeed differ in how we respond to stressful life events. We all use our wonderfully evolved brains to respond, and there appears (in my judgement) to be little evidence that genetic differences between us explain much in the way of those differences. But there are other possible reasons for such differences.

Psychological Vulnerability

Humans have evolved to learn. We learn simple things (not to put our fingers in the fire) and more complicated things. We learn high-level conceptual rules about the nature of the world in which we live. Even very young children swiftly learn complex information, vital to their survival, but also key to their mental health. This shapes our resilience or vulnerability.

A recent study hinted at how early we learn, and how complex and deep that learning can be. Francesco Margoni and colleagues at the University of Trento[17] found that even two-year-old children could tell the difference between legitimate power (when someone is chosen to be leader or has natural talents) and power based on bullying and fear. They showed the children little cartoon videos with scenarios illustrating these kinds of interpersonal behaviour. One, for example, began with three cartoon figures playing with a ball meeting a character wearing a flamboyant hat. This figure carried a stick that it used to strike the floor, apparently triggering a greeting ritual in which the first three characters bowed and murmured respect. The children seemed to be uninterested when these three characters then later obeyed the 'leader', but surprised when they showed disrespect. The opposite pattern was observed when the flamboyantly-hatted character acted aggressively (hitting the other characters on the head). Then, the children were surprised if the characters showed respect and were uninterested if the three little cartoon figures were disrespectful.

The point is that even young children can learn complex rules about our social lives, and these rules have implications. The example above concerned our social interactions, concepts of leadership and obedience and the consequences of doing what you're asked (or told). But the principle is generalisable to other issues. We learn (and we can assume that we learn from a very early age) what might be termed 'rules' for navigating the world. We learn about whether people (adults) do what they promise or whether they are not to be trusted. We learn whether our effort tends to be rewarded or not; many people learn, quite quickly, that it often doesn't really matter how hard we work or whether we're honest, we'll fail anyway. Many people (very sadly) have experiences that tell them that they're not competent, not loved, not valued. Other people, fortunately, have other experiences, and learn different things; that effort is rewarded, that things generally turn out positively, that even if you fail at something, the people around you will love you.

These highly abstract beliefs are important. They shape our emotional response to events. Throughout history, humans in all cultures have expended a great deal of effort on developing, celebrating, and promoting religious views. We have tended to codify and instruct young people on moral and interpersonal behaviour, how we should act (and think) about each other and the appropriate way to respond to disappointments. It matters to us how we answer the eternal question at the heart of Voltaire's great comic philosophical novel 'Candide'; why do bad things happen to good people? My colleague at the University of Liverpool, Philip Davis, Professor of Literature, believes that great literature throughout the ages; the Viking sagas, Greek myths, the great poetic stories such as the Epic of Gilgamesh, the works of Shakespeare and Cervantes, even religious works, are all examples of understanding how the world works and how we may best respond to life's challenges.

We might assume that the differences between us are genetic. That is, we do know that many of us are abused, bullied, assaulted, evicted, homeless or unemployed, but in each case, not all of us experience mental health problems. Explanations based on genetic differences are superficially attractive, but there's little evidence. On the other hand, our psychological 'schemas' also differ. We all differ, as a result of the things that happen to us, as a result of the upbringing and education we've been exposed to, in terms of how we understand, and respond to, adversity. The events don't mean the same thing to everyone. And this, at least as much as genetics, represents an understandable source of individual differences in vulnerability and resilience.

Inflammation: The new Hot Topic

There has been some recent interest in the idea that mental health problems, and particularly depression, might be associated with inflammatory processes in the brain.[18] Inflammation is a complex biological response to any bodily threat from infection, physical damage or chemical irritant. The biological functions are to eliminate the threat (including the removal of any dead or damaged cells) and to begin the process of tissue repair. To achieve those aims, chemicals released by damaged or stressed cells trigger a response of the immune system and other biological mechanisms. This, therefore, is a signalling mechanism in response to threats. But the inflammatory responses can be seen following non-physical threats such as adversity in childhood or loneliness. We all have the genetic 'blueprint' for out inflammatory mechanisms. When exposed to stress, of various kinds, we 'switch on' those genes; we activate, genetically, the mechanisms that produce the relevant chemicals and trigger the immune response. It is inevitable that social and environmental factors will affect us by perturbing neurochemical pathways. It is also possible both that these inflammatory processes might have an effect on our mental health and that this therefore represents at least one biological mechanism by which environmental stressors have their effect.

The research into the mental health implications of inflammatory processes has yielded a great deal of media attention. It has been suggested, for instance, that this kind of research '...will be life-transforming...'.[19] But, especially in media accounts of these ideas, sometimes the ideas get distorted a little. Instead of discussing the mechanisms that must, logically, mediate between stressors and our understandable reactions to these stressors, we start to read about 'causes'. That is, the mediating mechanisms (the inflammatory response, in this case) seem to be re-defined as 'causes'. Which is irritating (pun intended), because—again—the real causes are ignored. My colleague Lucy Johnstone addressed these issues in a tweet, saying: '*If we start by deconstructing the term "depression" & ask "What causes people to feel miserable, desperate, hopeless & suicidal?" it becomes obvious the only sensible answer is "Lots of things". Let's deal with them before these wild guesses about genes*'. I agree. If we were to move away from the 'disease model', if we were to stop assuming that emotional distress is merely a symptom of biological illness, we could instead embrace a psychological and social approach to mental health and wellbeing that recognises our essential and shared humanity.

A Personal Story

I wrote about the complex interplay of genes and environment in a blog about my own mental health.[20] I commented on whether or not I possess a 'phenotype', a pattern of observable characteristics or traits, resulting from the interactions of my genes and experiences. I have close relatives who have quite serious mental health problems, and I commented that I am occasionally emotionally labile; my self-esteem and emotions are, at times, fragile and very much dependent on what

I imagine other people are thinking. I frighten myself (given my relative's experiences) when I fantasise about winning Nobel prizes, winning Pulitzer prizes, being elected to this and that, being awarded knighthoods… frightening because I've seen self-referent fantasies ruin other people's lives. My selective attention is poor, and I find it difficult to avoid distractions. Those who know me well will know that I work with the BBC rolling news constantly running in the background, and I frequently play games while on the phone. I appear to have problems with face-recognition; I find it almost impossible even to recognise the faces of people whom I know well.

I find it difficult maintain eye-contact when in conversation, and look to the side to line-up images in the distance. And, perhaps most saliently, I lurch forwards and jump to conclusions in my mental logic. So, if you give me the sequence 'A, B, C' and ask me to complete the sequence, I'll say Z. Maybe that's a bit of a joke (a pun on 'complete'), and it's unequivocally good for me in my academic career. A creative professor is a good professor. I also and simultaneously make abstract and surreal connections. It's a recognised part of my teaching style; I occasionally veer off on a tangent. This may well be very useful for an academic whose career depends on innovative thinking. It is possibly engaging or at least entertaining for my students (if they can follow me…). But jumping to conclusions, tangential connectivity and abstract, 'clang' associations all have very interesting connotations in the field of mental health.

My parents had very strong religious beliefs. There was a degree of emotional repression and our family relationships were somewhat complicated. Just one example: my parents' belief system included the need to love God more than anything or anyone else, including one's children. So, after my mother's death, we discovered that, when she had confessed to a religious mentor that she was in danger of loving her children more than God, there was a subsequent process of re-adjustment. She was encouraged to practice loving her children less. My parents rejected the material world as merely a stepping-stone to heaven (or hell) and paid little attention to worldly pursuits. I remember opening a letter from Cambridge University confirming an offer of a place as an undergraduate. I told my mother, whose reply was; 'Very nice dear, now, do you want baked beans on toast for breakfast?' Pride was a very worldly emotion. I guess that experiences like that must have had an effect on my siblings and me.

So, I am very interested (and, I hope, open-minded) about what it is, if anything, that I may have inherited. How do I differ from other people? What proportion of the variance in these traits can be accounted for by genetic differences? What proportion of the variance in these traits comes from my upbringing? What proportion comes from being reinforced, through my childhood, for being academic? Which elements of my upbringing were different other people's anyway?

My childhood had at least as many oddities and peculiarities as would capture the attention of any competent psychotherapist. My professional eye has identified interesting phenotypes in my close family that reflect potentially heritable traits. These traits may well put me at risk of many emotional problems. Incidentally, they may well also make me difficult to live with, and I must give credit to those who do.

For some people, interactions of these heritable and environmental factors cause problems. For others, like me, a presumably very similar pattern of interactions has observable similarities but different outcomes. It's perfectly possible to be rational and open-minded about the contribution of genetic and environmental factors in our mental health. We can intelligently and respectfully discuss how experiences and heritable traits can interact to produce the wonderful variety of human experience. This is a much more accurate and helpful way to conceptualise what's going on than to say that some of us, but only some of us, have 'mental illnesses'. Labels such as 'schizophrenia' not only suffer from the validity problems that we've discussed, but also obfuscate these important considerations. It isn't helpful to consider how I have managed to avoid developing 'schizophrenia', or whether I might have 'attenuated psychosis syndrome'.

For many of us, there are echoes of blame, of stigma, when we identify the pathology within the genetic substrate of the person. I'm reminded of Eric Pickles' notorious throw-away comment to a voter campaigning about the abuse she'd experienced that she should; '...*adjust her medication*...'.[21] If the pathology lies in the person, and particularly if it is a biological problem, we can dismiss any further troubling considerations.

Rather than talking about 'abnormality', we are now really talking about normal psychological processes. It is generally seen as good and useful to be creative, to make connections between events, to see something and make a mental connection to something else. It's generally considered a valuable human trait to feel emotions (especially when the situation objectively justifies such emotions). It's also generally considered good for people to be personally involved with, or engaged in, their social lives. If a person is uncreative, makes no connections between distantly related ideas, is emotionally detached and unperturbed by events, there may well be something wrong. On the other hand, if a person makes spurious connections between unrelated ideas, is emotionally overwhelmed and sees personal salience and relevance in circumstantial events, they may well be at risk from this 'pattern of vulnerability'. What we appear to be looking at is less a 'gene for schizophrenia' or even a 'genetic abnormality', and more the normal variance in human characteristics, with all the positive and negative consequences that naturally follow.

An Envelope Falls on the Mat

The stoic philosopher Epictetus anticipated the basic principles of the cognitive behavioural therapies when he said (something like): '*It is not events that disturb people, it is their judgements concerning them*'.

So, when a slim white envelope drops on the mat, our emotional response is necessarily complex. A letter detailing a promotion has one effect; a letter giving notice of intended prosecution has a very different effect. In physiological terms, the processes of these two events are close to identical... up to a point. More photons bounce off the white paper than the black ink. Rod and cone cells in our retinas respond, sending electrical signals through an almost unbelievably complex system of information processing that successively recognises patterns of light and dark, edges and simple shapes, more complicated shapes, until those shapes are matched to stored representations first of letters and then of words. The words are recognised and sequenced in context until meaning is inferred. And that, in itself, is a hugely complicated process which involves quite a lot of controversy among academic psychologists.

We perform this analysis of the external world extremely quickly, almost automatically, but it is of course the personal meaning of the words on the paper (rather than anything to do with the biology) that makes the difference between happiness and depression. The biological systems support that meaning-making, but it's at the psychological level, not the biological level, where the significance lies. The letter, the ink on the paper, the photons, the biological systems…. they are all important in many ways. But what makes the difference, what triggers either a cascade of 'happiness' related biology or a cascade of 'depression' related biochemical, neurological, consequences, is the ordinary, human, meaning of the words.

Notes

1. References to 'the marshmallow test' are easily found on the internet, including a video at: http://www.cbsnews.com/video/watch/?id= 6419327n&tag=related;photovideo. The original paper is: Yuichi Shoda, Walter Mischel, and Philip K. Peake, "Predicting adolescent cognitive and self-regulatory competencies from preschool delay of gratification: Identifying diagnostic conditions," *Developmental Psychology* 26, no. 6 (1990): 978–986.

2. The (rather uncritical) report on the marshmallow tests in the *New York Times* can be found here: https://www.nytimes.com/2014/01/12/magazine/we-didnt-eat-the-marshmallow-the-marshmallow-ate-us.html.

3. The more recent investigation of the marshmallow test, incorporating social aspects, is: Tyler W. Watts, Greg J. Duncan, and Haonan Quan, "Revisiting the marshmallow test: A conceptual replication investigating links between early delay of gratification and later outcomes," *Psychological Science* 29, no. 7 (2018): 1159–1177. http://journals.sagepub.com/doi/abs/10.1177/0956797618761661.

4. Eric R. Kandel, "A new intellectual framework for psychiatry," *American Journal of Psychiatry* 155, no. 4 (1998): 457–469.

5. Carmine M. Pariante, "A parallel universe where psychiatry is like the rest of medicine," *Epidemiology and Psychiatric Sciences* 27, no. 2 (2018): 143–145. http://europepmc.org/articles/PMC5842894/.

6. Jay Joseph and Carl Ratner, "The fruitless search for genes in psychiatry and psychology: Time to re-examine a paradigm," in Sheldon Krimsky and Jeremy Gruber (eds.), *Genetic explanations: Sense and nonsense* (Cambridge, MA: Harvard University Press, 2013), 94–106.
7. Samuel B. Guze, "Biological psychiatry: Is there any other kind?" *Psychological Medicine* 19, no. 2 (1989): 315–323.
8. John Read, Roar Fosse, Andrew Moskowitz, and Bruce Perry, "The traumagenic neurodevelopmental model of psychosis revisited," *Neuropsychiatry* 4, no. 1 (2014): 65–79. https://doi.org/10.2217/npy.13.89.
9. This statistic is widely quoted and derives from a range of neurodevelopmental work. For at least one take on such issues (and references to this astonishing figure), try: Jeffrey Schwartz and Sharon Begley, *The mind and the brain: Neuroplasticity and the power of mental force* (New York: HarperCollins, 2007).
10. Jim van Os, Gunter Kenis, and Bart P.F. Rutten, "The environment and schizophrenia," *Nature* 468, no. 7321 (2010): 203. https://www.nature.com/articles/nature09563.
11. See note 10 and Jim van Os, "'Schizophrenia' does not exist," *British Medical Journal* 352 (2016): i375. https://www.bmj.com/content/352/bmj.i375.
12. Michael A. Nader, Paul W. Czoty, Susan H. Nader, and Drake Morgan, "Nonhuman primate models of social behavior and cocaine abuse," *Psychopharmacology* 224, no. 1 (2012): 57–67. https://www.ncbi.nlm.nih.gov/pmc/articles/PMC3469766/.
13. Avshalom Caspi, Karen Sugden, Terrie E. Moffitt, Alan Taylor, Ian W. Craig, HonaLee Harrington, Joseph McClay, et al., "Influence of life stress on depression: Moderation by a polymorphism in the 5-HTT gene," *Science* 301, no. 5631 (2003): 386–389.
14. Kenneth S. Kendler, Jonathan W. Kuhn, Jen Vittum, Carol A. Prescott, and Brien Riley, "The interaction of stressful life events and a serotonin transporter polymorphism in the prediction of episodes of major depression: A replication," *Archives of General Psychiatry* 62, no. 5 (2005): 529–535. https://doi.org/10.1001/archpsyc.62.5.529.
15. Neil Risch, Richard Herrell, Thomas Lehner, Kung-Yee Liang, Lindon Eaves, Josephine Hoh, Andrea Griem, Maria Kovacs, Jurg Ott, and Kathleen Ries Merikangas, "Interaction between the serotonin transporter gene (5-HTTLPR), stressful life events, and risk of depression: A meta-analysis," *Journal of the American Medical Association* 301, no. 23 (2009): 2462–2471.

16. Donatella Marazziti, Hagop S. Akiskal, Alessandra Rossi, and Giovanni B. Cassano, "Alteration of the platelet serotonin transporter in romantic love," *Psychological Medicine* 29, no. 3 (1999): 741–745. https://doi. org/10.1017/s0033291798007946.

17. Francesco Margoni, Renée Baillargeon, and Luca Surian, "Infants distinguish between leaders and bullies," *Proceedings of the National Academy of Sciences* 115, no. 38 (2018): E8835–E8843. https://doi. org/10.1073/pnas.1801677115.

18. Edward Bullmore, *The inflamed mind: A radical new approach to depression* (Picador, 2018).

19. The 'life-transforming' speculation can be found in this newspaper article: https://amp.theguardian.com/commentisfree/2018/apr/29/ revolution-in-our-understaning-of-depression-will-be-life-transforming.

20. My blog about my own mental health, and the complex pathways involved, can be found here: https://www.madinamerica.com/2015/03/ brain-baked-beans/.

21. Eric Pickle's unpleasant statement can be found here: https://www. independent.co.uk/news/uk/politics/eric-pickles-tells-survivor-of-alleged-child-abuse-adjust-your-medication-8846503.html.

4

Making Sense of Things

We are born as natural learning engines, with highly complex but very receptive brains, ready to understand and then engage with the world. As a consequence of the events we experience in life, we develop mental models of the world, including the social world. We then use these mental models to guide our thoughts, emotions and behaviours. Our social circumstances, and our biology, influence our emotions, thoughts and behaviours—our mental health—through their effects on how we have learned to make sense of, and respond to, the world. This puts psychology at the centre of discussions about mental health, but also adds something to the 'nature-nurture' debate. Seeing our mental health as the consequence of normal, understandable, psychological processes, rather than ill-defined and elusive 'illnesses', offers an opportunity radically to re-conceptualise mental health services.

Since the 1950s, psychologists, neuroscientists and anthropologists have learned a great deal about how people understand the world. We know a great deal about how our perceptual system makes sense of the huge volume of visual and auditory information hitting our eyes and ears every second. We understand how we make sense of this information and how the brain stores information in memory. Psychologists understand (and use) basic principles of reward and punishment, and the implications of such technical issues as 'discriminant stimuli' and 'intermittent

© The Author(s) 2019
P. Kinderman, *A Manifesto for Mental Health*,
https://doi.org/10.1007/978-3-030-24386-9_4

reinforcement'. Complex theoretical models such as the 'interacting cognitive subsystems' model[1] are highly unlikely to be perfect, but they might give helpful insights into how our minds progressively trans-form structural data about the world (the patterns of light and dark, edges and corners) into useful information concerning objects, people, actions, relationships, and finally we infer intentions and meaning.

Psychologists have published detailed (and constantly evolving) hypo-thetical models of the ways in which people understand their relation-ships with parents, with peers, partners and others. We conduct research into how we understand and explain events in the outside world, and into how we identify and appraise our own thoughts. Psychologists have studied how we form and maintain beliefs, relevant to a wide range of serious mental health problems. Psychologists and economists (because these issues inform our financial decision-making) have won Nobel prizes for studying 'heuristic reasoning', the mental 'short-cuts' that we use to act in a complex and uncertain universe.[2] Psychologists, especially from the behavioural tradition, understand how people and animals respond in circumstances of unremitting punishment (so-called learned helplessness). More recently, cognitive psychology (that is, psy-chological models based on our thinking processes) has explored our sense of self-efficacy (what we believe we can do, and why) and the neg-ative cognitive schemas (sets of related thoughts) that accompany (or possibly even cause) depressed mood.

We are born with highly complex but very receptive brains, ready to understand and then engage with the world. As a consequence of the events we experience in life, we develop mental models of the world, including the social world. We then use these mental models to guide our thoughts, emotions and behaviours. This puts psychology at the centre of discussions about mental health, but also adds something to the 'nature-nurture' debate. What we understand about the world, our beliefs, our psychology, has real causal value. If I believe I'm a worthless person, my mental health will suffer. Of course, there are reasons why I may think I'm worthless, but that is not unusual (many things in life have their own causes, but nevertheless have consequences). Our beliefs, whatever their origins in either nature or nurture, are a vital extra com-ponent to the 'nature-nurture' argument.

Levels of Explanation

We are living, biological, organisms and can do nothing to escape the laws of organic chemistry. Our brains are governed by gene expression, anatomy, neurochemistry and even electromagnetism. But for me, psychology—or how we think about the world—is at the centre of human life. Biological, social and circumstantial factors affect our mental health when they disrupt or alter psychological processes. We may be the product of an interaction between genes and environment, but humans are more than that because we make sense of the world.

Simple explanations are attractive because they imply that there might be a straightforward solution. Perhaps these explanations are also appealing because they appear to attach no blame to the individual or those around them; it's nobody's 'fault' that there's a chemical imbalance. Maybe they are attractive because the remedy (taking medication) requires little or no effort: the patient merely needs to obey the doctors, adhere to the regime, and the medicine will do the work. Perhaps this is also attractive because it also implies that the rest of society doesn't have to change; we don't have to put extra effort into protecting our children, or changing our homophobic and misogynistic society, or reform employment laws or, God forbid, redistribute wealth and power. We just have to sympathise with those of us unfortunate to fall ill and keep taking the pills. But life is more complex than that.

The European Commission Green Paper—'A Multiplicity of Factors'

In 2005, the European Commission published an important document discussing the kinds of actions and policies that European governments might be expected to undertake to improve mental health care across the continent.[3] In the preamble, the authors attempted to define the problems before moving on to discuss solutions. The European Commission concluded that: '… *for* **citizens**, *mental health is a resource which enables them to realise their intellectual and emotional potential and to find and fulfil their roles in social, school and working life. For* **societies***, good mental* *health of citizens contributes to prosperity, solidarity and social justice'*. The document continues: '*... The mental condition of people is determined by a **multiplicity of factors** including biological (e.g. genetics, gender), individual (e.g. personal experiences), family and social (e.g. social support) and economic and environmental (e.g. social status and living conditions)...*'.

It's widely accepted that most mental health (and, indeed, physical health) issues are best explained in terms of some form of complex interactions of biological, psychological and social factors. The UK's National Health Service offers online information about depression that echoes this: stating that 'there is no single cause of depression', and that 'different causes can often combine to trigger depression', before going on to list stressful life events, illness including coronary heart disease, cancer and head injuries, personality traits, social isolation, the use of alcohol and drugs and childbirth (as a risk for the mother, not necessarily the child).[4]

The Biopsychosocial Model

The 'biopsychosocial model' stems from the work of George Engel, published in 1977 in the journal *Science*.[5] Engel commented that many descriptions or explanations of both mental health problems and physical illness reduced the problems to very simplistic biological explanations, and he felt that this was particularly true for our mental health. Depression, anxiety and psychosis were all too frequently described simply as brain diseases (even if nobody could be too sure what that brain disease actually was). Rather than discussing parenting, love, hopes, fears, relationships, learning and traumatic life events, Engel thought that too many doctors were thinking of mental health purely in terms of neurones, synapses and neurotransmitters. For Engel, this excessive biomedical focus characterised physical illness too. A heart attack involves vascular problems in the coronary arteries, but Engel was concerned that social factors in the development of physical health problems (diet, exercise, access to health care) and in the consequences of illness (anxiety, depression, losing your job, impact on your family) were being ignored.

Engel explicitly hoped his model would provide a scientific account of mental health that could challenge these 'reductionist' biological approaches. And, to a large extent (and perhaps particularly in physical health) many of Engel's aims have been met. Across a wide range of threats to our physical health and wellbeing, we now recognise the importance of taking a public health, even political, perspective. We understand the causal roles of biology (for instance, the way in which the body metabolises lipids) and we understand how to intervene in these processes (e.g. through the use of statins). But we also recognise how our 'obesogenic' lifestyles, and, behind them, the laws and regulations on such issues as taxation policy, advertising regulation, the sale of schools' recreation grounds (a minor scandal in the UK), can impact on our health. We also recognise how 'interventions' such as dietary changes and increased exercise can more than supplement the prescription of statins.

Engel's biopsychosocial model has been extremely influential. The original article has been cited at least 11,000 times in scientific papers and yields an impressive 2.6 million Google hits on the Internet. The model is simple and flexible, which means it can absorb a wide variety of evidence supporting biological, social or psychological influences on mental health (in other words, a very comprehensive picture). It also means that different schools of thought pushed and pulled the model in different ways after its publication.

In 2005, Steven Sharfstein the incoming President of the American Psychiatric Association commented on the *extraordinary presence of the pharmaceutical industry* at the Association's conference.[6] He drew the attention of delegates to the annual profits of $19.9 billion from the sale of antidepressant and antipsychotic medication. Dr. Sharfstein argued that '… *financial incentives and managed care have contributed to the notion of a "quick fix" by taking a pill and reducing the emphasis on psychotherapy and psychosocial treatments…*'. He warned that pharmaceutical companies '… *have allowed the biopsychosocial model to become the bio-bio-bio model. In a time of economic constraint, a "pill and an appointment" has dominated treatment…*'. This phrase—'the bio-bio-bio model'—attracted my friend and colleague John Read, who referred to this pressure as the '*colonisation of the psychological and social by the biological*'.[7]

The biopsychosocial model is an entry-point to a debate about the causes of mental health problems, but it doesn't represent a final answer. As an explicit scientific proposition, the biopsychosocial model doesn't explain how the relationship between the three types of variable, biological, psychological and social, works in practice. Engel merely suggested that psychological (or, in his word, 'psychophysiologic', and that, too, is significant) responses to life events interact with 'somatic' or biological factors. This was, in 1977, a timely acknowledgement of the important contribution of psychological and social factors in many psychological and physical problems (since his paper did not only focus on mental health issues). However, Engel's phrasing also reflects an assumption that there is a biological or disease primacy—the responses are 'psychophysiologic' rather than 'psychological'—which ensures that psychological factors are linked to physiological ones. Moreover, in Engel's words, these responses serve to *alter susceptibility* to *diseases* which are assumed to have a genetic predisposition and a physiological basis. Phrasing such as this predates Read's *colonisation of the psychological and social by the biological*, but similarly encourages the reader to assume that mental health problems following deprivation, loss or trauma are best thought of in terms of altered susceptibility to a recognised 'disease' that has a genetic basis rather than, as they might otherwise assume, a normal and purely psychological response to the situation. Finally, as I've said, this statement fails to account scientifically for how these entirely different classes of phenomenon interact with each other.

We are more than mere biological machines and are more than unthinking clay, simply moulded by social and circumstantial pressures. We are more than the biological products of our genes and of the inevitable consequences of contingencies of reinforcement. We make sense of our world. Our beliefs, emotions and behaviours—including our mental health—are the product of the way we think about ourselves, other people, the world and the future. And this framework of understanding the world is, in turn, the consequence of our learning: the social circumstances, life events and experiences that we have been exposed to and the ways in which we have understood and responded to them. Our brain is a supremely efficient machine for learning, and we make sense of our experiences.

Although psychology is a relatively young scientific discipline, the insights of psychological science over the past few years allow us to understand ourselves in unprecedented clarity. Biological psychology tends to suggest that we are best understood as being the slaves of our brain and, ultimately, our genes. Behavioural psychologists have acknowledged that we learn, and that we are in large part shaped by the events in our lives, but traditional behavioural accounts tend to see human beings as mechanistic robots, shaped by patterns of punishment and reward. More recently, cognitive psychology has emerged as a dominant discipline, offering a much more optimistic vision of the human condition. This sees us as intelligent, enquiring, inquisitive creatures who construct active models of the world; forming and developing complex frameworks of understanding and acting accordingly. We are more than the raw products of their biology and are not mere pawns of the vicissitudes of life. We are born as natural learning engines, with highly complex but very receptive brains, ready to understand and then engage with the world. We develop, as a consequence of the events and examples we experience in life, mental models of the world that we then use to guide our thoughts, emotions and behaviours.

Learning

Although all human behaviour involves the brain, we don't need to look for differences in brain functioning to explain differences between people. The 'job' of the brain is information processing. If two identical twins, with identical genes and therefore brains, had learned to understand the world in different ways, they would behave differently. Yes, of course it's true to say, as Eric Kandel argued, that different behaviours represent different brain states. That is equivalent to saying that different laptop computers will have different configurations at the microscopic level. To be precise, information is encoded in computers via the magnetic status of billions of tiny elements of the storage device, each one independently magnetised or demagnetised to represent 0 or 1 in the binary number system. There is a physical (in the sense of magnetic) basis to the storage of information and hence, in that sense, my laptop (with my information on it) is very subtly different—physically—to every other otherwise identical model. If my laptop has a flower as its screen saver, and yours has a photo of your daughter, then at one level the pattern of magnetised and demagnetised storage units will reflect this difference. But it would be very odd—even misleading, certainly confusing—to notice the two pictures and say something like: '*Is that an image of your daughter? I see your laptop has been physically magnetised to a different configuration of crystalline direction of magnetic moment*'. You'd say: '*I'd like to choose a photo, too*'. And it would just as odd to reply: '*Yeah, you need to take steps to re-configure the matrix of moment of magnetisation of the 1600 MHz DDR3*'. If we want to use words like 'because', then the explanation for such a difference is not 'because' the magnetisation matrices are different, but 'because' I haven't bothered to choose a decent photo. The fact that your laptop is physically different to mine is not an adequate explanation for the difference; a more satisfactory explanation lies in the choices that we have made, and the information that we have stored on them.

Similarly, the things I have learned are encoded in the physical structure of my brain (no reasonable person would assume that this doesn't happen) and more specifically in some kind of physical, synaptic, connectivity. But what my thirteen years of schooling, two years of professional training, three years researching a Ph.D., and twenty-five years as an academic have given me, and what the life experiences of each one of us have given us, is not helpfully thought of in terms of biology. What we've learned in conceptual, implicational, teleological, terms—what this means at the human, more than the biochemical, level—is what matters.

Psychological understandings have moved on from the reductive biomedicine of the eighteenth-nineteenth centuries. Some of this psychology has, itself, been simplistic. A while ago, psychologists focussed on learned associations; the 'classical conditioning' of Pavlov. This led quite swiftly to the 'law of effect'; the basic principle of behavioural psychology which states that, if an action is followed by a reinforcing, positive, consequence, it is *more* likely that it will be repeated; whereas, if an action is followed by a punishing, negative, consequence, it is *less* likely that it will be repeated. That has helped shape all kinds of policies and practices, from childcare and education to criminal justice.

But modern scientific psychology does not just limit itself to behavioural psychology and the various technical extensions of the law of effect. Cognitive psychology focusses on the idea that human beings are born as natural learning systems. We have brains that are unique in the animal world, absorbing and incorporating information at an amazing rate. To develop the adult vocabulary of 20,000 words, children have to be able to learn up to 20 new words a day. But we learn more than just words; we learn complex, nuanced meaning. Within cognitive psychology, learning is understood as the development of mental models of the world. These are complex (and often largely unconscious) constructions that depend on the simultaneous manipulation of abstract representations of the world. To make sense of the world, we have to construct frameworks of understanding that include concepts such as 'he is trustworthy'. These are abstract in the sense that we can't physically touch the 'trustworthiness', but it's clear that our everyday behaviour is influenced by these kinds of cognitive models. It's also clear that most humans have highly complex representations of the world and are constantly processing information on many levels simultaneously. So, our mental models of the world are built up from the simultaneous manipulation of enormous numbers of complex abstract representations of the events, objects, people, relationships and interactions that we observe. These models have enormous significance, as they explain how we think, feel and behave; and if you can understand these mental models, you will understand people's behaviour, emotions and beliefs.

We Are All Imperfect Learners

We develop our understanding of the world via what is largely a constructive process. Rather than 'seeing' an image of the world projected onto our brains, we build up—develop or construct—a picture or the world.

The human brain has an enormous potential for learning. We also, uniquely among all animals, made a huge evolutionary leap by developing the ability to use abstract concepts. We don't merely understand where things are and make predictions about what might happen next (although we do this too, of course). We also understand what the meaning or implications of these predictions are. We use complex, abstract, concepts such as 'trust' or 'love' and manipulate these abstractions. These things matter because they have important consequences. Imagine a long-term relationship: the two people would probably say that they love each other and trust each other. If it turns out that one person has been stealing money from their partner on a regular basis, we would expect this to have an impact on the relationship. People behave differently because 'trust' is degraded. Human reasoning is based on the simultaneous processing of multiple abstract representations of the world, and many of our most important behaviours, especially in relationships, are shaped in part by these complex and abstract ways of understanding our social world.

Of course, this is fiendishly complicated. So complicated that much of our day-to-day human thought is not based on mathematical logic, but on 'heuristics'. These are simple rules of thumb that permit rapid, if inaccurate, action. People make many (perhaps most) important decisions using precious little logic but instead relying on 'rules of thumb' and rapid, practically useful, near-guesses. Our picture of the world is a very effective and usually accurate 'best guess'. The evolutionary pressures on our ancestors mean that if they weren't largely accurate (or useful), they wouldn't have survived to give birth to us. And research into eyewitness testimony tells us that our memory is fallible. The famous 'invisible gorilla effect' (where people can miss the most obvious events, even a man in a gorilla suit, if their attention is directed elsewhere)[8] tells us that we often fail to perceive dramatic events, essentially because we are not expecting them.

Our perceptions of ourselves and the world will be shaped, like all perceptions, by a constructive process. We even construct our sense of self. We understand who we are and how we function by making working models of ourselves in our own minds. We become depressed or anxious for completely understandable reasons to do with how we think about ourselves, other people, the world and the future. We can become convinced that we are being persecuted and that we can hear disembodied voices. However, since we are all merely struggling to make sense of a complex and constantly shifting world, such occasionally distressing experiences are also entirely understandable, in both senses of the word.

There Is No 'Normal' and 'Abnormal' Psychology

In other branches of the physical sciences, we describe the functioning of the natural world through universal laws. Like many people, I occasionally travel abroad. My flights (like everything else in life) depend on the operation of the laws of physics. Although air travel is very safe, there are occasional tragedies. When these happen, the authorities investigate the probable or likely cause of the incident for national security, legal and insurance purposes. Their analysis includes human factors, but also includes complex physics. To work out why a tragedy has occurred, investigators will calculate things like the wear and erosion of the components in the aircraft engines, metal fatigue and corrosion, and the role of weather events. They will calculate trajectories using equations of acceleration and deceleration. They will consider the role of centrifugal forces, lift, the fuel mixtures. They will measure elements of the physical world; the weight of the aircraft and its cargo, climatic conditions, the temperature, tyre pressures, the condition of brakes and the nature of the runway surface. All these aspects of physics are important; they explain why accidents happen. But air crash investigators don't use a special branch of physics called 'abnormal physics'. We don't expect scientists to apply one special branch of physics to aircraft crashes and differentiate this from the laws of physics that apply to 'normal life'. There is not an 'abnormal coefficient of friction' that leads to crashes on an airport runway and a 'normal coefficient of friction' that keeps us safe. Instead, and wisely, we recognise that it is important to understand the universal laws of physics, and then use that understanding to help design safer airports and aircraft.

The laws of psychology are similarly universal. There simply isn't an 'abnormal psychology' that applies to distress or explains 'illnesses' and a different 'normal psychology' that applies to everything else. There is just psychology. Everybody makes sense of their world and does so on the basis of the experiences that they have and the learning that occurs over their lifetime. We all use the same basic processes to understand the world, even if we come to very different conclusions. The patterns and contingencies of reinforcement, rewards and punishments shape us all:

the basic psychology of behavioural learning is universal. We all learn to repeat those things that are reinforcing, and we all withdraw from things that cause us pain. We all construct more or less useful frameworks for understanding the world, and we all use those frameworks to predict the future and guide our actions. That's true for someone who has learned to trust people, and it's true for someone who has learned to distrust them. We're all using the same processes of learning and understanding, and those processes have similar effects on our behaviour and emotions. However, because no one is exactly the same as anyone else, or has exactly the same experiences, we all make sense of the world in slightly different ways, with different consequences. But that's entirely different from suggesting that there is some kind of 'abnormal psychology'. We all share one psychology; it's misleading to try to separate 'abnormal' from 'normal' psychology.

A New Account—The Mediating Psychological Processes Model

In 2005, I published a short article in the *Harvard Review of Psychiatry*[9] in which I argued that we needed a more rigorous and coherent approach to the biopsychosocial model. Instead of merely suggesting that biological, psychological and social factors are coequal partners in the development of mental health problems, I suggested that biological and social factors lead to mental health problems through their combined effects on psychological processes. This model brings together several of the points I've made earlier in this book.

Nearly everybody recognises that there are multiple, simultaneous, interacting factors leading to the development of mental health problems. In statistical analyses (not in narrative arguments) cases, scientists often use the statistical technique of 'multiple regression' to test the degree to which each factor (each 'variable' in statistical terms) contributes to the outcome. To make sense of the pathways to mental health problems, I find it helpful to imagine a theoretical multiple regression analysis, predicting mental health from the biological, psychological and social components of the biopsychosocial model. A simple statistical model of those relationships might see biological factors, psychological factors and social factors all, collectively, predicting mental health.

There is a problem, however, in regarding all the different variables to be similar in kind or nature. But, as we've seen, genetic or biological and environmental factors (whether social or circumstantial) are always in dynamic relationship with each other. The same is true for the relationship between environmental factors, biological factors and psychological factors. We need to tease out the nature of those causal relationships, rather than merely stating that they combine in some ill-specified manner.

Biological factors impinge on experiences such as hearing voices, because biological factors (genetics, cerebral lateralisation, individual differences in dopaminergic pathways) impact on the brain structures and mechanisms related to source monitoring. The final, inescapable pathway to hearing disembodied voices is a psychological process. Biological factors are hugely important here because they can affect your ability to make that discrimination.

The same is true for the relationship between social or environmental factors and hearing voices. Source monitoring is affected or influenced by factors such as noise, stress, experience of traumatic events, and indeed by those kinds of phenomena that complicate the definitions of biological or environmental, such as street drugs. When stress or noise leads to hallucinations, they do so because they affect the brain's ability to perform the same function. When people experience hallucinations following traumatic events, it seems reasonable that the consequent intrusive, automatic, negative thoughts (which are very common indeed) are misinterpreted as voices. The events we have experienced will make it more (or less) likely that those intrusive thoughts occur; circumstantial, environmental factors will affect the likelihood of hearing those intrusive thoughts as voices. Both biological and environmental factors influence mental disorder through their impact on psychological processes. And how we have learned to make sense of, and respond to, challenges in our lives will affect how we respond to and deal with such experiences.

This type of analysis is not limited to hallucinations. As we saw earlier, abnormalities in serotonin metabolism have been implicated in depression. To give one example of this: the amino acid tryptophan is a dietary precursor of serotonin (the body manufactures serotonin from tryptophan). If we eat a specially designed tryptophan-reducing diet, this can have the knock-on consequence of affecting serotonin levels and inducing depression (a rather unpleasant experience). Again, biological factors have psychological consequences. Serotonin is implicated, in turn, in the neurological mechanisms supporting various important appraisal processes. When we are happy, our serotonin levels appear to rise… a reverse of the normal cause and effect relationship of psychiatry. More importantly, serotonin is an important neurotransmitter related to processing of information to do with social status, impulsivity, and reward and punishment. All of these issues, our social status, in particular, are key to how we see ourselves, our world and our future; the negative cognitive triad of the cognitive model of depression. So, the biological tryptophan/serotonin system is indeed implicated in depression. Equally, when other factors (such as negative life events) have a similar effect—changing the way we think about ourselves, our world and our future—low mood naturally follows. In other words, what matters is the effect of all these different factors on psychology. Therefore, biological factors appear to have their effect on mental health through psychological processes.

Again, this is true for social or environmental factors. Living in poverty and in conditions of social deprivation can indeed lead to problems such as depression, but living in such a disadvantaged environment may also lead to disillusionment, hopelessness and learned helplessness; to a realisation that there is little or nothing that can be done to improve the situation and that your actions have no effect or purpose. Depression is the direct consequence of this disruption of psychological processes. The same applies to particular life experiences or circumstances. Being assaulted by your parents would obviously lead to problems, but psychologists would argue that the association between cause (assault) and the effect (later problems) is, again, mediated by the disruption of psychological processes. Abuse changes the ways in which the children (and later the adults) make sense of themselves, the people in their lives, their own actions and their consequences.

The conclusion of all these arguments is that psychological health and wellbeing are essentially psychological phenomena, the consequence of biological, social and circumstantial factors disrupting or disturbing psychological processes (Fig. 1).

This approach places particular priority on psychological factors. It suggests that mental health and mental wellbeing are quintessentially a psychological issue. It means that psychological factors are always implicated in mental health issues. Another way of putting it is that psychological factors are a 'final common pathway' for the development of mental health problems. This is a statement that some might find a little arrogant, but mental health, whatever else it is, involves the behaviour, thoughts and emotions of human beings.

These 'psychological factors' include a wide range of quite basic processes, many of which may be relatively unconscious. Consequently, the impact of social or biological factors on these psychological processes often happens without any conscious attention towards the mechanism itself. This applies equally to social or biological factors. So, a person whose genetic inheritance has led to less well-lateralised language areas in the brain might have difficulty monitoring the source or origin of mental events. That inheritance could be related to the pattern of making creative and personally salient connections between events that I discussed earlier in the context of Jim van Os's research. Exposure to high levels of stress, street drugs and excessive

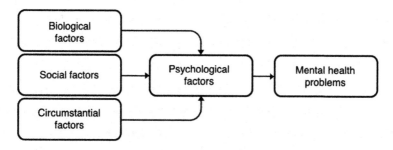

Fig. 1 A psychological model of mental health © Peter Kinderman (2014)

caffeine intake might also be factors. In these circumstances, as we've seen earlier, the person might be at risk of auditory hallucinations, mistaking internal mental processes for external voices.

It is extremely difficult to see how these factors could lead to hallucinations without affecting psychological processes. The 'point' of a hallucination is that a person comes to the (automatic, often unconscious) conclusion that the experience is 'voice-like' when in fact there is no external voice. If it were suggested that biological factors could lead to hallucinations without affecting some form of psychological process, that would be essentially the same as saying that there is no mental processing involved in coming to that conclusion, which is difficult to imagine. Even more interestingly, if there are no psychological processes involved, that's rather akin to saying that the brain isn't involved (since that's what the brain is for) and it's rather difficult then to imagine how brain-based biology could be involved.

The idea that biological factors affect our mental health through their effect on psychological processes is entirely compatible with the broad thrust of neurological research. Jim van Os and colleagues argued that this interaction is associated with psychotic problems though the effect on how children develop 'social world representations' or 'mental representation of the social world'.[10] Forming representations of your social world is a quintessentially psychological issue, involving psychological processes; the 'evaluation of self-related stimuli', 'hypervigilance to threat' or 'generating an internal representation of reality'. For these neuroscientists, it is important to identify how the neurological abnormalities that have associations with mental health problems might achieve their effects. They do that by making reference to those psychological processes that have, in turn, been associated with mental health problems. So, in the case of anxiety, researchers discuss such things as how the amygdala is associated with hypersensitivity to subtle or unconscious sensory and visceral stimuli; in other words, responding more strongly to subtle signs of threat. All psychological processes—or at least all those psychological processes in the material world open to scientific scrutiny—must involve some grounding in neurology, but the psychological processing of information remains the key part of the puzzle.

Similarly, we might think about a person growing up in socially deprived circumstances, exposed to traumatic or stressful events, and whose genetic heritage may involve subtle anomalies in serotonin metabolism. In these circumstances, people may also tend to feel their actions will have little effect, to imagine themselves to be ineffectual and to find day-to-day experiences rather unrewarding. This helps to understand how depression might have psychological processes as a 'final common pathway'. It's very difficult to imagine how either biological or social factors could conceivably lead to mental health problems without invoking psychological processes.

It is certainly true that people frequently experience problems such as lethargy or agitation; these are well-known physical conditions that can affect our mood. One example is anaemia, which is common in women after childbirth and can result in very significant lethargy; a condition that is relatively easily treated by iron tablets. What is interesting about this phenomenon is that there is a qualitative difference between the physical effects of such physical problems (such as lethargy), and the psychological consequences (such as depression) that follow when these biological processes start to affect how a person is making sense of their world; how they think about their ability to cope with family life, or worry about their health, for instance. When biological factors make you depressed, that's because the psychological processes that you use to make judgements have been affected and your thoughts about self, world and future have been altered.

We are Shaped by our Thoughts

Our mental health is largely determined by how we make sense of and understand the world. This is a broad concept, but the most important issue in mental health seems to be our 'cognitive triad' of thoughts about self, world and future. While all animals make some kind of sense of their world, human beings appear to be unique both in manipulating abstract representations of the world and in being self-aware. What we believe about ourselves, our abilities, strengths and weaknesses, what we hope—or fear—for the future, and our beliefs about the nature of the world, especially the social world, is crucial to our mental health.[11]

These ideas lead to the revolution of CBT or cognitive behavioural therapy, developed and popularised by the American psychiatrist Aaron (Tim) Beck.[12] I like the ideas of CBT and apply them in my clinical work. For me, this is less of a therapy to which I feel I should owe allegiance, and more of a practical, useful, application of cognitive psychological science. Indeed, modern developments have taken CBT and improved it. My close colleague, Sara Tai, in particular, has taken psychological therapies beyond the idea that our emotions are simply the product of 'negative thinking'. Applying the very general principles of 'Perceptual Control Theory' (a comprehensive model of how organisms organise and control their behaviour), Sara and colleagues have developed a novel therapeutic approach, the 'Method of Levels'. This doesn't so much aim to 'restructure' 'negative automatic thoughts', but instead uses therapeutic questioning to help people become more aware of conflicts between incompatible goals, and the control strategies they are using to try and achieve these goals.[13] What links these novel approaches to psychological therapy with CBT and with psychological science is the idea that our psychological health depends on how we are making sense of our world, appraising, responding to, and (hopefully) resolving the challenges that face us.

Testing This Idea

Scientific ideas are only useful when they can be tested, and when they pass that test. If our theories are remotely correct, there should be a relatively straightforward set of relationships between biological factors, social and circumstantial factors, psychological factors and mental health and wellbeing. With the help of the BBC, Sara Tai and I were able to test these ideas using an online mental health experiment on the BBC LabUK website.

Over 40,000 people participated in the experiment, which looked at how each of the main factors of the model (biological, circumstantial and social factors, psychological processes and both mental health problems and wellbeing) related to each other. I am strongly of the opinion that peer-reviewed, scientific journals are the right place to dissect and explore scientific experiments, so I won't go into details of that experiment here. I was, of course, immensely reassured that the (extraordinarily complicated) statistical analysis substantially supported our theories. All of the key factors that were believed to be important in our mental health and wellbeing were indeed significant.[14] Most importantly, however, the best way of explaining how these factors interrelated was with psychological factors (how we respond to challenges, and how we explain negative life events) mediating the process.... almost exactly what we had predicted eight years earlier.

We are shaped by thoughts, and our thoughts are shaped by events. The developments in psychology, particularly cognitive psychology, over the past twenty years make it clear that our thoughts, emotions and our behaviour (and, therefore, our mental health) are largely determined by how we make sense of and understand the world, which is, in turn, largely determined by our experiences and upbringing. These biological, social and circumstantial factors affect our mental health through their effect on psychological processes.

This relatively simple idea is the essence of clinical psychology as a profession and is—or should be—the basis of psychotherapy. Clinical psychology has grown rapidly as a profession. It didn't exist before the twentieth century and was still a small profession in 1989, when a report recommended that by the year 2000 there should be as many as 4000 'healthcare psychologists' employed in the UK's NHS. Now, there are over 10,000 clinical psychologists in the UK, and about 6000 psychologists in other branches of the profession (such as forensic psychology, counselling psychology and health psychology). It is no accident that this growth in the profession has paralleled the developments in cognitive science described in this book. Clinical psychologists pride themselves on applying the psychological theory they have studied as undergraduates to their work in the clinic. It's a sign of the success of the scientific developments, understanding better the ways in which people make sense of the world, and how that can sometimes lead to mental health difficulties, that the profession has been so successful.

We often talk as if discussing 'therapy for depression' is conceptually the same as 'antidepressants for depression', but the ideas presented here suggest a rather different approach. Since people's mental wellbeing is dependent (at least in large part) on the framework of understanding and their thoughts about themselves, other people, the world and the future, helping people think differently about these things can be helpful and should be the basis of therapy. We do not need to assume we're treating illnesses, but, instead, helping people think effectively and appropriately about the important things of life.

Notes

1. Philip J. Barnard and John D. Teasdale, "Interacting cognitive subsystems: A systemic approach to cognitive-affective interaction and change," *Cognition & Emotion* 5, no. 1 (1991): 1–39. http://www.tandfonline.com/doi/abs/10.1080/02699939108411021.
2. Daniel Kahneman, Stewart Paul Slovic, and Amos Tversky, eds., *Judgment under uncertainty: Heuristics and biases* (Cambridge: Cambridge University Press, 1982).
3. European Commission, *Promoting the mental health of the population: Towards a strategy on mental health for the European Union* (Brussels: European Commission, 2005).
4. The NHS website, describing 'depression' can be accessed here: https://www.nhs.uk/conditions/clinical-depression/causes/.
5. George L. Engel, "The need for a new medical model: A challenge for biomedicine," *Science* 196, no. 4286 (1977): 129–136.
6. Steven S. Sharfstein, "Big pharma and American psychiatry: The good, the bad, and the ugly," *Psychiatric News*, American Psychiatric Association, 40, no. 16 (2005): 3. https://psychnews.psychiatryonline.org/doi/10.1176/pn.40.16.00400003.
7. John Read, "The bio-bio-bio model of madness'," *The Psychologist* 18, no. 10 (2005): 596–597.
8. Many psychologists have studied change blindness. Christopher Chabris and Daniel Simons are responsible for the 'invisible gorilla' effect, and have used this engaging approach to good effect on their website www.theinvisiblegorilla.com/videos.html and in print: Christopher F. Chabris and Daniel Simons, *The invisible gorilla: And other ways our intuitions deceive us* (Harmony, 2011).

9. Peter Kinderman, "A psychological model of mental disorder," *Harvard Review of Psychiatry* 13, no. 4 (2005): 206–217.

10. Jim van Os, Gunter Kenis, and Bart P.F. Rutten, "The environment and schizophrenia," *Nature* 468, no. 7321 (2010): 203. https://www.nature.com/articles/nature09563.

11. Peter Kinderman and Sara Tai, "Empirically grounded clinical interventions clinical implications of a psychological model of mental disorder," *Behavioural and Cognitive Psychotherapy* 35, no. 1 (2007): 1–14.

12. Aaron T. Beck, ed., *Cognitive therapy of depression* (Guilford Press, 1979).

13. See: Sara J. Tai, "Using perceptual control theory and the method of levels to work with people who experience psychosis," *The Cognitive Behaviour Therapist* 2, no. 3 (2009): 227–242. https://www.cambridge.org/core/journals/the-cognitive-behaviour-therapist/article/using-perceptual-control-theory-and-the-method-of-levels-to-work-with-people-who-experience-psychosis/6F1F61F2C2D37E7DB-D82D3F63A08F574; and Timothy A. Carey, Warren Mansell, and Sara J. Tai, *Principles-based counselling and psychotherapy: A method of levels approach* (Routledge, 2015).

14. Peter Kinderman, Sara Tai, Eleanor Pontin, Matthias Schwannauer, Ian Jarman, and Paulo Lisboa, "Causal and mediating factors for anxiety, depression and well-being," *The British Journal of Psychiatry* 206, no. 6 (2015): 456–460. https://www.ncbi.nlm.nih.gov/pubmed/25858180.

5

Labels are for Products, not People

The assumption or assertion that our distress is best understood merely as a symptom of diagnosable 'illnesses' is only one perspective. Instead, more appropriate systems for describing and defining people's emotional problems are available. Traditional psychiatric diagnoses are arbitrary and invalid and do not map onto biological processes or describe real illnesses. They are also circular concepts, attempting to explain our behaviour, emotions and thoughts merely by labelling them as pathological. This reinforces a reductionist biological view of mental health and wellbeing and encourages negative attitudes, discrimination and the use of inappropriate medical treatments. Scientific and humane alternatives are needed, both for individual care planning and in the design and commissioning of services.

Across the physical and social sciences, we clearly, simply, appropriately and objectively define the phenomena that we're studying. Accurate, objective, definition of terms is a key part of the scientific approach; we define the phenomena, carefully observe and logically analyse the data.

But when we try to define the phenomena of mental health, we can see a clear schism. On the one hand is what we might want to think of as the careful definition and observation of the nature of our thoughts, emotions and behaviours. On the other is the diagnostic system, based

© The Author(s) 2019
P. Kinderman, *A Manifesto for Mental Health*,
https://doi.org/10.1007/978-3-030-24386-9_5

on the flawed assumption that distress is best thought of as a 'symptom' of an 'illness'.

According to a survey[1] of 4,887 psychiatrists from 44 countries, 79% reported that they 'often' or 'almost always/always' used a formal classification system as part of their day-to-day clinical work. But, when I discuss the use of diagnosis with my psychiatric colleagues, I observe a curious phenomenon. Occasionally, diagnosis is described as, for example, being 'invaluable'[2] or both 'valid' and 'essential'.[3] When this is challenged, however—whether on the statistical grounds of reliability and validity, or on the more pragmatic grounds that we can actually do better using alternatives—my colleagues often take a rather different line, pointing out that they rarely actually make diagnoses. This sometimes goes further, with colleagues arguing that any decent clinician would base clinical decisions on a formulation, not a diagnosis… until someone in my position argues that, therefore, we could stop using diagnosis and instead rely on formulation… whereupon the argument entirely flips.

In his unfinished masterpiece 'Billy Budd',[4] the American author Herman Melville wrote about the complex relationship between 'sanity' and 'insanity'. The literary device is the military trial of Billy Budd, accused (unjustly) of 'mutiny' and then sentenced to death by hanging, with his future dependent on the possibility that his Captain might decide that he can be excused on the basis of 'insanity'. The Captain wrestles not only with his conscience but also with the whole concept of distinguishing between sanity and insanity.

Who in the rainbow can draw the line where the violet tint ends and the orange tint begins? Distinctly we see the difference of the colors, but where exactly does the one first blendingly enter into the other? So with sanity and insanity. In pronounced cases there is no question about them. But in some supposed cases, in various degrees supposedly less pronounced, to draw the exact line of demarkation few will undertake tho' for a fee some professional experts will. There is nothing nameable but that some men will undertake to do it for pay.

Melville deliberately (the phrase is repeated) mentions that some people are prepared to '… *draw the exact line of demarkation… for a fee*'. It is perhaps unsurprising that professionals involved in traditional mental health services will defend diagnosis. But, based on my many years of research and clinical experience, I am forced to conclude that we can do much better than relying on the superficially attractive, but ultimately inappropriate and unhelpful, practice of diagnosis.

A Peculiar Circular Logic

Psychiatric diagnoses convey the idea that people's emotional difficulties can be understood in the same way as bodily diseases. That is, the experiences are symptoms caused by and indicative of an underlying pathology. That pathology is both an explanation for the experiences and the target for treatment. I disagree with pretty much all of this analysis.

One consequence of the 'disease-model' idea, and the reliance on diagnosis, is that we fail to look for meaning in people's 'disordered' responses and experiences. The phenomena, according to the 'disease-model', are the symptoms of an illness and, in this framework of understanding, can be interpreted as little more. They are not (in this model) ordinary psychological phenomena, occurring for meaningful reasons and playing roles within our lives. It also implies that people need 'expert' help and that their own skills and resources are not enough.

Worse, diagnoses are inappropriately, misleadingly, used as pseudo-explanations for troubling behaviours. Take, as an example, the experience of hearing voices. Many people, perhaps even most people, who hear voices don't find them distressing. But for others they *are* distressing, and these are the people who might seek help from mental health services and receive a diagnosis. Within the disease-model approach, the voices (themselves rendered into technical, professional, medical, language as 'hallucinations') are seen as symptoms of 'schizophrenia'. The assumption, either implicit or explicit, is that the 'schizophrenia' is causing the hallucinations. But that's a circular argument; the dog is chasing its own tail. The hallucinations are caused by the schizophrenia; 'why is that person hallucinating?', 'because she has schizophrenia'. But at the same time, the diagnosis of 'schizophrenia' is dependent on those very phenomena it's assumed to be causing; 'how do we know she has schizophrenia?', 'because she's experiencing hallucinations'.

Why, and How, Do We Diagnose 'Mental Illnesses'?

Like most people, I accept professional or expert opinions on quite a range of issues. My trust is that the peer-review process, the 'research integrity' checks that we have at universities, and even the competition between academics (where we tend to try to find flaws in our colleagues' work) mean that I can rely on much of what's published as 'fact'. The whole point of scientific discovery is that we constantly find out new things, reveal mistakes and find that our theories need to be revised.

Given this reasonable trust of experts, many people mistakenly believe that psychiatric diagnoses reflect real 'illnesses', things that 'really' exist. This is exactly what our traditional approach tells us. But scientific analysis of the problems that people experience and the nature of those diagnostic labels suggests that this is a mistake. And this mistake compounds others.

Some people do find diagnostic labels reassuring or helpful because they appear to recognise, explain and validate their problems, and (currently at least) they often unlock help. Some professionals and policy-makers mistakenly assume that we therefore need to use diagnoses in order to allocate resources to those who need them. Many medical and legal professionals, and in particular medical researchers, mistakenly believe that diagnoses are needed in order to allow people to communicate efficiently with one another. However, many public and social services achieve these aims without the need for 'diagnoses'.

We can do much better than this medicalised, pathologising, diagnostic, approach. These kinds of diagnoses are misleading and unnecessary; a simple and direct list of a person's actual experiences and problems in their own terms would provide more information and communicate much more than a diagnostic label. Certainly, we need to research into the nature, causes and remedies of problems, but again that does not mean that diagnosis is necessary; researchers would be better advised to study the nature of, causes of and proper response to specific, easily identified problems rather than looking for differences between groups of people with different 'diagnoses'. But in order to understand the extent to which psychiatric diagnoses are mistaken and unhelpful, we need to look at how 'mental illness' is currently classified.

There are two major international classificatory systems for the classification and diagnosis of mental health problems.

The World Health Organization's International Standard Classification of Diseases, Injuries and Causes of Death—ICD-10

Almost immediately after the Second World War, the newly formed United Nations established the World Health Organization. One of its first actions was to publish a comprehensive list of the world's diseases and illnesses, with the aim of measuring and thereby improving the world's health. The International Standard Classification of Diseases, Injuries and Causes of Death[5] (or 'ICD') included psychiatric 'conditions', as we might have expected. This confirmed the almost universal assumption that these kinds of problems fell under the aegis of medicine and ensured that diagnosis, classification and categorisation were the method of choice. This diagnostic manual has been extensively revised over the years, and we are now using ICD-10, the tenth and most recent revision, with ICD-11 in draft form. ICD-10 is the international standard classification system, recommended for administrative and epidemiological purposes and forms the basis of statistical procedures in the UK National Health Service.

American Psychiatric Association's Diagnostic and Statistical Manual—DSM-5

The immediate post-war period also saw the publication of the American Psychiatric Association's Diagnostic and Statistical Manual, DSM.[6] This developed from a 'National Conference on Nomenclature of Disease' at the New York Academy of Medicine in 1928, but was also strongly influenced by the administrative scheme used by the US Army in World War II, and the need to unify the Academy's system with the different schemes used by the American armed forces and, confusingly, that of the Veterans Administration. The committee undertaking the development of what was to become DSM-I was well aware of the existence of the ICD and expended a great deal of attention in ensuring the compatibility of the two systems.[7] Nevertheless, there was clearly a desire to develop a bespoke American system. It is difficult to determine exactly why the American Psychiatric Association decided not merely to accept the international system. It may well be the case that international cooperation was less well developed outside of military matters, and the USA was in a process of remarkable nation-building. But it is also possible that some matters of professional self-interest were involved. While the experts concluded that deaths should be classified according to the international system, they also commented that '*adjustments must also be made to meet the varied requirements of vital statistics offices, hospitals of different types, medical services of the armed forces, social insurance organizations, sickness surveys, and numerous other agencies*'.

Scientifically positive and definitive statements fit uneasily with compromises in nomenclature made for administrative purposes. Indeed, the original DSM-I contains many of the seeds of the continuing complex, shifting, tensions of biomedical and social psychiatry seen subsequently. The nomenclature is first described as a list of 'Diseases of the Psychobiologic Unit'. To me, this is a slightly ominous phrase, as well as appearing to be an attempt at inclusion. I would not want to consult a psychiatrist or psychologist who regarded me as a 'psychobiologic unit', and I don't regard our subject matter to be 'diseases'. DSM-I is also interesting because it describes as 'reactions' a wide range of problems more recently labelled as 'illnesses' or 'disorders'. Remembering that these are first subsumed under 'diseases of the psychobiologic unit', DSM-I therefore lists 'manic depressive reaction, manic type', 'manic depressive reaction, depressive type' and a range of 'schizophrenic reactions'. None of this language is either scientific or humane, but it is interesting that these experiences were then seen as 'reactions'.

It's difficult to make sense of this, in all honesty. In DSM-I and sub-sequently, in diagnostic taxonomies, in position papers and in books both promoting and critiquing traditional psychiatry, our mental health problems are described almost interchangeably as 'reactions', 'disorders', 'illnesses', 'conditions', etc. In DSM-I, we see a common pattern; the phenomena are described as 'reactions' and 'diseases' in the same document. When I'm in a grumpy mood, I comment that it's a little like the fair-ground game of 'whack-a-mole' (the little stuffed mole pokes its head up through the first hole, and you try to whack it with a stick, then it pokes its head up somewhere else...). Here, the problems are described as 'diseases', 'illnesses' and '...like any other illness', but when the logic and evidence supporting that assertion are challenged, the problems are described as 'reactions', and it's pointed out that biological systems are necessarily deployed in any normal response to environmental stress. When that, new, position is challenged (e.g. by arguing that, therefore, there's no reason to use a medical framework to understand or address issues that are not in that definition 'disorders' or 'illnesses'), the argument shifts back, to point out that, for example, there are recognised neurotransmitter abnormalities addressed by medication such as antidepressants, that not everybody living in poverty becomes depressed... When these ideas are challenged on scientific grounds, the argument shifts back again, pointing out that psychiatrists always have recognised the social context of their work and have always considered the social determinants of mental health problems....

When I'm not so grumpy, I think that these documents (the diagnostic taxonomies, the position papers, the books explaining or justifying psychiatric practice) are almost deliberately internally inconsistent so as to appeal to all perspectives on the issue. Coldplay are immensely popular (and I like them, too), but their lyrics are hardly precision scientific expositions. You can sing along at festivals... '*I swam across, I jumped across for you. Oh what a thing to do. 'Cause you were all yellow...*'. Well; quite. You can enjoy it, and sing along, ... and you can read almost anything you want into it. If you want to write a diagnostic manual that stands the test of time, given that there are so many different voices within mainstream psychiatry, it makes sense to cover all the bases.

As with ICD, the DSM system has been revised and re-edited over time, meaning that the current edition is the fifth, DSM-5. Although the ICD system is the World Health Organization's standard and recommended text, the dominance of American culture means that, because DSM is used for research classification as well as epidemiological and statistical purposes, and because most researchers want to publish their results in US-based, English language publications, it has become common for researchers, even in Europe, to use DSM criteria. The two systems, ICD and DSM, have run in parallel ever since their inception, and there is considerable overlap, and increasing convergence, between the two systems.

The fact that there are two separate classification systems itself raises some questions for a diagnostic model. It is problematic if it is argued that an objective illness of 'depression' (or 'schizophrenia' or 'attention deficit hyperactivity disorder' or whatever) exists if we follow an American tradition but not a European nomenclature. Scientists and clinicians recognise this, which is why one of the principal reasons for the latest revision of DSM (from DSM-IV to become DSM-5) was to permit easier 'read-across' between the two systems. However, the two codes are not identical. A good illustration of this is in the diagnostic criteria for depression. The DSM-5 diagnostic guidelines are more complex, more detailed and more prescriptive than the ICD-10 criteria. It is possible for a person to meet the ICD-10 criteria for a diagnosis of depression, but fail to meet the DSM-5 criteria. For example, if you have been experiencing low mood, loss of interest and enjoyment and reduced energy for the past three weeks, you would meet the ICD-10 criteria for a diagnosis of 'depressive episode'. But unless you are also experiencing weight loss or sleep disturbance, feel agitated, worthless or guilty, are unable to concentrate or having thoughts of suicide, you would not qualify for the equivalent DSM-5 diagnosis of 'major depressive episode'.

There have been many specific changes as DSM-IV has been revised to become DSM-5. One controversial change[8] was the decision to drop a specific exclusion criterion. The fourth edition suggested that people should not be diagnosed with 'major depression' if they had been recently bereaved. In technical language, it was not appropriate to record a diagnosis of 'major depressive episode' if '...the symptoms are not better accounted for by Bereavement...'. We all feel low when a loved one has died and so, the logic went, we don't need to label people in that situation as 'ill'. But this requirement was dropped in DSM-5. That means it now *is* possible to receive a diagnosis of 'major depressive episode' if you experience low mood following the death of a loved one.

Many people worldwide were concerned by this development and the idea that someone grieving for a loved one could be diagnosed with a 'mental illness'. I agree. But here are, strictly within the logic of psychiatric diagnosis, sensible or at least understandable reasons for this odd decision. First, the ICD-10 diagnostic criteria for depressive episode don't include an exclusion for bereavement, so it could be argued that this brings the two manuals closer together. And, technically, DSM is not designed to identify the causes of or reasons for a person's problems. If a person is experiencing low mood, they are experiencing low mood. The fact that a loved one has died is a very good reason for such low mood, but it doesn't mean the low mood isn't there. The problem is not really whether bereavement is, or is not, included as an exclusion criterion for a diagnosis of 'major depressive episode'. My concern is a larger one. I simply don't think we need to be asking these kinds of questions in the first place.

Reliability

The first scientific test of a diagnostic system is to ask if it is reliable. To be reliable (in this context), a diagnostic system would need to ensure that two professionals would both agree on which diagnosis to use. One of the reasons that the diagnostic manuals (DSM and ICD) were developed in the first place, and one of the reasons they have been revised, is to ensure reliability. Several years ago, research suggested that clinicians in different countries (the researchers particularly studied the USA and UK) tended to make rather different diagnoses when presented with identical sets of problems.[9] What would lead to a diagnosis of, say 'schizophrenia' in one country would lead to a diagnosis of say 'bipolar disorder' if you were to consult with a clinician in another country. There are many reasons why this might happen (the people reporting the problems might behave differently or say different things, the person making the diagnosis might interview people in a different manner, the environment might be different, etc.), but a central issue was that different countries tended to have different diagnostic systems, different rules for combining symptoms and different systems of naming the 'disorders' that were diagnosed. The DSM and ICD diagnostic systems were drafted specifically to address these kinds of problems; the issue of reliability was addressed by international agreement on criteria, and rules for which 'symptoms' would count towards which diagnosis.

The reliability of psychiatric diagnosis is rather poor. In fact, reliability appears to be getting progressively worse with each new edition of DSM.[10] Although we do change over time, a reliable diagnostic system would mean that we would get the same result each time. That doesn't deny the reality of personal capriciousness; rather, it accepts that reality and concludes that, therefore, a diagnostic system is inappropriate.

Supporters of psychiatric diagnosis sometimes point out that the reliability of some diagnoses in the arena of physical health is also poor. So, for example, pathologists may be mistaken about the cause of death on as much as a third of occasions when their expert judgements are compared with the results of post-mortems, and even diagnoses of illnesses like tonsillitis can be less reliable than those for 'schizophrenia'. However, there is one important difference: in the arena of physical health, post-mortem examinations and laboratory tests can confirm or refute clinical impressions. There are no such laboratory tests for mental health problems.[11] It is, moreover, a poor defence of unreliable practice to point out that other people are equally unreliable. And, even if psychiatric diagnoses were reliable, that wouldn't be enough. Diagnoses also need to be 'valid'; that is, to be meaningful and to represent real 'things'.

Validity

It is quite possible for a diagnosis to be completely reliable, but still not be valid. For example, we might suggest that there exists a disorder called 'Kinderman Syndrome'. Kinderman Syndrome might be diagnosed if someone possesses all of the following 'symptoms': having thinning brown hair, a south–east English accent and protruding ears. This diagnosis would probably be quite reliable. Although some interviewers (especially ones from a different culture to mine) might be poor at discerning a 'south-east English' accent, and some might be uncertain as to the exact definition of 'thinning' hair, I suspect a rigorous investigation would establish that any panel of suitably selected and trained clinicians would be able to agree at least 75% of the time as to whether these criteria are met. We might have to develop the criteria carefully; we might have to define 'protruding' in relation to ears, and even define the exact shade of 'brown' we meant. There might be some work needed to refine the definitions, and we might need to train our clinicians. But at least in theory we could get high reliability.

But is it valid? Is there in any real sense a syndrome, a disorder, a mental illness that—validly—exists merely because we can define it? Of course not. I am sure a few of the people I have encountered in my professional life would leap at the idea of 'Kinderman Syndrome'. But we cannot accept that 'mental illnesses' exist merely because we can name them. We can't accept that reliability alone makes a 'disorder' a valid concept.

There have been plenty of invalid diagnoses and indeed many diagnoses that psychiatrists have unhesitatingly and correctly rejected. In the nineteenth century, an American doctor called Samuel Cartwright seriously suggested that slaves who attempted to escape from their captors were suffering from the illness of 'drapetomania'[12] (the Greek word drapetes means a runaway slave). According to Cartwright, men and women with a desire for freedom were merely exhibiting the symptom of an illness. Cartwright wrote an attempt at a scientific paper (the *diseases and peculiarities of the negro race*') in which he hypothesised that the aetiology of his newly identified 'illness' involved slave-owners treating their possessions as if they were human beings. Unsurprisingly, Cartwright suggested that the 'treatment' for 'drapetomania' was whipping.

Of course, not only is this nonsense, it was recognised as such by the psychiatrists of the day. But those psychiatrists of the time did, like pretty much everybody else at the time, think it was appropriate to medicalise and pathologise (some of) our sexual preferences. In my professional opinion, we need to question the validity of all mental health diagnoses. As colleagues and I said in a recent paper, we should '*drop the language of disorder*'.[13]

'Oppositional Defiant Disorder'...Really?

People unfamiliar with psychiatric diagnostic practices are surprised to learn that the DSM-5 includes a diagnosis of 'oppositional defiant disorder'. This diagnosis, used with children, is defined by 'a pattern of negativistic, hostile, and defiant behaviour lasting at least 6 months'. The specific diagnostic criteria include: actively defying or refusing to comply with adults' requests or rules, deliberately annoying people, blaming other people for his or her mistakes or misbehaviour and being angry and resentful. If you believe DSM-5 (I don't), these can be grouped into three types: angry/irritable mood, argumentative/defiant behaviour and vindictiveness.

Our children can sometimes be painfully unhappy. And children can sometimes be entirely unresponsive to their parents, or, indeed to other authority figures. I certainly would not want to imply that such problems don't exist or that they are trivial. The consequences can be life-changing and may well point to very substantial underlying issues. I just don't think they are 'illnesses'. I am—to be clear—absolutely convinced that children and young people can be negativistic. They can be hostile. They can actively refuse to comply with adults' requests or rules. These kinds of problems are often indications that the child has experienced some significant trauma. I do not wish to make light of real, painful, problems. These kinds of difficulties can have terrible consequences for children and their parents. But it simply isn't sensible, useful, scientifically appropriate or clinically justifiable to suggest that the children have a 'disorder'. Apart from anything else, this kind of labelling makes people think that these problems are not really normal human problems at all, but instead are 'symptoms of mental illness'. I don't like it when my children are defiant or refuse to comply with my requests. But I don't think they are mentally ill.

Another example of the problems with the idea of 'mental illnesses' is the contentious issue of 'personality disorder'. 'Personality disorders' are defined as 'long-standing patterns of maladaptive behaviour that constitute immature and inappropriate ways of coping with stress or solving problems'. It is fascinating and horrible how a person's whole character can be rendered into a 'disorder'. Examples of personality disorder include: 'antisocial personality disorder', 'paranoid personality disorder', 'narcissistic personality disorder', 'schizoid personality disorder', etc. Antisocial personality disorder is particularly interesting in the context of the validity of diagnoses of mental disorder, because it illustrates the weird circularity of these ideas. Do people do bad things because they are suffering from 'antisocial personality disorder' or do they get labelled with 'antisocial personality disorder' because they do bad things?

So-called 'personality disorders' also illustrate how the authors of diagnostic manuals are undecided as to how many of these 'disorders' there are. The DSM and ICD systems do not agree, and there are very significant differences between ICD-10 and ICD-11 (between the 10th and 11th editions of that manual). There are frequent debates as to whether 'personality disorders' could be entirely expunged from the diagnostic manuals (replaced, perhaps, with a description of personality traits). They appear to have a fleeting, ghost-like reality—written into existence; potentially deleted—as the committees deliberate. But, despite their oddity, their circularity and their tenuous claimed validity, it can be significant if you receive a diagnosis of 'personality disorder'. The UK government linked an entire offender management programme—the Dangerous and Severe Personality Disorder programme, designed to help manage very seriously dangerous offenders—to the concept.

On Being Sane in Insane Places

The 1973 experiment by David Rosenhan, 'on being sane in insane places',[14] has been widely reported and indeed criticised. But it remains informative. Rosenhan arranged for eight ordinary people from conventional backgrounds to go to hospitals in the USA and tell unsuspecting psychiatrists that they had heard disembodied voices saying the words 'empty', 'hollow' or 'thud'. Other than reporting this entirely fictional experience (if true, a conventional criterion for the diagnosis of schizophrenia, but only one of several necessary elements), the eight undercover researchers were told to answer all questions honestly. All eight were admitted to hospital, the majority of them with a diagnosis of schizophrenia. Once they were admitted, each 'pseudopatient' continued to behave normally. But the fact that they had been admitted to hospital and given a psychiatric diagnosis appeared to change the way they were regarded by the staff. Staff saw one pseudopatient pacing the corridors—the individual was bored—and suggested that they were experiencing 'anxiety'. One pseudopatient was seen to be writing—in fact, writing notes of their experiences—which was recorded as 'patient engages in writing behaviour'. The scientific or medicalised language ('writing behaviour') subtly changes our understanding of what is happening; the observed behaviour, described in detached, clinical, terms, suggests something unusual or pathological is going on. Rosenhan reports that it was only the other (genuinely distressed) patients in the hospital who realised that there was something odd going on; one challenged a researcher, saying: 'you're not crazy, you're a journalist or a professor. You're checking up on the hospital'.

The pseudopatients received appalling treatment from a professional, legal and human rights perspective. Once in hospital, the undercover researchers reported that they no longer heard any voices and behaved entirely conventionally. And indeed, after an average of 19 days (with a range of 7–52), the staff agreed that they were now well enough to be discharged. All were discharged with a diagnosis of 'schizophrenia in remission' (and a book could be written about that alone), but, by then, the pseudopatients had been prescribed a total of 2100 pills. We should be careful not to read too much into Rosenhan's research. It was conducted in 1973 and things have undoubtedly changed. But we should note that staff members only spent 11% of their time interacting with patients in Rosenhan's study, and that comments like 'Come on, you mother f – – -s, get out of bed' were reported as common. We can compare this with the stories we are told about residential mental health units today, from both users of mental health services and staff, some of which I have included in this book.

It is inappropriate (and insulting) to suggest that the psychiatrists in Rosenhan's study were unable to tell the difference between sanity and insanity. This research demonstrates that it is as simple to lie to a psychiatrist about psychiatric symptoms ('*I heard a voice saying "thud"*') as it is to lie to a rheumatologist about pain ('*I feel intense grating pain whenever I flex my shoulder*'). It isn't particularly odd for a medical practitioner to make the most appropriate diagnosis on the basis of the information given to them, even if the pseudopatient is lying. Within the logic of the 'disease model' of psychiatric diagnosis, the psychiatrists apparently duped by Rosenhan's pseudopatients had reasonable grounds for making their diagnostic decisions, and subsequent decisions to admit to hospital and prescribe medication. In the standard diagnostic manuals, hearing voices (auditory hallucinations) is a symptom of 'schizophrenia'. And the disease model dictates to psychiatrists that 'schizophrenia' exists, has particular well-recognised symptoms and warrants hospital treatment and medication. Within this flawed system, diagnosis, the diagnostic classification, hospitalisation and prescription are justified with the simple caveat that sometimes people fail to tell the truth. My point is that there is little scientific justification for the 'disease model', and so the diagnostic and treatment decisions that follow are equally flawed. Again, what we need is paradigmatic change.

Utility; What Utility?

Many professionals, including many clinical psychologists, see some merits in the diagnostic approach. About a third of the people involved in the taskforce drawing up DSM-5 were psychologists. For many, their decision to accept a diagnostic approach is purely practical; they see DSM as a tool for categorising problems and suggesting what might help. However, dispassionate and objective scientific evidence suggests that diagnoses are in fact unhelpful.

It is very difficult to predict what treatments people will find helpful on the basis of the diagnosis they receive. In physical medicine, specific types of drugs are helpful for specific problems. For example, penicillin is a specific treatment for bacterial infection and not for viral infection.

It is different with psychiatric medication. Proponents of diagnoses usually stress that diagnosis is needed to decide the right treatment. But, in reality, psychiatric diagnosis appears almost irrelevant in this regard. I shall discuss the role of medication later, but it's worth reflecting on the fact that, while we know quite a lot about what psychiatric medication does to the brain and the effects they have on our thinking and moods, there is precious little evidence that they actually treat the disorders named in their names. The psychiatrist Dr. Joanna Moncrieff comments wisely on this issue.[15] In essence, Dr. Moncrieff recommends a 'drug-centred' rather than 'disease-centred' approach to the use of medication. This slightly surprising-sounding phrase refers to the fact that the drugs have known effects, some helpful, some unhelpful, which should (in Dr. Moncrieff's opinion) be the correct basis for prescription. Some drugs raise mood; some drugs calm anxiety; some drugs sedate us. If we understand what the drugs do, we can better decide whether or not they may be helpful things to prescribe in any particular situation. This contrasts with the fact that the effectiveness of these drugs does not appear to depend on the diagnosis. In other words, some drugs raise our mood, and other drugs calm our anxieties (at least in the short term), but that is not at all the same as saying that any particular drug is an effective treatment for, say 'major depressive disorder', because people whose problems meet the criteria for such a diagnosis may be experiencing either low mood, or anxiety, or both. Dr. Moncrieff concludes that diagnosis should not be used as a basis for prescribing. This is a fatal problem for the diagnostic approach.

Diagnoses also have little practical utility for prognosis, predicting the future course of an illness (in medical terms) or predicting someone's future behaviour (in psychological terms). In psychology, we know the truth of a well-worn mantra: 'past behaviour predicts future behaviour'. People who have been violent to an intimate partner on one occasion are more likely to offend again. People who have been to the gym regularly for the past year are likely to keep up the habit. In mental health, people who have been depressed or anxious before are likely to be depressed again. But the diagnostic labels are extremely poor at making any useful predictions beyond that. A valid diagnosis, a diagnosis that means something in the real world, should say something about the outcome that people given the diagnosis should expect. Again, however (with the exception of neurological diseases and learning disability, which are rather different) the outcomes for people given nearly every diagnosis are highly variable. Moreover, each person's outcome appears dependent much more on their social situation than on their diagnosis, whether they are in a relationship, whether they have friends, whether they have a job, whether they have somewhere decent to live. Healthcare professionals, quite correctly, tell people that there is a huge range of possible outcomes, and (again correctly) that many things can be done to affect their prognosis. Arguably this all makes diagnosis rather redundant.

There is a perception that people with psychiatric diagnoses are more likely than others to be violent. However, in fact, very few acts of violence are committed by people with a history of mental health problems. The most important factors predicting violence are: having a history of violence, being male, and using alcohol. Specific diagnoses like 'schizophrenia' do not predict dangerousness. Some specific experiences and beliefs, such as a conviction that others intend to do you physical harm, or hearing voices telling you to do something violent, are associated with a small increased risk. But even among people who have these experiences, few actually end up acting on them. Even where people do, the association is with the specific experiences or beliefs rather than with a particular diagnosis. And that is precisely my point. The specific experiences are useful indicators; the diagnoses are not.

Despite this story of failure, many of my colleagues who advocate the use of diagnosis in mental health care appear still to rely on the myth of utility, the idea that diagnoses are useful. One medically qualified contributor to an online blog (hosted by the well-respected Oxford University Press) tried to defuse this row by saying that: '*clinicians need to communicate to each other, and even a wrong diagnosis allows them to do so*'. I try very hard not to be rude to fellow professionals, but his statement is not only foolish, it's dangerous. It suggests not only that clinicians expect their care to be guided by 'wrong' diagnoses, but they believe that they should (perhaps need to) share their errors with colleagues. Another contributor suggested that we need to understand diagnoses such as schizophrenia as 'heterogeneous diagnoses'. We have one influential proponent suggesting that diagnoses are useful even if they are 'wrong', and another suggesting that they can be catch-all or 'heterogeneous'. While it seems very strange to suggest that something that is wrong can also be necessary, it is truer to say that psychiatric diagnoses are 'heterogeneous'. That is precisely what I have been saying; research suggests that the treasured psychiatric diagnosis simply does not represent discrete phenomena.

Statistical Relationships are not Diagnoses

There are regularities and patterns to our behaviour. Scientists use powerful statistical techniques to understand the ways in which people's experiences of psychological health problems cluster together, and whether they cluster in the ways predicted by the diagnostic approach. The central idea of diagnosis is that particular psychological problems cluster together, and in most biomedical explanatory models, this is further explained by invoking an underlying pathological process. Diagnosis depends on a particular 'disorder' or 'illness' having shared characteristics that make it distinct from other 'disorders' or 'illnesses'. In general, the results of this approach have not been supportive of the diagnostic model. There do appear to be patterns and relationships between problems, but these relationships tend to cut across diagnostic categories.

This applies perhaps more powerfully when we explore the role of biological factors. It was with some fanfare that researchers announced[16] that they had identified some genetic factors associated with a range of common mental health problems. This is important, and significant, work. However, these genetic characteristics, the associated biochemical pathways and the psychological processes that affect and are affected by them are not specific to particular diagnoses. Quite the reverse, the biological and psychological pathways cut across these diagnostic categories.

Continua

There is a widespread idea that there is a fundamental distinction between normal emotions and 'mental illness'. People talk about 'clinical depression' and distinguish it from 'ordinary' depression. One influential journalist in the field of popular science recently decried how people fail to distinguish everyday feelings of depression from (real) 'depressive symptoms'. The disease model of mental health tends to reinforce the idea that the experiences and emotions of people whose problems are placed in diagnostic categories such as 'depression', 'schizophrenia' and 'bipolar disorder' are qualitatively different from 'normal' emotions and experiences. Traditional psychiatry, the 'disease model' of mental health and the diagnostic approach all conceptualise, or at least present a vision of, 'mental illnesses' as qualitatively different to and separable from normality. Research suggests something rather different: that it is very difficult indeed to discern a dividing line between 'normal' and 'abnormal' emotions, experiences or behaviours.

Many people, especially clinical psychologists, have suggested that these supposed 'symptoms' of mental illnesses in fact lie on a continuum with normality. Sometimes experiences and emotions become problematical, but this is the same with any human experience or tendency. Our behaviours, thoughts, even emotions can become problems if they are extreme. This idea is neither new nor unusual. I opened this chapter with a quote from Herman Melville's novel *Billy Budd*, and quoted from the editorial in the *Times* from 1854. I can see why the idea that there is such a dividing line is popular: it reassures us that mental health problems are discrete, diagnosable entities, experienced by people who are different to us. But in truth, all these experiences lie on continua.

The Times editorial in 1854 commented that: '... *nothing can be more slightly defined than the line of demarcation between sanity and insanity...*'. My colleague Alex Langford (whom I mentioned in an earlier chapter) decided to entitle his blog about diagnosis '*categorically ill*'. The point he was trying to make was that there is a 'categorical difference' between being ill and not being ill. Unfortunately for this argument, we observe something completely different that psychological health problems lie on continua. And this, in turn, implies that we are not observing something categorically abnormal or disordered, but rather the way in which humans respond to the hugely variable experiences and challenges that we face in life.

Some of us are mildly anxious, and others are so crippled by obsessions and compulsive rituals that our lives are very difficult indeed. Most of us will have had unusual perceptual experiences from time to time, but some of us are plagued by continual psychosis. We all get down from time to time, but low mood is so extreme for some people that they contemplate suicide. Everyone has experienced anxiety at some point in their lives. Some of us have experienced sheer terror or perhaps become extremely anxious very frequently. Many more of us are frequently anxious, but to a lesser degree. Only a few of us (fortunately) will ever experience extremes of anxiety such as a series of panic attacks, crippling obsessions or compulsions to do certain things that would be recognised in the diagnostic textbooks as justifying a diagnosis of an anxiety 'disorder'. Many of us will have had unusual perceptual experiences from time to time, but most of us will have not been disturbed by them and will have dismissed them as transient and trivial events. Others are plagued by continual psychosis. Some people hear disembodied voices, but regard the experience as 'normal' or for other reasons are not troubled by them. Some people welcome such voices as either helpful or supportive, or see them as spiritually valuable. Other people are terrified by what they hear. We all feel low from time to time, but some people feel so guilty, depressed, fatigued or pessimistic for the future that they contemplate suicide. And—and this is important—all shades of experience fall in between.

Madness and sanity are not qualitatively different states of mind, but can instead be seen as lying at the extreme ends of several spectra of experience. If madness lies at one end of a continuum, the opposite end will be a never-experienced utopia where we are gloriously happy, rational at all times, clear-sighted and with the acute and precise hearing of an owl. In the words of the *Times* editor; free from all passion, prejudice, vice and vanity. Each of these, and many more, is individual dimension. The ways in which we manage anxiety will speak to dimensions that may well not be the same as those dimensions on which we respond to threats to motivation and pessimism. Fear and pessimism may well be closely related, explaining, perhaps, why depression and anxiety often co-occur. But each phenomenon also relates to a wide variety of psychological processes that also represent continua in human experience.

The inescapable fact that those phenomena which constitute the field of 'mental health' lie on continua is important because this is a pattern that better resembles an understandable set of human responses to life's adversities than it does a set of discrete illnesses. It is perfectly true to point out that many ailments in the conventional medical realm also lie on continua, blood pressure, lipid levels, etc. But in the field of psychology, the pattern doesn't support a simple 'disease-model' approach. The observation that these very understandable patterns lie on continua also supports the idea that these are human responses to environmental pressures.

These continua are not simple, straight-line, relationships. We should not expect a one-to-one correlation between our income (e.g.) and our levels of depression. An important element of how psychologists understand a wide range of mental health problems is based on understanding vicious cycles and feedback loops. When something bad happens—maybe somebody gives us a piece of bad news—we tend to feel a little low. And the way that human psychology works means that, when our mood drops, there is a range of consequences. We might be less likely to keep physically active, if the drop in our mood is particularly serious or long-lasting. That will affect our mood, both directly (exercise makes us feel good, probably in part through the effect of endorphins on our brain) and indirectly (we feel a sense of achievement, we know we're doing ourselves good, we might even look better for it). Similarly, if we become depressed, we might stop seeing our friends so much, and our relationships are good for our psychological health (meaning another feedback loop or vicious cycle). We might have to take time off work, and that in turn will have negative consequences. We might find that a drop in our mood makes it more likely that we think about other negative things (other, that is, than the issue that sparked the episode of depression). This might lead us to feel even worse, and perhaps to interpret subsequent events in a more negative light than we would do otherwise.

All these feedback loops and vicious cycles might drive our mood down further. When we become depressed, we feel fatigued, lethargic and 'anhedonic' (we are no longer able to enjoy the things we used to). It is then natural to withdraw, to withdraw from social events, to stop doing those things we used to do (but which we no longer enjoy so much), to let our self-care slip. When we do that, we are cutting ourselves off from things that offer us the possibility of reward and enjoyment. And so, our mood drops further. And a vicious cycle ensues, pulling us down into depression. Many problems that involve anxiety also show these kinds of feedback loops. If we are anxious about something (performing in public, perhaps), it is very easy to end up avoiding situations that might expose us to our fears.

These vicious cycles mean that our psychological health problems do sometimes escalate. If, for example, we deal with our anxiety (or, more precisely, with our intrusive and obsessive anxious thoughts) by deploying some compulsive rituals that make us less anxious (washing, cleaning or checking are common, but we can also deploy compulsive cognitive rituals—styles of thinking—that can be very problematic), we can find ourselves effectively addicted to the compulsions to cope with future anxiety. The fact that many emotional problems are driven at least in part by such vicious cycles means that our journey along the pathway—down the continuum—is not a linear progression. Once the process starts, we can accelerate progressively downwards ... like a snowball, as we roll downhill, we pick up speed and our problems can escalate.

These processes mean that problems are not distributed evenly. Since understandable psychological and social mechanisms mean that there's a tendency for depression to leverage more depression, without counter-vailing forces (without, that is, mechanisms that act against the 'snowballing' tendencies) protecting us. We recognise this in the common experience of panic attacks, where a trigger can lead to a rush of anxiety. But, importantly, we can see how normal psychological and social mechanisms can lead to a wide variety of sometimes quite extreme experiences and states.

We can see (non-linear) continua in every area of psychological health and wellbeing. As children, we differ in our ability to learn, to pay attention at school, to focus our attention and to regulate our emotions. For parents, these are all part of the business of childhood, of parenting, of education. When I was a child, I found it difficult to remain focussed and attentive for the full range of the school day and into the evening. I wouldn't claim to have had significant problems as a result—I managed to concentrate well enough to do OK at school and go to university—but my attentiveness was certainly not 100%. Even now, I am still distracted by squirrels outside the window, by conversations in the corridor, by the nagging suspicion that there is something interesting in the kitchen. It is simply an inevitable part of the human condition, and the fact that we all differ, that some of us have more difficulty in that regard than do others. Occasionally our problems with concentration as children cause our parents and teachers great concern. Sometimes there is real disruption to school life. Unsurprisingly, therefore, such problems tend to be associated with other problems and difficulties later in life. Equally unsurprisingly, there is a wide range of biological and social factors that can affect our ability to concentrate. But all that is hugely different to the way in which we currently often approach these problems—by invoking the idea of an 'illness' called 'attention deficit hyperactivity disorder' or 'ADHD' which only some children 'suffer from'. As Professor Sami Timimi (who is, incidentally, a child and adolescent psychiatrist) has eloquently argued, we should think of these issues much more as developmental and educational problems than as 'illnesses', or even less accurately, as 'diseases'.[17]

Attempts to Define 'Bullshit'

In 2013, the American Psychiatric Association published its revisions of the DSM franchise. The changes represented an increased emphasis on the supposed biological underpinnings of psychological distress; the language is couched in terms of biological illness. This is worrying, since it does not reflect the widespread scientific consensus that distressing experiences are the result of complex, individual interactions between biological, social and psychological factors rather than the result of a disease process. By using the language of 'disorder', diagnostic manuals (and DSM-5 is merely the latest and possibly the worst example) undermine a humane response; they imply that these experiences are the product of an underlying biological defect. The publication of DSM-5 in 2013 provoked something of a minor revolution. We saw the growth of a significant community of opposition drawn from a range of groups. Psychiatrists, psychologists, scientists and users of mental health services alike voiced their opposition to many of its proposals and particularly the pathologising of grief.[18] When someone close to us dies, many of us suffer profound, long-lasting, grief. That is not an illness, it's the price we pay for love. Traumatic experiences of all kinds change the way we see the world and our part in it, and the traumatically emotional memories are encoded in our minds in ways that cause understandable problems into the future. But it is not a 'disorder' to remain distressed by bereavement after three months. It is humane and appropriate to offer help and support. But it isn't an 'illness'.

This does not—absolutely not—mean that I, and those colleagues who share my views, believe the problems do not exist. It does not mean that we consider them to be trivial. There are many social problems that are not illnesses. Debt and crime are not illnesses. Certainly, we need to understand how and why children can manage their emotions and focus their attention. We need to study the neuroscience of these phenomena just as much as we need to study the social and cultural aspects. But they are not 'illnesses'.

Weirdly, even the supporters of the diagnostic model—even key players in the development of the major manuals—don't seem fully to believe in the project. To be fair, their argument would probably be similar to Winston Churchill's famous quote about democracy, in effect that it's a terrible system of government ... apart from all other possible models. But their pragmatic support for diagnosis is half-hearted at best. Dr. Allen Frances, Chair of the committee drawing up DSM-IV, said that: '*DSM-5 will radically and recklessly expand the boundaries of psychiatry... there is no reason to believe that DSM-5 is safe or scientifically sound*'.[19] Now, given that Dr. Frances was responsible for the fourth edition, and not for its revision (DSM-5), it might be the case that his criticism of the revision reflects his pride in his original work. But he should know the ins and outs of the process. And he's not the only critic. Dr Steven Hyman, former director of the US National Institute for Mental Health, said that DSM-5 is '*totally wrong, an absolute scientific nightmare*' and a fellow NIMH Director, Thomas Insel, said: '*Patients ... deserve better... The weakness is its lack of validity*'.[20]

My favourite quote, however, is another of Allen Frances's comments: *'There is no definition of a mental disorder. I mean, you just can't define it. It's bullshit'*. Which may well be true; Dr. Frances should know. He did chair the process that led to the publication of DSM-IV, the American Psychiatric Association's official diagnostic manual, the device designed specifically to define mental disorder.

Our Lives in Context

The traditional system of psychiatric diagnosis is demeaning and dehumanising. When we are in distress, we are not simply a set of symptoms to be assessed and classified. At the point when we most need, and deserve, to be shown compassion and understanding, when we need our individual circumstances to be recognised and taken into account, we are instead merely given a label and allocated to a category within a flawed and out-dated system.

The 'disease-model' approach and its principal practical tool—diagnosis—tend to minimise and ignore issues such as poverty, deprivation, social isolation and childhood abuse. All these, and more, lead to distress, and our natural and understandably human responses are then (mis)diagnosed as mental disorders. Giving us a diagnosis of an 'illness' when we are distressed is essentially futile; merely giving something a name doesn't make it easier for us to deal with the issues and doesn't offer any hope of a solution. We need to drop the labels and start thinking about psychological health issues in a different way, with less emphasis on what is 'wrong' with us and more on how and why we feel or act the way we do.

Real Experiences but Non-existent Illnesses

The experiences that we have are very real, even if the pathologising language of diagnosis obscures, rather than explains, their meaning. And the experiences that we have, of course, reflect the biological reality of our lives, the fact that every thought, and every emotion, emanates from the brain. It should be obvious, as we think about our loved ones, what we want to eat for lunch, feel contentment when the sun falls on our faces, that we cannot simply leap from an understanding of the biological basis of psychology to an assumption that every manifestation of this fact is, in itself, an illness.

One consequence of this is a curious paradox. When I discuss the limitations of medical diagnosis in mental health, colleagues frequently point out a range of biological processes that can lead to psychological health consequences. The 'chemical-imbalance' theory of depression seems largely to be officially discredited these days (although it also seems to be used more commonly in professional consultations than in academic journal articles) but the idea that inflammatory processes might lead to depression is currently popular. I have also been reminded on more than one occasion that traumatic brain injury is very frequently followed by depression. There is, unsurprisingly, a rather large list of medical conditions that affect our moods or our thinking styles. So, for instance, B12 deficiency, DiGeorge syndrome, temporal lobe epilepsy, porphyria, Wilson's disease, lupus, HIV infection; these are all associated with emotional or cognitive consequences. I myself was recently identified as being deficient in vitamin D, like a large number of people in Northern Europe (where the sunshine is a little weak, and few of us have jobs that take us outdoors for long periods). Equally, we know that a large number of chemicals are psychoactive, from alcohol, to mushrooms. Even lettuce, it appears, contains chemicals that affect our mood.[21]

The fact that head injuries can lead to depression is supremely unsurprising, especially if there is mileage in the idea that inflammatory processes are involved. It is equally unsurprising that what we eat or drink can affect our moods. But it is odd is that these observations are used to back up the idea that the diagnosis of illnesses or disorders is appropriate. For me, they tend to suggest the very opposite. If depression, as a phenomenon, is a common consequence of head injury or, for example, DiGeorge syndrome, that suggests to me that it is best thought of as exactly that, a consequence (or symptom, if you like) of another condition. But it doesn't suggest that depression is also a disorder in its own right. We experience depression as a result of many different challenges, psychological as well as physical. It is a tautology, simply misses the point and passes the buck, to suggest that the experience of depression occurs as a consequence of 'major depressive disorder'.

Notes

1. Geoffrey M. Reed, Joao Mendonca Correia, Patricia Esparza, Shekhar Saxena, and Mario Maj, "The WPA-WHO global survey of psychiatrists' attitudes towards mental disorders classification," *World Psychiatry* 10, no. 2 (2011): 118–131. https://www.ncbi.nlm.nih.gov/pubmed/21633689.
2. Robert Kendell and Assen Jablensky, "Distinguishing between the validity and utility of psychiatric diagnoses," *American Journal of Psychiatry* 160, no. 1 (2003): 4–12. https://www.ncbi.nlm.nih.gov/pubmed/12505793.
3. Allen Frances, *Essentials of psychiatric diagnosis, revised edition: Responding to the challenge of DSM-5®* (Guilford Publications, 2013).
4. Billy Budd is now out of copyright and freely available on the internet, for instance at: http://www2.hn.psu.edu/faculty/jmanis/melville/billy-budd.pdf.
5. ICD-10 is described well on the WHO website: www.who.int/classifications/icd/en/. The full reference is: World Health Organization, *International classification of diseases and related health problems, 10th revision* (Geneva: World Health Organization, 1992).
6. American Psychiatric Association, *Diagnostic and statistical manual of mental disorders* (DSM-5®) (American Psychiatric Publications, 2013).
7. The original DSM-I can be found here: http://displus.sk/DSM/subory/dsm1.pdf and includes within its text considerable discussion of the process of its development and the debates and political context that surrounded its production.
8. The Lancet, "Living with grief" (2012): 589.
9. World Health Organization, *Report of the international pilot study of schizophrenia* (Geneva: World Health Organization, 1973).
10. There is an excellent on-line article by Jack Carney on the declining reliability statistics for the DSM franchise: http://www.madinamerica.com/2013/03/the-dsm-5-field-trials-inter-rater-reliability-ratings-take-a-nose-dive/.

11. There are various biological correlates of different psychological states, whether neural activity detectable by fMRI technologies or biochemical correlates of inflammatory processes, but these are not diagnostic tests. Indeed, it's difficult to imagine how any such laboratory tests would be meaningful. Depression and other mental health issues are essentially problems of experience, not biology. If you were to be experiencing major problems, a negative test result would still leave you with problems, and they'd need to be addressed. A positive test would tell you nothing more than you already knew, although it might offer spurious scientific confirmation. There is the theoretical possibility that positive biological data could indicate a raised risk of developing mental health problems in the future, but again, we are a long way from such successful technologies being available. There's an interesting, if slightly densely written, historical account of the search for biomarkers in this paper: Richard Noll, "The blood of the insane," *History of Psychiatry* 17, no. 4 (2006): 395–418. https://doi.org/10.1177/0957154x06059440 or https://www.researchgate.net/publication/6472404_The_blood_of_the_insane.

12. Cartwright set out his ideas in a journal article: "Report on the diseases and physical peculiarities of the Negro race," *The New Orleans Medical and Surgical Journal* (1851): 691–715. A modern discussion of this idea can be found in: Arthur Caplan, James J. McCartney, and Dominic A. Sisti, eds., *Health, disease, and illness: Concepts in medicine* (Georgetown University Press, 2004), 28–39.

13. Peter Kinderman, John Read, Joanna Moncrieff, and Richard P. Bentall, "Drop the language of disorder," *Evidence Based Mental Health* (2013): 2–3. Doi: https://doi.org/10.1136/eb-2012-100987, https://ebmh.bmj.com/content/16/1/2.

14. David L. Rosenhan, "On being sane in insane places," *Science* 179, no. 4070 (1973): 250–258.

15. Joanna Moncrieff, *The myth of the chemical cure* (London: Palgrave Macmillan, 2008).

16. Cross-Disorder Group of the Psychiatric Genomics Consortium, "Identification of risk loci with shared effects on five major psychiatric disorders: A genome-wide analysis," *The Lancet* 381, no. 9875 (2013): 1371–1379. https://doi.org/10.1016/s0140-6736(12)62129-1.

17. Sami Timimi, *Naughty boys: Anti-social behaviour, ADHD and the role of culture* (London: Palgrave Macmillan, 2005); and Sami Timimi, Neil Gardner, and Brian McCabe, *The myth of autism: Medicalising men's and boys' social and emotional competence* (Palgrave Macmillan, 2011).

18. The Lancet, "Living with grief" (2012): 589.

19. Allen Frances's quote can be found here: https://www.newscientist.com/article/dn23490-one-manual-shouldnt-dictate-us-mental-health-research/.

20. The quotes from Hyman and Insel can be found here: http://ahrp.org/two-nimh-directors-debunk-dsm-deplore-psychiatrys-unscientific-mo-dus-operandi/.

21. Wild lettuce, and lettuces grown historically, used to contain relatively high levels of opioid-like chemicals, now reduced through selective breeding, but still a topic of discussion both among historians and aficionados of naturally-growing mind-altering chemicals.

6

Appreciating the Functions of Diagnoses

Alternatives to biomedical diagnosis in mental health care must address the functions diagnoses set out to serve. To implement a shift from a solely biomedical to a psychosocial approach, and to help deliver better, more responsive, more effective, services, we need to reform our systems for identifying, recording and responding to our problems. Significant change is needed, but despite the overwhelming influence that biomedical approaches have on our understanding of the nature of our psychological health, the various laws and policies underpinning our health and social care systems could easily accommodate such changes.

We must stop regarding our very real emotional distress and clear problems as merely the symptom of diagnosable 'illnesses'. But, what could we do differently?

Psychologists and others have recommended simply leaving behind all the assumptions of the disease model of psychiatry. This doesn't mean actively inventing new systems, it means returning to a less complicated, simpler and approach. It is noticeable that many proposed alternatives to the clear unreliability, invalidity and lack of utility of traditional diagnoses are themselves complex, multi-dimensional and structures of taxonomy. Thus, the RDoC system (the Research Domain

© The Author(s) 2019
P. Kinderman, *A Manifesto for Mental Health*,
https://doi.org/10.1007/978-3-030-24386-9_6

Criteria project—a highly biomedical proposed taxonomic structure) and the resolutely bio-reductionist and unambiguously pathologising (by definition) 'Hierarchical Taxonomy of Psychopathology', attempt to deal with the undeniable complexity of our mental health with multiple different themes or threads, covering biochemical mechanisms, the impact on personal life, etc. These are brave attempts, but also an unconscionable mess.

People are Reassured by Diagnoses

Giving a name to our distress serves a function. Naming something (whether a child, a pet or a moon of Jupiter) is an important psychological event. Many people actively want their doctor to give a diagnosis. People are dissatisfied when they do not receive a diagnosis and often describe their 'struggles' in obtaining a diagnosis from an unresponsive system. Many people comment that it wasn't until they received a diagnosis that help started to be provided.

There are different things happening here. There is the process of naming the problem, and there is the process of identifying that problem as a symptom of an 'illness'. These two issues are confused in many discussions of diagnosis. There are massive benefits to the former (defining and naming the issue at hand). It opens the door to the application of the scientific method, and therefore, to understanding and help. But we do not need, also, to assume that everything we name is an 'illness'. It helps to name racism and sexism when we see them, and it helps to know what we're talking about when we use these terms… but racism and sexism aren't in any real sense 'illnesses'.

Classifying things as 'illnesses' changes our sense of personal responsibility and that may have major benefits. If I am plagued by thoughts of being a terrible parent whose children would be better off without me, hearing that I am 'ill' and that what I am experiencing has a name and can be treated, could be very reassuring. *'You're not going mad, you're not a bad father, you're not mistaken… you're just ill and can be fixed'*.

Conventional, physical and medicine include some hugely valid and important medical diagnoses. Government campaigns urge us to look out for blood in our poo. This is important, because blood can be a symptom of bowel cancer. Recognising that I may have bowel cancer is something that is not merely synonymous with having blood in the toilet, it is entirely the province of medicine; the diagnosis (of cancer) is clearly more than the symptom (the blood itself); and the underlying condition—the cancer—is unequivocally caused by a pathology. But in mental health care, the logic falters. The 'diagnoses' often appear to be little more than a very brief repetition of the problems that the person took to the doctor, with the addition of an explicit clause that those problems are interfering with a person's daily life, and an implicit assumption that they derive from an illness, a pathology, a disorder. This happens occasionally in physical health, too. I might go to a doctor complaining that my hair is falling out and get told that I have 'alopecia'. I may say that my hair has started falling out after a period of considerable emotional stress and be told I have 'stress-related alopecia' or perhaps 'alopecia not otherwise specified'. I have gone to my doctor reporting that my hair is falling out, the doctor has translated that into 'alopecia', and I feel somehow reassured by this. It's significant that the diagnoses are often in Latin or Greek. The languages of tradition, of academic authority, of antiquity and (by extension) of the clerics carry a lot of symbolic weight.

The diagnosis, but also the tone of voice, the non-verbal behaviours, and so on, all tell the patient that the doctor has heard and, to a degree, understood their problems. The technical, slightly obscure, language, the setting (a medical clinic) and our expectations all tell us that the doctor is an expert in the field and conveys confidence. However, despite these potential or possible benefits, a cool and dispassionate look at the data suggests it may be difficult to make valid, reliable or useful diagnoses of psychological problems.

The Apparent Unavoidability of Diagnosis

The idea that psychiatric diagnoses represent real entities pervades our thinking. So, it is unsurprising that many legal, and other professionals mistakenly believe that diagnoses are needed in order to allow people to communicate efficiently with one another. In a similar vein, we need to research the nature, causes and remedies of problems, and many colleagues seem to think that diagnoses are essential in this regard. Similarly, many medical professionals and policymakers mistakenly assume that we need to use diagnoses in order to allocate resources to those who need them.

Because diagnoses are misleading and unnecessary, a simple list of a person's actual experiences and problems would provide more information and be of greater communicative value than a diagnostic label. In research, 'diagnoses' are again misleading: rather than trying to investigate hypothetical 'illnesses', researchers would be better advised to study the nature and causes of specific, identified problems, and what can help. And we can see from how resources are successfully allocated in a vast swathe of other public services that this simply isn't true.

The preamble to DSM5 states: '*DSM is... a tool for clinicians, [and] also a tool for collecting and communicating accurate public health statistics on mental disorder morbidity and mortality rates*'. The unfortunate fact that psychiatric diagnosis is presently central to health care was also acknowledged in a recent discussion document I co-authored, published by the British Psychological Society and the Power Threat Meaning Framework.[1] This is an ambitious document that uses psychological perspectives to explain mental health difficulties, with a particular focus on the dynamics of power operating in our lives; the kinds of threat we are exposed to and the ways we have learned to respond. While welcomed by some people, it was seen as threatening (or just plain wrong) by others. In particular, some people found the document's rejection of a diagnostic model disempowering of their own understanding of their difficulties, which they were perfectly happy to see as 'illnesses'. The evidence (and logic) of psychiatric diagnosis means we could do much better; we could be much more effective invalidating people's experience by referring to their actual experience rather than a putative illness. But the fact that people find alternatives to diagnosis such as the 'Power, Threat, Meaning Framework' so threatening illustrates how much of a hold this approach has over our thinking.

We need to be able to describe our difficulties and secure helpful responses. We rely (or we appear to rely) on psychiatric diagnosis in a large variety of ways. It is widely argued that the provision of psychiatric care depends on diagnosis, but the diagnostic approach is seen in other areas. Across a swathe of policies and laws, the dominant disease model and its associated diagnostic systems dominate. When we need to take time off work, our family doctors need to provide an appropriate reason (because, in the ultimate analysis, our contracts of employment require a good reason to take time off work, at least if we expect to be paid and keep our jobs) and the diagnostic framework is the go-to solution. Admittedly, many family doctors use euphemisms or anachronisms, such as 'nervous exhaustion', but nevertheless, a diagnostic approach dominates. If, then, we were to stop using this approach, would we find it impossible to take time off work if we're depressed, or anxious or hearing voices? For some of us, personal circumstances mean that we can no longer work on a permanent basis. If we're fortunate enough to have an occupational pension, then psychiatric diagnosis seems to be an inevitably necessary mechanism to retire 'on ill health grounds'. If, then, we were to move away from the use of psychiatric diagnoses, many people are worried that they would be unable to access their pensions.

Most worrying, for many people, is the potential threat to our benefits, support for people unable to work. Many people with serious psychological health problems, quite understandably, find it either difficult or impossible to work, and there are complex rules governing our access to financial and practical benefits. These are, many people argue, based on psychiatric diagnoses. Many people fear that they would lose benefits if we were to deliver services on a non-diagnostic basis.

Diagnosis and Gate-Keeping

Dr. Kate Allsopp and I recently explored the ways in which diagnoses are used in the delivery of health care. Policymakers are very keen to see us collect reliable data on the kinds of problems being addressed and are therefore very frequently encouraging us to use systems such as DSM and ICD. Indeed, both ICD and DSM are clear in their own preamble that diagnosis is vital for modern health care. Kate and I therefore wanted to explore scientifically the ways in which psychiatric diagnoses are used within UK mental health services. Our research questions were quite simple; is it the case that diagnosis dominates both the way we talk about mental health problems and our access to services, or is the true picture a little different?

To explore these issues, we used Freedom of Information Act requests to each of the 17 NHS mental health Trusts in the North of England. Although the UK has a National Health Service, with national standards, each local NHS Trust (covering a specific geographical region) has the responsibility to determine how best to deliver those standards. Hence, even NHS services' entry and eligibility criteria are locally decided. For our research, each request asked: '*What are the service entry criteria for each of the adult mental health services (community & specialist) within the trust? I.e. on what information is a decision based when accepting an individual to each service (e.g. the service entry criteria for CMHTs, early intervention, eating disorders services and so forth)?*'.

Although not every NHS Trust gave full information (even with the use of the Freedom of Information Act), a clear pattern emerged. Across the North of England, according to the information we received, there were four different ways of planning services. What we termed 'broadly diagnostic services' made reference to medicalised terms, but not in a form that matched the recognised and formal ICD or DSM diagnoses. Services need to explain what specialist skills are available and help clinical colleagues (and members of the public) work out where the most appropriate referral should be. But that, we found, tended to rely on broad quasi-diagnostic terms, not the carefully crafted 'official' terms. The majority of services, in our research at least, identified broad bands of diagnoses, such as 'learning disabilities', 'personality disorders', 'mild to moderate mental health difficulties' or 'early intervention in psychosis'. The impression of a system that is only extremely loosely based on diagnostic terms is supported by the detailed inclusion or referral criteria themselves. One Trust said explicitly that: '*... acceptance will be based on symptom presentation rather than diagnostic criteria*', another that: '*...acceptance is irrespective of potential diagnosis*'. Echoing calls for a phenomenological approach, some Trusts mentioned specific experiences, rather than diagnoses, such as, '*...distressing hallucinations or delusional beliefs of sufficient intensity and frequency*'.

When diagnoses were mentioned, they were frequently used to reassure potential users of the services or referring colleagues that they offered a comprehensive approach. It was noticeable, however, that one diagnostic term stood out. Services frequently suggested that they were inappropriate for people with a diagnosis of 'personality disorder'. This is worrying for many reasons. That particular diagnosis (or cluster of diagnoses) is notorious as a misogynistic, pathologising, insult to people surviving childhood abuse and has been pilloried as an excuse to deny people the services they need (illustrating how diagnoses can pathologise and stigmatise, rather than liberate). In 2003, the then National Clinical Director for Mental Health Services optimistically described 'personality disorder' as 'no longer a diagnosis of exclusion'.[2] In 2019, it clearly remains just that.

The dominant picture was of a large group of NHS Trusts, and individual services within Trusts, that had an extremely loose relationship with psychiatric diagnosis. This was also true for the second broad category of services identified. These, which we called 'problem-specific but non-diagnostic' services, provided specialist help for people experiencing recognisably similar problems (meaning that the specialist skills were available in an expert multi-professional team), but did not use diagnostic categories. Examples of these services were specialists working with psychosexual problems or alcohol and substance misuse problems. These services offer an example of teams working together with specialist skills and are clearly both descriptive and specific, but also indicate how, in practice, NHS Trusts can design, commission and manage services without necessarily relying on diagnoses.

A third group of services were more clearly identified as offering support within the NHS system for specific life circumstances. For example, Trusts offered specific mental health teams who worked with veterans of military service, for homeless people, for people in the traveller community, for new mothers (a perinatal mental health service), for young people, and variants of these (such as '*families in temporary accommodation and refugees*' and '*pregnant women and adults in temporary accommodation and hostels*'). It's perhaps worth stressing that these are extremely valuable services, using our professional skills highly appropriately… the point is that we don't need diagnoses to access them.

This was most clearly true for the largest group of NHS services, which we labelled simply 'needs led services'. In retrospect, this shouldn't have been at all surprising. In most cases, members of the public or family doctors have sufficient awareness of the issues to decide what kind of referral to make, but there are several reasons to avoid making a diagnosis at the point of referral. By definition, the services to whom the referral is being made have the expertise to make appropriate diagnoses (even if one were to accept that the diagnoses are, indeed, appropriate). The person making the referral is usually requesting exactly that kind of service from their colleagues. Not that long ago my GP made a referral for me to attend an oncology/dermatology clinic (I was worried about a lump). It is precisely because neither he nor I had a particular diagnosis in mind that we needed to access the skills of an oncologist. If he, or I, knew enough to make a diagnosis of that lump (it was completely benign, by the way), we would have acted differently. Equally, if the oncology clinical had required a diagnosis (for instance 'malignant melanoma') before I was able to access their lists, the whole system would have collapsed.

Similarly, in mental health, the large majority of services (or, at least, the ones we studied) offered help to those members of the local community who needed it. These included the majority of commonly recognised mental health services: community mental health teams, home treatment teams, inpatient services, including psychiatric intensive care units and liaison psychiatry services. None of these services relied—in their inclusion criteria, as revealed in our research—on diagnostic terms for inclusion. Instead, the majority of these services used a combination of criteria. They specified the (entirely understandable) fact that their business was general mental health difficulties ('*substantial and complex mental health needs*' or '*complex presentations with a significant risk of self-harm, harm to others, risk of harm from others or serious self-neglect*') which required '*skilled or intensive treatment, multi-agency approach*', with geographical criteria. In fact, rather than relying on diagnostic criteria, many services instead explicitly commented on how diagnoses were not relevant. One Trust reported that: '*decisions on whether someone should be accepted for services are based on their health and social care needs as a whole and not on diagnosis alone*'.

Medical Records

Record-keeping is arguably the function most legitimately served by conventional diagnostic frameworks. Both the World Health Organization's 'International Classification of Diseases and Causes of Death' (ICD) and the American Psychiatric Association's 'Diagnostic and Statistical Manual' (DSM) make it clear that their systems are designed to facilitate valid, reliable and useful record-keeping.

There are very real reasons to doubt whether any record-keeping system based on unreliable and invalid diagnostic categories could be useful. In 1973, the psychological scientist Kurt Salzinger became so frustrated by the inability of his colleagues to see the wood for the trees that he wrote: '*Imagine that... you are to describe the unicorn, explain where it comes from, and specify how to capture it. If you know anything about unicorns, you will immediately go to the library and start looking under mythology. There you will find descriptions of a fabulous animal with one horn and, in the more expensive books, you will find coloured illustrations. The pictures and verbal descriptions will show you that the unicorn comes in assorted colours and sizes, and that it has a single horn in the middle of its forehead. If you stop at that point you will have arrived at a satisfactory description, but if you delve further you will find that the unicorn cannot be captured except by a virgin, and even then, only rarely...*'.[3]

Giving something a name, and even reaching consensus on a definition, doesn't mean that it exists in reality. Unicorns are not real. The existence of the label can give us the misleading impression that the 'thing' exists. As psychiatrist Jim van Os puts it: '*The complicated, albeit ultimately meaningless, Greek term suggests that schizophrenia really is a "thing", i.e. a "brain disease" that exists as such in Nature. This is a false suggestion*'.[4]

There is good cause for us to record the reasons for our problems, how they present, what help is offered and what the outcomes are. But counting the number of times a clinician has used a term like 'emerging emotionally unstable personality disorder' tells us nearly nothing.

Today, because of the dominance of the medical, disease model, thinking, mental health care is planned, audited and commissioned on the basis of diagnosis. I am constantly proud of the UK's National Health Service, a comprehensive system ensuring world-class health care available to all, free at the point of need and predicated on the principles of universal and equitable provision. Other nations are less fortunate and still rely heavily on either commercial provision or on services funded through insurance. In these latter schemes, diagnosis is often important in gaining access to services, and people attempting to access those services therefore suffer. In the UK, the role of diagnosis is somewhat different; in that we tend to use diagnostic information for records systems, rather than for service provision. In the UK, services are currently commissioned on the basis of a wide range of parameters, in liaison with local authority social services through the joint Health and Wellbeing Boards.

We need to know the extent of the problems that we have to address, and the scale of the response needed. We need to know how many psychological therapists, how many clinical psychologists and how many psychiatrists to employ. We need to know what type of residential services to commission, and how many people will be needed to staff them. We need to know the extent of the problems; how many working days are lost each year to emotional problems, how many children are finding it difficult to attend to their school work (and who might need the help of educational psychologists). Commissioners and planners of services need answers to questions that are unrelated to diagnosis. They need to know how many people experience certain problems, the economic costs associated with those problems and the recommended interventions. It is a perfectly valid question to ask how many employment advisors are needed in our psychological health services, but knowing how many people have a certain diagnosis doesn't tell us that. Once again, we need information about specific problems, specific needs and specific circumstances, not diagnoses, to plan for care.

Not all public services, and not all medical specialists, rely on diagnostic categories and criteria. Examples include education (where pedagogical research and educational provision are not predicated by the 'diagnosis' of educational 'disorder', but instead respond to learners' needs), social work (where decades of sociological, economic and geographic research, as well as local government agencies, respond to the needs of citizens), the criminal justice system (where the operations of the police, legal, judicial, penitential and probation services are not, outside of the occasional incursions of diagnostic psychiatry, but instead, quite naturally, follow a more ecologically valid mechanism for responding to societal requirements) or even the work of spiritual and religious communities (where the services of rabbis, priests, imams and pastors are in no sense dependent on diagnostic theory). Within medicine, prevention relies on accurate record-keeping and data collection, but does not rely on the identification of putative illness entities. Medical professionals offer health care aimed at keeping well people well without diagnosis. We offer 'well-man' and 'well-woman' services, provide health care for children and young people and encourage vaccination and preventative healthcare checks, medical support for pregnant women. All these groups benefit from appropriate health care, but are in no sense 'ill'.

This is an 'applied science' rather than a medicalised diagnostic approach. It emphasises clear and replicable definition of the subject matter (which includes, but is not limited to, experiences and phenomena included within psychiatric diagnostic criteria), and then developing and testing hypotheses as to the origins and maintenance of, and appropriate intervention to address, those phenomena. All these perspectives meet the appropriate aspirations of data collection, measurement, definition, communication, etc., thereby meeting the legitimate aspirations of a scientific approach, but do not assume the presence of putative 'illnesses', indicated by complex combinations of experiences, avoiding most of the problems identified above.

The Equality Act 2010

There are many links between the law and psychological health. In the UK, the 'NHS Constitution' and a large number of local policies govern the care offered by the National Health Service. These echo the service entry criteria discussed earlier that individual need, rather than the presence or absence of a diagnosis, should dictate what help is offered. In the UK, however, the Equality Act 2010 offers an overarching legal framework.[5] The Equality Act 2010 prohibits discrimination across a range of 'protected characteristics'. One of these is 'disability', which covers the provision of goods, facilities and services, the exercise of public functions, premises, work, education and associations.

People with disabilities are eligible (at least in the UK) to a range of services, concessions, schemes and financial benefits. These include, for example: local authority services for disabled people; the Blue Badge parking scheme; tax concessions for people who are blind; and disability-related social security benefits. Each of these schemes has its own individual eligibility criteria, but the Equality Act offers a great deal of protection. When it comes to psychological health services, there are two interesting points. First, a psychological health problem can lead to a person meeting the criteria for disability In the Equality Act, someone is regarded as having a disability if they: (a) have 'a physical or mental impairment' and (b) the 'impairment' has a substantial and long-term adverse effect on their ability to carry out normal day-to-day activities (which is not the same as meeting the criteria for any particular mental health diagnosis). Second, the Equality Act means that someone cannot be legally refused services because they do or do not have a particular diagnosis.

The point here is perhaps a subtle one, but it's an important one. We've already seen how NHS services do not (contrary to expectations) rely on diagnostic criteria to control access. The addition of the Equality Act to the picture means that not only are diagnosed less relevant than our functional needs, but that, in fact, it would be illegal to deny services to anyone with an identified disability on the basis of the presence or absence of a diagnosis.

The Mental Health Act

It might ordinarily be thought that the use of diagnosis would be most obvious in the application of the Mental Health Act; the legislation that permits people to be detained in hospital and treated for mental health problems without their consent.[6] Once again, however, the legislation does not refer to diagnosis at all.

The criteria for detention and treatment under the Mental Health Act clearly relate to our mental health (and, shockingly, do not at present address the issue of our ability to make decisions for ourselves, something I'll discuss in a later chapter), but they echo the Equality Act in being formulated on the basis of need, not diagnosis. These, again, can be utilised by clinicians to work in the best interest of their clients, without using specific diagnostic labels.

Section 2 of the UK Mental Health Act (as amended in 2007) allows for a person to be admitted to hospital, whether or not they consent, for assessment for up to 28 days. Section 3 of the Act is very similar, except that it permits detention in hospital for up to six months and for the purposes of treatment as well as assessment. In the words of the Act: '...*detention can last for up to six months after two doctors have confirmed that the patient is suffering from mental disorder of a nature or degree which makes it appropriate for the patient to receive medical treatment in a hospital, the treatment is in the interests of his or her health and safety and the protection of others and appropriate treatment must be available for the patient*'.

In this context, it's worth pointing out that the wording refers to '... *mental disorder...*', rather than '... *a mental disorder...*' (I was responsible for contributing to the debate that removed the indefinite article (the '*a*') from this wording[7]), and the Act itself makes clear that '... "*mental disorder*" means any disorder or disability of the mind'. This circular language ('*mental disorder means a disorder of the mind*') is very common in legal circles, and I find it personally frustrating. But, once again, this definition does not refer to any of the recognised diagnoses in DSM or ICD (or any other diagnostic manual). It refers to the nature or degree of the problems, the appropriateness of care, safety and protection, etc. It is also interesting, as a psychologist, that one of the amendments brought in by the 2007 amendments was to remove the two words '...or brain...' from that definition.

There are many problems with the Mental Health Act, and with our approach to compulsion in mental health (as I'll discuss later in this book), but here it's once again worth pointing out that these are functional, needs-based, criteria, and not diagnoses.

The Mental Capacity Act

Paralleling the Mental Health Act, the UK's Mental Capacity Act 2005 provides a legal framework for making decisions on behalf of people who lack the capacity to make particular decisions for themselves.[8]

This is not widely used in mainstream mental health services, but is relevant in this context because, once again, the criteria for application of the Act are non-diagnostic. It is certainly true to say that the Mental Capacity Act (like the Mental Health Act) applies only when person is determined to have an *'impairment of their mind or brain'*, and indeed, this is often referred to as the 'diagnostic' test. This terminology presumably reflects the ubiquity of the diagnostic, biomedical, model in both society and legislation. However, the central issue of the Mental Capacity Act is the question as to whether a person is able or unable to make a specific decision when they need to. Protection is extended under the Act in both cases; a person capable of making a decision will have that decision respected, and a person unable to make a particular decision is protected by a legal framework for the decision-making by others designed to protect our best interests.

What is important in this context is that the issue of capacity—the judgement as to whether a person possesses or lacks capacity in any particular situation and about each particular decision—cuts across diagnosis. The presence of any particular diagnosis ('major depressive disorder', 'schizophrenia', 'bipolar disorder') does not tell us whether a person therefore lacks capacity. It is certainly true that the current wording of the Act means that, first, a person must be determined to have an *'impairment of their mind or brain'*, but the assessment of capacity is not included within, nor follows from, a diagnostic decision. Whatever a person's psychiatric diagnosis, capacity must be independently assessed… and the threshold is high. We must unequivocally demonstrate the lack of capacity, and autonomy is assumed until incapacity is proven. In other words, once again, a key part of UK legislation is not defined by clinical, psychiatric, diagnosis, but by functional need.

Pensions and Occupational Benefits

There are complex rules for the application of various occupational benefits such as pensions and time off from work. In the main, these derive from disability law, and hence the provisions of the Equality Act apply.

This is important, because the most common assumption is that these kinds of quasi-legal (and very important) decisions are not only medical ones but depend absolutely on diagnoses. It may very well be true that professional decisions are required; in that we may very well need a properly qualified professional to attest to a particular issue. We may, for instance, be in discussions with our employer about the psychological consequences of workplace bullying. Because there no sensible physical tests for the impact of such behaviour, we do need to rely on professional judgements themselves based on interviews and observations. It would be unreasonable (and rapidly ineffective) if we were to award employment tribunal damages on the basis of a claimant's unsupported testimony. But professional judgements are not always diagnoses.

Many people assume that we need a diagnosis to take legitimate and protected time off work. While there are many reasons why a health professional might wish to make a diagnosis (although I would recommend a different approach), this is not strictly necessary. Employers may differ in terms of the policies the individually adopt for their employees, but family doctors can, and regularly do, offer their professional opinion on a person's temporary suitability for work without using diagnoses. Once again, a simple description of a person's experiences and needs—backed by professional judgement—suffices perfectly.

Things become a little more complex when people are seeking retirement 'on ill-health grounds'. Here, we are again told that we need a diagnosis if we wish to (or, more properly, if we need to) retire on the grounds of 'sickness' or 'ill-health' (the terminology differs). And it is very complex indeed. But… because the regulations derive from disability law, and because the Equality Act applies to this area of law, again the dominance of a strict diagnostic regime is overstated.

The regulations for claiming occupation pensions on ill-health grounds are strict, and care is taken to ensure there is no fraudulent or slip-shod practice. Occupational pensions are typically worth more than our houses and the cash value of a UK occupational pension for a middle-class professional is often worth well over £1,000,000. Great caution is needed. And medical expertise is key. But the criteria are not exactly diagnostic. As an example, the criteria for the pensions scheme that covers most UK university employees (USS; the Universities' Superannuation Scheme[9]) states: '*In order to be eligible for early payment of benefits on the grounds of partial or total incapacity you must: be under age 65; and have completed two years' active membership in USS at the date it is proposed that the relevant employment should end; and be in the opinion of your employer suffering from long-term sickness or infirmity'.* This does, to be fair, use language with which I am somewhat uncomfortable, but (as yet) we're dealing with 'long-term sickness or infirmity', without mention of any diagnostic criterion. As we look in more detail, this becomes clearer: *'Medical evidence:... In order to approve an application we must be satisfied that you are suffering from long-term sickness.... We will require a medical report from your doctor to assist the trustee's medical advisers in assessing your fitness to attend work and carry out your duties'.*

This is complex and circular language, but the combination of the terminology used ('infirmity' and 'fitness to attend work and carry out your duties'), and the overarching protection of the Equality Act, makes it clear that functional, not diagnostic, criteria are important.

I have personal experience of this. A member of my own family found herself unable to work as a result of the psychological consequences of a traumatic birth (a medical mistake meant that she experienced a hugely traumatising and dangerous complication). Subsequently, on returning to work after maternity leave, she found that intrusive thoughts and memories of the experience, and fears for the welfare of her child, made it impossible to work. After some deliberation, and with the support of her family doctor, she decided to retire on 'ill-health' grounds. Unfortunately, however, her application was not initially approved. It was not rejected, per se, but was challenged under a variant of the rules above (she was in a different scheme to the USS system) to provide medical evidence. Specifically, she was told that she could not avail herself of the retirement scheme unless she could provide a specific diagnosis. We challenged this decision and were asked to navigate an appeals system that relied on her family doctor's professional judgement and an interview by a panel of three medical assessors. The interview was anxiety-provoking for her, but was in truth relatively straightforward; she was asked about her experiences and what had caused them and a panel of three medical assessors (family doctors earning extra income) made their decision.... that she was indeed entitled to claim an occupational pension under the established rules of the scheme which she had joined. In other words, an expectation of a system dictated by medical diagnosis, but in fact a system that (with some pressure) responded to the legal requirements to assess our circumstances on the basis of need.

Welfare Benefits

The UK has a bewildering array of benefits for people out of work, on low income, or with disabilities. The current government (as I write this book) has made reform of the benefits system a political priority, and (in addition to a right-wing agenda of reducing the support available to people) have planned to revise the complex system with a more streamlined approach (called 'universal benefit').

Many people (including me) would like to see fewer means-tested benefits and indeed support a system of 'universal basic income'; where the wealth of a nation is shared among its citizens through a basic income, received by all adults regardless of whether they are working or not.[10] However, at present at least, there are complex sets of criteria for the receipt of State benefits, and even more complex rules for assessing whether psychological health issues qualify as reasons for the award of financial support.

Central to the assessment of a person's eligibility for benefits is a Work Capability Assessment. This is a quasi-medical assessment, conducted by employees of the Department for Work and Pensions (or, more properly, of commercial organisations contracted by them to do their work for them) to assess a person's medical or psychological capability for work. There is very strong political opinion that the entire system is failing and is in fact designed to minimise the cost of benefits to the State. The political and scientific failings of the system are numerous and significant. The British Psychological Society[11] has argued that the Work Capability Assessment: '… *is failing to assess people's fitness for work accurately and appropriately, with people who are seriously physically and mentally ill being found fit for work*'. However, in this context, the question is whether (as is commonly assumed) people require a diagnosis to obtain benefits. And the answer is a resounding 'no'. The system for 'Personal Independence Payments', for instance, (rather ruthlessly) requires the collection of 'points' reflecting the degree of difficulty each person experiences dealing with everyday tasks. These cover such issues as: *'preparing food... eating and drinking... managing your treatment... washing and bathing... dressing and undressing... communication... mixing with other people... making budgeting decisions... planning and following a journey'* and *'moving around'*.

There are huge problems with this approach. It is an attempt to limit, not to provide, support. Governments, especially right-wing governments, are often staggeringly malign. It (perhaps therefore) sets a very high threshold; many people with very serious problems are left without support (and expected to work when they cannot) and it seems particularly poorly aligned to the needs and disabilities of people with psychological health problems. For many people, this seems merely an attempt to punish poor and disabled people for being poor and disabled. If the assessments used do not mention the crushing effect of low mood on our motivation, the daily impact of obsessions and compulsions, the consequences of paranoid fears or hearing voices, then people will be judged as 'fit for work' and ineligible for benefits. There have been reports of people interviewed as part of the benefits system, who, when discussing their low mood, have been asked *'Why haven't you killed yourself yet?'*

It's possible to argue that a genuinely diagnostic system—particularly one that respects the views of medical professionals—would protect people who use mental health services. My view is different. I appreciate that politicians with reprehensible views are likely to seize any excuse to cut benefits. That may well include misrepresenting doubts about the validity and utility of a pathologising, biomedical, perspective on mental health as suggesting that people aren't 'really' ill and don't need benefits. This reflects the views of some junior psychiatrists I commented upon earlier. But the fact that unscrupulous politicians misrepresent the evidence shouldn't stop us discussing the issue. And the present system for allocation of benefits does not, currently, rely on a diagnostic model. It's impossible, therefore, to say that diagnoses protect our benefits. In my opinion, the best way to organise services is on a non-pathologising basis, and the best way to allocate benefits is on the basis of need.

Criminal Justice

Sometimes our low mood, risk of suicide, confusion or disturbed behaviour puts us at extreme risk or, in very unusual cases, renders us a risk to others. In addition to both the Mental Health Act and the Mental Capacity Acts, mental health professionals occasionally find themselves asked to offer expert advice on a range of issues; on the risks posed by someone, for instance, who may have committed a violent crime and has a history of psychological health problems, on whether a particular crime was, perhaps, committed as a consequence of unusual beliefs or under the instructions of a hallucinatory voice, or whether a person is able to control their temper when angry. It is important to legislate for people whose difficulties put them at significant personal risk or who pose a risk to others. But this is a social and psychological problem, not a medical one. Diagnosis and even severity of an 'illness' do not relate to risk and dangerousness.

In terms of the law, such decisions do not have to be based on diagnoses. Courts have wide latitude in terms of the expert evidence on which they can rely when determining guilt or when considering a sentence. However, the dominance of the medicalising, diagnosis-driven, current system means that mental health professionals are frequently called upon by lawyers to answer questions such as: '*Does Mr X suffer from a mental disorder, and if so, which one? Was Mr X suffering from a mental disorder, and if so, which one, at the time of the index offence?*'

In my experience, despite all the scientific doubts about the reliability and validity of psychiatric diagnosis; despite the fact that such diagnoses don't explain anything, don't map onto any form of biological or psychological pathology, don't predict the course or outcome of so-called disorders, don't predict how we might respond to treatment, aren't actually included in service entry criteria and are specifically illegal (not just irrelevant) if you were to use them to deny someone public services, aren't part of the criteria for the Mental Capacity or Mental Health Acts and aren't included in any sense at all in the criminal justice legislation; despite all that, my colleagues tend to interview their clients and decide whether or not their problems meet the criteria for one or more of the currently listed clinical diagnoses.

This is unhelpful, and I have serious professional doubts about the validity of such labels. There is a complex professional dilemma here. In my professional opinion, given the overwhelming dominance of the diagnosis-driven 'disease-model' in mental health, it's entirely unsurprising that Courts and lawyers ask diagnostic questions and believe that this is a meaningful enquiry. Therefore, when asked such questions, I make it clear that labels such as 'personality disorder' may indeed currently be recognised diagnoses in manuals such as the World Health Organization's International Statistical Classification of Diseases and Related Health Problems, but I make sure that I add that this cannot be equated to a simple conclusion that any individual has a 'mental illness'. I ensure that any conclusion I make about diagnosis is contextualised in both mental health care and legal perspectives. In my legal reports, I say things like: '…*diagnoses, and especially diagnoses of so-called personality disorders, are essentially shorthand labels for complex behaviours. To say that your client's problems are consistent with a diagnosis of 'personality disorder' is synonymous with listing their observed difficulties (eating problems, self-harm, emotional instability etc.). It is also important to note that most psychiatric diagnoses, and especially diagnoses of 'personality disorder', reflect social conventions and are subject to change over time'*.

Notes

1. Lucy Johnstone and Mary Boyle, with John Cromby, Jacqui Dillon, David Harper, Peter Kinderman, Eleanor Longden, David Pilgrim and John Read, *The power threat meaning framework: Towards the identification of patterns in emotional distress, unusual experiences and troubled or troubling behaviour, as an alternative to functional psychiatric diagnosis* (Leicester: British Psychological Society, 2018).
2. National Institute for Mental Health in England, *'Personality disorder: No longer a diagnosis of exclusion', Policy implementation guidance for the development of services for people with personality disorder, Gateway reference 1055* (London: NIMHI, 2003).
3. Kurt Salzinger, *Schizophrenia: Behavioral aspects* (New York: Wiley, 1973).

4. Jim van Os, Richard J. Linscott, Inez Myin-Germeys, Philippe Delespaul, and Lydia Krabbendam, "A systematic review and meta-analysis of the psychosis continuum: Evidence for a psychosis proneness–persistence–impairment model of psychotic disorder," *Psychological Medicine* 39, no. 2 (2009): 179–195.

5. The Equality Act 2010 can be found online here: https://www.legislation.gov.uk/ukpga/2010/15/contents.

6. The Mental Health Act 2007 can be found online here: https://www.legislation.gov.uk/ukpga/2007/12/contents.

7. Some of my evidence can be found here: https://publications.parliament.uk/pa/cm200607/cmpublic/mental/memos/ucm6802.htm.

8. The Mental Capacity Act 2005 can be found online here: https://www.legislation.gov.uk/ukpga/2005/9/contents.

9. One pension scheme's guidance can be found here: https://www.uss.co.uk/~/media/document-libraries/uss/member/member-guides/post-april-2016/your-guide-to-universities-superannuation-scheme.pdf.

10. One argument in favour of a universal basic income, written by the group 'Psychologists for Social Change', can be found here: http://www.psychchange.org/uploads/9/7/9/7/97971280/ubi_for_web_updated.pdf.

11. The British Psychological Society's position on 'work capability assessments' can be found here: https://www.bps.org.uk/news-and-policy/bps-call-action-reform-work-capability-assessment.

7

A Phenomenological Approach

Rather than employ medical, pathologising, language and methods, we can and should use effective, scientific and understandable alternatives. Both of the major diagnostic systems contain the kernels of alternative systems for identifying and describing psychological phenomena and distress, and an improvement upon diagnosis would be simply to list a person's experiences as described by that person. Such a straightforward phenomenological approach—the operational definition of our experiences—would enable our problems to be recognised (in both senses of the word), understood, validated, explained (and explicable) and initiate a plan for help. This would meet the universal call for appropriate, internationally recognised, data collection and shared language use and avoid the inadequacies of reliability and validity associated with traditional diagnoses. Such phenomenological codes offer a constructive, radical way forwards.

The Oxford English Dictionary defines the scientific method as: 'a method or procedure that has characterized natural science since the seventeenth century, consisting in systematic observation, measurement, and experiment, and the formulation, testing, and modification of hypotheses'. Scientists use precise operational definitions of relevant concepts. Clinical psychologists are 'applied scientists'; we develop hypotheses about the factors and variables that lead to and maintain

© The Author(s) 2019
P. Kinderman, *A Manifesto for Mental Health*,
https://doi.org/10.1007/978-3-030-24386-9_7

the phenomena of human nature. Why we hear voices, why we become depressed, why we get anxious and why we get trapped in obsessional thoughts and compulsive responses. We test out these hypotheses scientifically. And we use the knowledge gained to plan better solutions.

Unfortunately, the diagnostic approach falls short of this rather effective system of clear, operational, definition. The individual components, the 'symptoms', can each be identified with some rigour. But when they are combined into 'disorders' through the application of the rules for combining 'symptoms', the rigour is lost. We can reliably and validly agree on the presence of 'auditory hallucinations', 'delusional beliefs' or 'thought disorder' (although it would be possible and preferable to use some less pejorative names). But that validity is lost when we try to identify 'schizophrenia'.

The use of Existing 'Phenomenological Codes'

A perfectly appropriate alternative to diagnosis would be simply to list a person's experiences as described by that person. The blogger Flo Bellamy described this from her experience.[1] Flo reported that someone she knew; '...said she was labelled as a personality disorder and experienced severe depression and suicidal ideation. She said no one understood what she meant when she said those words and everyone would go silent or change the subject. Another in the group asked, "What did you say before you had any experience of the mental health world?" to which she replied, "Well I said I felt like shit and that I wanted to kill myself." To which the other person said, "And did people understand that?" She had to admit that they did'.

The American Psychiatric Association's manual evolved over time, across swathes of psychodynamic, behavioural, cognitive and biological assumptions about the nature of mental health problems and for the pragmatic benefit of clinicians. The World Health Organization's ICD system evolved for slightly different purposes, being more closely oriented to public health needs and the monitoring of both health and threats to health.

The history of these diagnostic frameworks is one of the medical dominances; the assumption has been that progress is to be made via increasingly detailed and complex diagnostic criteria, focussing on the presumed 'disorders'. This has left the development of precise operational criteria for phenomenological entities relatively ignored. Nevertheless, imbedded within both the DSM and ICD systems are the prototype of a system approximating the 'phenomenological' approach to identifying and responding to mental health problems.[2] ICD-11 is still (at the time of writing) in draft form, but the specific 'phenomenological codes' that have been proposed would permit the recording of a wide range of relevant and potentially extremely useful phenomena. These include: non-suicidal self-injury (MB23.E), defined as '*intentional self-inflicted injury to the body, most commonly cutting, scraping, burning, biting, or hitting, with the expectation that the injury will lead to only minor physical harm*', anxiety (MB24.3), depressed mood (MB24.5), elevated mood (MB24.8), feelings of guilt (MB24.B) and auditory hallucinations (MB27.20). Helpfully, ICD-11 even differentiates between a 'suicide attempt', defined as 'a specific episode of self-harming behaviour undertaken with the conscious intention of ending one's life' (and with its own code) and 'suicidal behaviour', defined as '*concrete actions, such as buying a gun or stockpiling medication, that are taken in preparation for fulfilling a wish to end one's life but that do not constitute an actual suicide attempt*'.

What this means is that the ICD system, at least in draft form, is rapidly evolving towards a relatively functional phenomenological recording system. We do not yet have a complete taxonomy of phenomenological terms, and we don't yet have well-developed operational definitions. But we have a workable system. Moreover, it's a system already embedded in official diagnostic manuals. We don't need a new system, we can use the best bits (but the rarely used bits) of the existing system.

Such an approach meets the universal call for appropriate, internationally recognised, data collection and shared language use. It avoids the well-known inadequacies of reliability and validity associated with traditional diagnoses.[3] With clearer links to social inequity, it would help establish a rights-based approach to care,[4] and it would meet the calls from clinical colleagues for a phenomenological approach which is more effectively informed by an individual's particular difficulties rather than diagnostic codes.[5] Looking back at the historical records tells us that we used to pay much more attention to the circumstances in a person's life than we do today; the creeping medicalisation of mental health care. Research (notoriously hampered by invalid diagnoses that correspond neither to biological nor psychosocial causal mechanisms) would benefit from objective clarity. Any record system in the modern world will use categorisation but we can, and should, avoid unnecessary pathologisation and welcome precision. Finally, this is a more valid basis for co-produced clinical case formulation, which, if linked to such codes, may have greater precision, validity and reliability than purely narrative accounts.

This partially developed, very rarely used, but officially sanctioned, system of phenomenological coding shows how many traditional diagnoses could be replaced with more appropriate language. It's easy to see how we could simply 'drop the language of disorder', as I and three colleagues argued in 2013. We understand what it means when someone is depressed, has intrusive anxious thoughts or feels compelled to carry out certain behaviours. We understand what it means to hear voices, and we know how to recognise when someone is harming himself or cutting herself.

In the present system, I could go to my GP or family doctor with a problem that defies description or diagnosis, and I would still get referred (although perhaps to the wrong service) but it would be tricky to categorise my difficulties. This is relatively common, at least in the UK, doctors make notes which include a wide range of comments and descriptions (some a little rude) that defy classification. Going to my family doctor with a problem which, as yet, nobody else had ever experienced, doesn't strike me as too much of an issue—we would simply describe and record that problem. I'm sure, for instance, that I am able to describe my problems in straightforward language, and I'm confident in my GP's ability to do the same. But there is good reason to suppose that a relatively short list of common problems would cover most people's experiences. While there are estimated to be hundreds of different psychiatric diagnoses, the number of individual problems is much smaller. That is not only counter-intuitive, it undermines a fundamental idea behind diagnosis—the idea that a bewildering variety of 'symptoms' cluster into a more manageable and limited number of 'disorders'.

In 2009, Gemma Parker, Simon Duff and I looked at the statistical validity of diagnoses using a statistical technique called smallest space analysis.[6] We were interested in whether, using this particular mathematical approach, individual experiences would associate with one another as predicted by the disease-model diagnostic approach. It's no particular surprise that they didn't, in fact, cluster in that fashion (just as previous cluster analyses and factor analyses have failed to support the diagnostic model) but instead the specific problems were best seen as distributed on a continuous basis. As a first step in this analysis however, we first had to extract the specific problems or phenomena themselves. Gemma identified only 65 different specific symptoms within DSM-IV (this was conducted before the revision of the franchise). More recently, my colleague Kate Allsopp, while conducting her Ph.D. studies into diagnosis, performed a similar breakdown of constituent elements of ICD-10 (before the draft release of DSM-11). She identified only 57 common problems.

This could support great individual flexibility. If people were to present with only three problems, each time they talk to a health professional, and these three problems were randomly distributed among the 57 possibilities from Kate's list, this would yield $57 \times 56 \times 55$ or 175,560 different combinations for each person. That is a huge number and highlights how flexible a problem-list approach could be. The system needs only require a mental health professional to record three key problems from a manageably short list, and we get over one hundred thousand possible combinations.

This helps to highlight important differences between a problem-list approach and a diagnostic approach, and important benefits of the former. When I recommend replacing diagnoses with simple problem-lists, supporters of diagnosis often suggest that they are essentially the same thing. If that were in fact true, nobody needs to be scared of the proposal that we adopt a phenomenological approach, but there are many essential differences. Diagnoses are generated by combining symptoms with 'if–then' rules. 'Schizophrenia', for example, is diagnosed when a person has one of a number of possible combinations of individual problems: <u>if</u> they hear voices <u>and</u> are frightened that people may do them harm, <u>but</u> have not recently experienced a bereavement, to give one of many possible combinations. A phenomenological or problem-list approach explicitly keeps these problems separate. Only a very small number of diagnoses have only one symptom. The vast majority of diagnoses in common use rely on the combination of symptoms, leading to what is (in mathematical terms) a commonly used subset of the (175,560) possible combinations. The medical, diagnostic, approach can be seen as a process by which some, the more plausible, of these combinations make it onto an approved list, whereas others don't.

Fortunately, we don't need to go through a complex process through which professionals (usually reflecting the dominant cultural powers: middle-class, male, White, Western, heterosexual) decide among themselves which particular combinations of experiences should make the shortlist. And we don't need to decide which of these combinations reflect 'real illnesses' on the basis of our assumptions about the underlying nature of psychological health problems. The scientific method is more than capable of answering such questions for us. If problems tend to co-occur, then straightforward epidemiological research will reveal that (we don't have to make assumptions) and we can then explore possible reasons. And these don't have to be reasons of pathology. Many psychological phenomena co-occur. Given that we tend to find things that relieve our anxiety rewarding, it makes perfect sense for us to occasionally find that we have become dependent on anxiety-relieving behaviours (otherwise known as compulsions). It's certainly not inevitable that we would develop compulsive behaviours even if we experience life-changing, anxiety-inducing and intrusive thoughts. But it is perfectly understandable how we might find ourselves dependent on those inappropriate quasi-solutions if they offer a way of managing our anxieties (even if these responses are ultimately unhelpful). Psychological phenomena are linked in all kinds of understandable ways. Epidemiological research can find these examples of co-occurrence, and more in-depth research can explore the mechanism of these links. That's really the basis of formulation as clinical psychologists understand it. In other words, the diagnostic categories are assumptions, unsupported by evidence, that are unnecessary if you study—rather than impose assumptions upon—the experiences themselves.

Why don't we just do it?

For those currently in positions of influence (with power, attractive salaries, job security, etc.) the medicalised, diagnostic, system serves a function. If we were to question the certainties of diagnosis, would the whole edifice come crumbling down? It certainly does seem to be the case that the desire to diagnose is strong. For example, ICD-11 permits us to identify and record 'MB24.5 Depressed mood'. This is defined as a *'negative affective state characterized by low mood, sadness, emptiness, hopelessness, or dejection'*. But we can also diagnose, '6A70 Single episode depressive disorder'. This is diagnosed by *'the presence or history of one depressive episode when there is no history of prior depressive episodes'*. Like all similar diagnoses, the presence of a 'disorder' is confirmed via the use of the additional criteria of (a) duration, '...*a period of almost daily depressed mood or diminished interest in activities lasting at least two weeks...*' and (b) additional or other symptoms such as '...*difficulty concentrating, feelings of worthlessness or excessive or inappropriate guilt, hopelessness, recurrent thoughts of death or suicide, changes in appetite or sleep, psychomotor agitation or retardation, and reduced energy or fatigue...*'.

I would approach things differently. A two-week criterion for diagnosis is useful for clinicians and health service planners. It helps to know if a person's problems are transient or persistent, and it would change what advice we might give. But a system in which the two-week issue was addressed not via a diagnostic inclusion criterion, but simply by specifying for how long a person has been experiencing MB24.5 (depressed mood), would be more useful still.

The diagnosis of '6A70 Single episode depressive disorder' requires the presence of certain 'symptoms' in addition to "*depressed mood*", but these are all, separately, identified ICD-11 phenomena. That means we can record, quite simply: difficulty concentrating (MB21A), hopelessness (MB22.3), guilt (MB24B), recurrent thoughts of death or suicide (MB26.A), both decreased (MG43.8) and increased (MG43.9) appetite, poor sleep (7A01), psychomotor agitation (MB23N) and fatigue (MG22). In other words, there is literally nothing in the diagnosis of 'single episode depressive disorder' that isn't already captured in the detailed phenomenological descriptors and a measure of duration.

This matters. Diagnoses have major unintended consequences. People are labelled as 'ill' and 'sick', and we tend to believe that there is, therefore, something wrong with them. We can and should avoid this. It is true to say that a single designator—6A70—is shorter than to specify the duration of my depressed mood and to detail any additional problems. But what a rich source of valuable information is lost!

What characterises depressed mood? What are the most common kinds of problems? Is there a consistent relationship between these experiences combined within the diagnosis? If there are patterns—may be, for example, a pattern of more 'physical' experiences, involving fatigue and appetite or a pattern of more 'cognitive' experiences, of rumination or thoughts of guilt or worthlessness—then do these relate to either identified causes or interventions? Is it the case, perhaps, that a pattern of negative thought might be associated with depressed mood after negative life events and respond well to psychological therapies, but physical interventions such as exercise might help people with other experiences? Interesting questions (at least in my opinion) which could be answered if we adopt a phenomenological approach but would be lost if we use a diagnostic approach.

Exactly the same arguments can be made in all other diagnoses. We would be able to offer much more appropriate care if we were to stop using quasi-medical diagnoses such as DSM-11's Moderate Personality Disorder (6D10.1), and instead record the specific problems that the individual is experiencing. We can record, in official terminology, such problems as anger (MB24.1), depressed mood (MB24.5), feelings of guilt (MB24.B) and non-suicidal self-injury (MB23.E). These phenomena might well co-occur (it makes a great deal of sense that they could), but that doesn't make 'personality disorder' a legitimate illness, and it's through the scientific deconstruction of the concept that we could start to understand better these kinds of problems. We can also (as I'll explain in a moment) record those adverse experiences that may have led to these problems. This would—just as in the case of depression—allow us to explore specifically, and individually, experiences such as sexual abuse, spouse or partner violence or poverty.

So… why don't we do it? Why don't we use those elements of the existing system that would allow us to identify our problems in non-pathologising language? Sadly, I believe it's because it's in the interests of some professionals (not the public) to retain the closed shop of medical psychiatry.

Recognising Causes in the Real World

We know that childhood trauma, poverty and social inequity are major determinants of our psychological health, and I have previously stressed how the United Nations Special Rapporteur[7] characterises mental health care not as a crisis of individual conditions, but as a crisis of social obstacles. It is important, therefore, that the circumstances that have given rise to distress—those 'social obstacles'—should be formally recorded alongside the distress itself. In the absence of that recognition, and that data collection, we're left identifying an 'illness' but not identifying a cause. In that case, and in the context of widespread messages about biological, genetic, causes, there's every chance that we will simply assume that—with no external cause—the problem must be the result of some pathology or flaw within us.

As well as offering diagnoses, the World Health Organization's ICD system was designed to permit health care planners to understand the root causes of ill-health; the factors that led to the incidence of disease '…and causes of death…'. That means that the ICD system comes with a whole variety of vitally important healthcare indicators issues that are not themselves illnesses, but which are necessary to record in order to help track and explain illness. It's mildly entertaining (at least for me) to look within the ICD system for obscure and amusing causes of injury (which are, I suppose, much less amusing if you're the one who's been injured). So, in ICD-11, we have XE69N, which is the code to be used if someone has received an injury from a 'parrot, parakeet, or cockatoo', and XE4AP is the code used if someone has injured themselves with 'nightclothes, pyjamas, nightwear, underwear, undergarment, or lingerie'. I have to confess to an adolescent amusement by the idea of a code for 'injury by underpants' (although I did, myself, once trip over and break my own toe in a XE4AP-related incident). But the point is that ICD is designed to collect data on the <u>causes</u> of injury.

Despite being rarely discussed, used or reported either in clinical practice or in the academic literature,[8] both ICD-11 and DSM-5 incorporate descriptive information regarding adverse life experiences and living environments. In ICD-11, these quasi-diagnostic codes document such factors as a personal history of sexual abuse (QE82.1) or a history of spouse or partner violence (QE51.1).

That seems clear and useful. These events in our lives are of great causal significance in the development of psychological health problems, and, therefore, vital information both for clinicians as we develop co-produced formulations and for health service planners. All of this emphasises the importance of the social context of mental health. And all this contextual information is perfectly recordable, within the 'official' World Health Organization's recommended statistical manual.

But the ICD-11 system goes further and allows us to record a long list of very significant factors: low income (Z59.6), inadequate housing (Z59.4), threat of job loss (QD82), burn-out (QD85) and separately, caregiver burn-out (QF27), illiteracy (QD90), conviction (QE40) and imprisonment (QE41), one's removal from home in childhood (QE90) or—very importantly—'...*a personal history of maltreatment*' (QE82). We can record not 'post traumatic stress disorder', but rather 'experiences of crime, terrorism, disaster, or war or other hostilities (QE80)'. We don't have to assume that our clients are depressed, or, worse, suffering from 'major depressive disorder', we can say what's actually happening; that they are receiving 'insufficient social welfare support (QE31)' and exploited because of 'unpaid work (XE8VF)'. DSM-5 generally mirrors the ICD system and therefore includes codes for a wide variety of problems related to family upbringing, and housing and economic problems.

Broadening routine data capture could target information regarding established social determinants of psychological health problems, such as inequality, poverty and trauma. This could then lead to more inclusive, social, systemic and psychologically comprehensive services. At present, it would be seen as a serious clinical omission if a professional working in mental health were to fail to record a diagnosis of a serious mental health problem. Imagine if it were equally serious to fail to document a history of childhood sexual abuse or to fail to pass on to the authorities evidence of 'insufficient social welfare support (QE31)', or exploitation through 'unpaid work (XE8VF)'.

Again, why don't we just do it?

I recently obtained the (fully anonymised) data for an entire year's caseload for a major NHS mental health Trust as part of a research project. The most striking finding was the fact that even diagnostic codes were rarely used. For the 21,000 people for whom healthcare records were available, only 4657 had received a diagnosis, 764 relating to alcohol or substance use and 1605 relating to organic diseases or dementia. This raises questions about the quality of record-keeping, but also throws into sharp focus the claim that diagnoses are invaluable tools for the clinician. In only 20% of cases were the diagnoses significant enough to warrant recording.

Our healthcare records are also shockingly inadequate, when compared to how rich they could be. In an economically deprived city, our mental health professionals made no formal mention of 'poverty'. There was one record of 'homelessness' and two of 'unemployment'… our unemployment rate in the city is currently 5%. Across the database of 21,000 people and more specifically within the 2288 receiving help for mental health problems, there were only 9 (nine) records of sexual abuse and in the 102 cases where 'post-traumatic stress disorder' was diagnosed, there was not a single record of any event that might have led to that diagnosis. Across the 21,000 people, the only record of 'assault' is the (frankly bizarre) single instance of '*assault by pesticides*' (which is not in ICD, as it happens). Clinicians did, in fact, avail themselves of experiential or phenomenological codes. There were 453 records of self-harm, by far the most common phenomenological record. Interestingly, and positively, the term 'depressive episode' (rather than '…disorder') was used very frequently, on 661 occasions. That implies, strongly, that when such codes are available (albeit as a quasi-diagnosis), psychiatrists will choose a quasi-phenomenological code, a finding that is important, interesting and positive. One final nugget was revealed from this data (which has many further stories to tell). Illustrating, perhaps, the wonderful flexibility of the ICD system, one person was recorded as exhibiting 'R46.2 Strange and inexplicable behaviour'. I find this mildly insulting and a little odd. But it does, perhaps illustrate how we can find non-diagnostic codes for pretty much anything.

We seem to be a long way from the routine recording of such vital data. I suspect that one reason is that there are subtle, unpleasant, but powerful reasons for avoiding looking too deeply into these issues. The World Health Organization very definitely would like to know about the social, circumstantial and material factors that impact on our health. That's just as true for physical illnesses as for mental health issues, by the way; the World Health Organization (and well-meaning governments) is very interested in tracking the social determinants of health across the board. Dainius Pūras, in his report for the United Nations (and the World Health Organization is an executive agency of the UN) stressed how we should move from mental health care systems focussed on 'chemical imbalances' to 'power imbalances'. And, to repeat myself, it's by recognising and recording these social factors that we might effect change.

But this may be difficult for some in power. We know—and politicians know—that political factors are relevant to our mental health. There is overwhelming evidence of the influence of poverty (QD50) and crime (e.g. sexual abuse [QE82.1] or spouse or partner violence [QE51.1]), low income (QD51), unemployment (QD80) and homelessness (QD71.0) on our mental health. It may well be convenient for politicians to downplay these issues, to leave mental health to medical professionals and effectively wash their hands of the problem. It becomes even more difficult for politicians (or at least, right-wing politicians) if we were to measure the impact on our mental health of other social factors included in ICD-11. The UK government programme of reassessing disability benefits using the Work Capability Assessment has been associated with an increase in suicides, mental health problems and prescription of antidepressants, as well as widespread mistakes and errors. If, then, we were to embark on a programme of recording such ICD-11 codes as QE31—'insufficient social welfare support'—we might see significant embarrassment for our politicians.

This all means that a much more appropriate approach than the use of quasi-medical diagnoses is within reach. Although it will remain possible, using ICD-11, to offer a diagnosis of Moderate Personality Disorder (6D10.1), it is possible instead to record formally one or more adverse or traumatic experiences and subsequent specific mental health difficulties. For example, personal history of sexual abuse (QE82.1), history of spouse or partner violence (QE51.1) and low income (QD51), leading (understandably) to: anger (MB24.1), depressed mood (MB24.5), feelings of guilt (MB24.B) and non-suicidal self-injury (MB23.E).

If we were to combine phenomenological data with social data, we would have a powerhouse of information. We could, if we used both coding sub-systems and stopped making diagnoses, be far more precise. We could also link specific social factors (unemployment or a history of childhood trauma) to specific experiences, low mood, guilt, anger, dissociation, hearing voices, etc. The potential for clinicians and researchers would be immense.

So, then, why don't my colleagues do this? Why ignore the ICD criteria for specific problems and why ignore the 'social codes'? The World Health Organization approves both, and they offer transformational levels of detailed information.

My medical colleagues don't do this because it's not how they're taught to think. It seems clear to me that the mental health care system (the clue is in the name) is dominated by medical, diagnostic and thinking. The training of most of our professionals works that way. I recognise that it's a major challenge to change established thinking, but it needs to be done. Here, because decades of medical education, across the world, have institutionalised the practice of diagnosis, that's what doctors do. When I raise the possibility of an alternative—simply identifying a person's problems, with an indication of duration (and with the possibility of additionally recording likely causes)—I tend to receive a puzzled shake of the head, and a comment to the effect that it's all wrapped up in the diagnosis and there's no real need for change.

Including the routine recording of these kinds of data within UK National Health Service records (and elsewhere) could establish more inclusive, social, systemic and psychologically comprehensive patterns of difficulties. We would be able to identify our problems clearly, precisely, and in readily understood language. This would avoid the deliberately obscure Latin and Greek phrases, which serve to distance us from our own experiences, ignore the causes of our difficulties, and collapse our individual stories into an agglomerated diagnosis. We would avoid labelling people as 'disordered' and implying pathology and flaw. We would avoid implying that the root cause of our difficulties is brain disorders or diseases and avoid the subsequent medicalised 'treatments' offered or coercively imposed. We could target help precisely to address the problems identified and conduct research on the problems, on their causes and on the mechanisms that lead to their onset, maintenance or severity.

If we were to use the existing, and officially approved, mechanisms for identifying not only the experiences themselves, but also the social context of those difficulties, we could better use the available information regarding established social determinants of mental health problems, such as inequality, poverty and trauma. As clinicians, we might be better able to serve our clients if we can use such data capture to apply more effective pressure on the political system and drive wider system reform. Such use of the existing and available psychosocial codes is presently very uncommon. It should become routine. We are aware in general terms of the links between social pressures and psychological health problems, but we seem to do very little about it in real terms.

We should not expect that clinicians are able to resolve such difficulties or that they should shoulder this responsibility; it is not the job of mental health professionals to end poverty. Nevertheless, proper recording of psychosocial ICD and DSM codes is imperative.

From time to time, we read of tragic cases where people miss out on the necessary assessments and referrals or interventions that professional policies and good practice guidelines recommend in their situation. In many of these reports, although the better journalists recognise the complexity and challenge of diagnosis, the idea of missing key information in a person's presentation (in physical health, that might be failing to recognise the presence of a child's rash which doesn't disappear when pressed; in mental health, it might be neglecting to enquire about 'suicidal ideation'), or indeed of making incorrect diagnoses. Despite the transparent concerns about the validity of psychiatric diagnoses, there is also a strong tradition of concern over mistaken or incorrect diagnoses. So, we are worried about the ability (and, to be honest, commitment) of some of our colleagues to accurately spot, and then use, symptomatic or diagnostic information. It really matters if a family doctor misses or ignores a two-week pattern of low mood and fatigue. So… imagine if it were as serious to fail to document extreme poverty as it would be for a clinician to fail to identify severe depression.

Changing Language

Not long ago, I gave a lecture on the theme of this book in Norway. A colleague of mine from the Norwegian Psychology Association was in the audience, and, when we went for lunch, he quizzed me about the issues I'd discussed. '*So, tell me, Peter*', he said. '*Your argument is that we should stop thinking about mental illnesses, and stop diagnosing disorders, and instead use detailed, phenomenological, scientific, descriptions of our problems and difficulties. Is that right?*' I told him he'd got it exactly right. '*Ah…*' he said. '*Well then… let me tell you something. Obviously, you gave your speech in English. But I had to translate it, in my head, into Norwegian. And, so, I had to find a Norwegian word to use for your "detailed, phenomenological, scientific, descriptions". And the best word is…. "diagnose"*'.

That conversation stuck with me. My colleague, gently, was pointing out that it might not be terrible to 'diagnose' … if that is what 'diagnose' meant.

If that were what 'diagnose' meant, I might agree. But we're not quite there yet. First, diagnosis isn't exactly the same as classification or description. Diagnosis is quite specifically the classification of something as an illness or disorder. People certainly do use the word 'diagnose' as a metaphor or an analogy; an engineer will 'diagnose' the fault with our car or an accountant might 'diagnose' the problem with a business proposal. But they are analogies.

The language of diagnosis is the language of pathology, of illness, of fault and of flaw. It implies that there's something wrong with us, that the underlying causes of our difficulties are brain disorders or diseases and implies that we need medical intervention. All these assumptions are unhelpful. We'd be better off not using the term 'diagnosis' and instead observe, record and describe.

Notes

1. This is from 'Discursive of Tunbridge Wells', an excellent blog site addressing some of the same issues I discuss in this book. http://discursiveoftunbridgewells.blogspot.co.uk/2014/01/flo-bellamy-does-diagnosis-simply.html.
2. Peter Kinderman and Kate Allsopp, "Non-diagnostic recording of mental health difficulties in ICD-11," *The Lancet Psychiatry* 5, no. 12 (2018): 966. https://www.thelancet.com/journals/lanpsy/article/PIIS2215-0366(18)30394-8/fulltext.
3. John Read and Rachael Mayne, "Understanding the long-term effects of childhood adversities: Beyond diagnosis and abuse," *Journal of Child & Adolescent Trauma* 10, no. 3 (2017): 289–297.
4. See Dainius Pūras's report: http://ap.ohchr.org/documents/dpage_e.aspx?si=A/HRC/35/21.
5. Peter Kinderman, John Read, Joanna Moncrieff, and Richard P. Bentall, "Drop the language of disorder," *Evidence Based Mental Health* (2013): 2–3. Doi: https://doi.org/10.1136/eb-2012-100987, https://ebmh.bmj.com/content/16/1/2.
6. Gemma Parker's thesis is available for public access but, unfortunately, only from the University of Liverpool Library, where it is lodged with the accession number: lvp.b2182260.
7. See Dainius Pūras's report: http://ap.ohchr.org/documents/dpage_e.aspx?si=A/HRC/35/21.
8. Kate Allsopp and Peter Kinderman, "A proposal to introduce formal recording of psychosocial adversities associated with mental health using ICD-10 codes," *The Lancet Psychiatry* 4, no. 9 (2017): 664–665. https://www.thelancet.com/journals/lanpsy/article/PIIS2215-0366(17)30318-8/fulltext.

8

Formulation and the Scientific Method

To understand and explain our experiences, and to plan services, we need to do a little more than simply make a list of those problems. This means developing co-produced 'formulations'. It is via these formulations that we can recognise the fact that psychosocial factors such as poverty, unemployment and trauma are the most well-established causes of psychological distress. It is, equally through such multidisciplinary formulations that we can acknowledge how other factors—for example, genetic and developmental—may influence the way in which each of us reacts to challenges. And it should be these formulations that form the basis for intervention.

Frustrated at the need for reform, we sometimes argue that we need a whole new way of thinking about psychological health care. But in truth, we don't really need to invent a new system. We have one already—we have applied science.

The scientific method is integral to the profession of clinical psychology. Early in my professional training, I was introduced to the work of Monte Shapiro, a pioneer in my profession. Back in 1947, at a conference in Boulder, Colorado, the modern profession of clinical psychology was born—as an applied science. In the UK, Shapiro pioneered the value of a psychologist as an applied scientist. Clinical psychologists use

© The Author(s) 2019
P. Kinderman, *A Manifesto for Mental Health*,
https://doi.org/10.1007/978-3-030-24386-9_8

validated methods of assessment and apply scientific principles of observation, hypothesis generation and hypothesis testing to the individual clients, systems, problems or issues. We welcome research which improves these methods of assessment, and which increases our understanding of the psychological mechanisms underpinning those problems that we try to address. It also means using such interventions—whether therapies or advice or any other kind of helpful intervention—as are demonstrably effective and which follow from an understanding of those mechanisms. Scientists try to avoid trial-and-error approaches, as a rule, and instead develop theories as to what might help, then systematically apply those possible solutions and carefully observe the results, modifying strategies as necessary.

We don't need to develop a new, hitherto undiscovered, alternative to diagnosis; we already have the ability objectively to identify and describe human psychological phenomena. The applied scientific method is the alternative to diagnosis, and to the disease model. It's worked incredibly well across all societies and in all areas of life for at least 200 years (arguably for 40,000 years before being systematically described) and has applied to clinical psychology since 1947. It seems quite simple and straightforward to me; operationally define your phenomena (that's not the same as diagnosis), generate hypotheses (based on the research literature) about the origins and maintenance of those problematic phenomena, collect relevant data to test those hypotheses, and (taking a precautionary principle) intervene, observe the results and adjust as necessary. And central to all of this is 'formulation'.

Psychological Formulations

Psychological formulations are hypotheses, tentative, co-produced, accounts of why people may be experiencing difficulties and what might help, based on psychosocial principles and with reference to psychological theories.[1] Formulations take as their starting point a problem that the person describes, rather than a diagnosis or a professional's opinion. This is how formulations fit with and derive from objective descriptions of such problems as low mood and lack of motivation, hearing voices, problems functioning at work, paranoia, etc. That would be different than, for example, formulations about 'schizophrenia'. Partly, that's because the diagnoses—in their heterogeneity, poor reliability and dubious validity—reflect entirely different causes, mechanisms, likely helpful interventions and outcomes for any of us with the same diagnosis.

Clinical psychologists are therefore informed by psychological science, as we work with our clients to develop hypotheses about what might have led to the development of these problems and, consequently, theories about what might be helpful. The more precise information we have about the exact problems for which the person is seeking help, the events and circumstances of their lives, as well as how they have responded and what things they have done to try to help, the better the formulation will be. Because all these issues are highly personal, each formulation should be very individual, tailored for each person and their specific problems. I've previously used an example of a civil engineer building bridges; the principles of architecture, and the physics of the construction (the tensile strength of steel, for example) are universal, but, because of the idiosyncrasy of the geographical topology of each canyon, each bridge will be unique.

Many professions in mental health care rightly emphasise the importance of formulations. Those developed by psychologists (as one would expect) place particular emphasis on psychological processes to explain and account for the problems. That means a focus on the way that people make sense of their world. In the words of the Health and Care Professions Council (the regulatory body for clinical psychologists in the UK), clinical psychologists must '…*understand psychological models related to how biological, sociological and circumstantial or life-event related factors impinge on psychological processes to affect psychological well-being…*'.

This is not just an academic issue, and it isn't necessarily a cause of so-called 'guild disputes'. But it is important. Diagnosis sends an inappropriate message about the fundamental nature of mental health problems. It is inappropriate to suggest that a 'disease' called 'depression' is responsible for the low mood and fatigue someone is experiencing. It is inappropriate philosophically, because it confuses a label with an explanation. It doesn't help to say that the label that we give to the experience of low mood is the cause of the low mood. It doesn't help us understand why a person is hearing voices to suggest that the cause of the voices is a disorder called 'schizophrenia'. 'Schizophrenia' is again merely a label we give to a variety of problems, including hallucinations. This is inappropriate because it's lazy thinking, and it's inappropriate because it pretends to offer an explanation, but doesn't actually deliver. This is probably most worrying when parents need to understand why their child has problems with attention or emotion regulation. To say: '...*he is having problems concentrating at school because he has ADHD...*' is circular and misleading to the point of being genuinely counterproductive.

Formulation is collaborative. Formulation includes: a summary of the client's core problems, hypotheses, developed on the basis of psychological theory, that account for the development and maintenance of the client's difficulties, therefore, suggestions as to how the client's difficulties may relate to one another, and a consequent plan of intervention. The problem list could include such things as: low mood and lack of motivation, hearing voices, problems functioning at work, paranoia, etc. Typically, a formulation will also examine key formative events in a person's life, and how they have interpreted and reacted to these. Formulations tend to change as the psychologists and their clients learn more about the problems: they are designed to be 'best guesses' about the problems, and these guesses are tested out over time. Everything is open to revision and re-formulation. Psychological case formulations are therefore complex and clinical psychologists draw on a large variety of psychological theories, each drawing on scientific research. Although each individual case formulation will not draw on all this research, each person may have a range of interrelated psychological difficulties, which can make formulation a complex, skilful, process.

Clinical psychologists develop formulations of problems involving individuals, couples and families. Occasionally, psychologists might develop formulations for multidisciplinary teams addressing shared problems for the group. Formulations may also be developed and shared concerning individuals or groups with other agencies and services: wards, hostels, schools, care homes, courts, etc. In such circumstances, there will be a range of interests, priorities and concerns that need to be accommodated in the formulation. Psychologists need to bear in mind the needs of all those involved, and this can be a difficult task.

The wider context of psychological wellbeing is important. People have very different values, spiritual and religious beliefs, as well as beliefs about health and psychological health, all of which must be incorporated in our formulations. We know that people from Black and minority ethnic groups are particularly likely to have psychological health problems, but are less likely to be referred to psychological services. Many citizens have experienced racism and discrimination, both directly and as a result of our history of colonialism and exploitation. Refugees and asylum seekers are particularly vulnerable to developing mental health problems as a result of their difficult and traumatic experiences. Language differences may create an additional complexity to the communication of distress (English, and Western, scientific, idioms are not necessarily statements of truth, and are not universal), and there can also be cultural variance in how distress is expressed. Western psychological approaches and, therefore, forms of therapy often stress independence and autonomy for good psychological health, whereas non-Western cultures tend to focus more on notions of spirituality and communality and tend to prioritise the needs of the family rather than the individual. Culturally appropriate psychological formulations need to be able to incorporate all these issues.

Formulations are certainly not perfect: as with offering a diagnosis, developing and then sharing a formulation with a client can be a powerful intervention in itself. I share the view of my psychologist colleagues, and indeed my professional body, that formulation is a powerfully positive tool, but it's also clear that clients themselves have a complex response to receiving a formulation. While people report finding formulations helpful, encouraging and reassuring, and increase the trust they feel in their psychologist, clients can also (sometimes at the same time) find formulations saddening, upsetting, frightening, overwhelming and worrying. Formulations are complex accounts of the origins of serious problems, frequently rooted in traumatic events and the person's response to these events. Just as the process of diagnosis can be open to bias and may occasionally lead to disempowerment, hopelessness and other negative consequences, so too psychological formulation can be used in insensitive or disempowering ways.

Formulation as a Multidisciplinary Skill

Many professional bodies stress the role of individual 'formulations' as either alternatives to, or supplements to, diagnoses. Formulation is fundamental to the training and practice of clinical psychologists, but is also practised by health, educational, forensic, counselling, and sports and exercise psychologists. It also appears in the curriculum for psychiatrists' training in the UK.[2]

There are, however, some significant differences between psychiatric and psychological formulations. In most cases, a psychiatric formulation will begin with a diagnosis, which is an account of the various biological, psychological and social factors involved in the development of the diagnosed disorder. Richard Bentall and others have suggested, however, that if a psychiatric formulation—an account of the various factors leading to a diagnosis—is conducted successfully, the psychiatric diagnosis itself becomes redundant.

As an example, we can think about some of the ways in which depression (for instance) is linked to biological processes. I mentioned earlier how traumatic brain injury is very frequently followed by depression, and quite possibly because inflammatory processes (as well as other forms of physical damage) affect our brains. That's a hugely unsurprising observation. When a mental health professional sits down with a client to discuss the various reasons that might explain why they have been feeling so depressed, the physical consequences of a recent head injury would come into the mix, as would other recent life events, the person's characteristic style of responding to events, sense of self and so on. If, in such a scenario, a recent head injury were to be seen as a key causal factor, the diagnosis of 'major depressive disorder' isn't so much wrong or right, but irrelevant. The experience of depression (as a phenomenon) is more than understandable, but it makes little sense to see this as a 'symptom' of an illness called 'major depressive disorder'. Indeed, even within criteria for that diagnosis, this would be inappropriate; because there is, technically, an exclusion criterion; that the experiences are not better explained by another medical condition, such as head injury. In other words, if we can find a plausible medical explanation for the low mood, it ceases to be 'major depressive disorder' and takes its place as a recognised and uncontroversial symptom of something else.

This doesn't mean we should disparage diagnoses. Since many people find psychiatric diagnoses helpful, it is merely respectful and appropriate to incorporate this perspective. In such cases, many psychologists tend both to explain the way in which a diagnosis may be used ('when people have these kinds of problems, we sometimes find it helpful to use the diagnosis 'major depressive episode', which describes, in technical terms, the kinds of problems you've described'), and to explain why a diagnosis might be seen as helpful ('you're able to retire on ill-health grounds') and offers a useful way of explaining your difficulties to family and friends. The process of developing a formulation, collectively with the client, offers an opportunity to discuss alternative, psychological, ways of looking at their difficulties.

Psychological formulations should always include those psychological processes that explain and account for the origin of the problems, which means a focus on the way that people make sense of their world. In the words of the Health and Care Professions Council (the regulatory body for psychologists in the UK), clinical psychologists must '*understand psychological models related to how biological, sociological and circumstantial or life-event related factors impinge on psychological processes to affect psychological well-being*'. It is in no sense a disparagement of the approach of psychiatrists; it's necessary and welcome that their focus will be slightly different.

Notes

1. The British Psychological Society's guide to formulation can be found here: https://www1.bps.org.uk/system/files/Public%20files/DCP/cat-842.pdf.
2. The UK's Royal College of Psychiatrists' guide to formulation: https://www.rcpsych.ac.uk/usefulresources/publications/collegereports/op/op103.aspx.

9

The Drugs don't Work: The Difference Between Curing and Helping

We would offer better care if we were sharply to reduce our reliance on medication. Our current heavy reliance on psychiatric medication is based on flawed logic. Many chemicals are known to affect our mood and thinking, and there is no clear evidence that psychiatric medication is correcting underlying biochemical abnormalities. Psychiatric medication, taken long-term, also appears to have some very distressing adverse effects. Rather than seeing mental health as a biological or medical issue and assuming that medication will 'cure' non-existent underlying 'illnesses', medication instead should be used sparingly and in response to specific problems. In practice, this means adopting Dr. Joanna Moncrieff's 'drug-based' approach in contrast to the more common 'disease-based' approach.

In late 2018, I took part in a 'question and answer' session following the screening of a movie about the possible use of psilocybin—a psychedelic drug—to help people who were experiencing depression and who had not been helped by other approaches. There's a lot to say about psilocybin, as it happens. Psilocybin is the psychoactive chemical in 'magic mushrooms' and has been used as a recreational and sacred drug for millennia. In chemical terms, it binds strongly to serotonin receptors, triggering a psychological response which can last for about 6 hours. It doesn't 'release' serotonin, but has a complex impact on the serotonergic

© The Author(s) 2019
P. Kinderman, *A Manifesto for Mental Health*,
https://doi.org/10.1007/978-3-030-24386-9_9

systems of the brain, including theories that it leads to 'neuroplasticity' (the tendency to break, make, and reform, synapses and the growth of new dendritic connections) and that it is associated with anti-inflammatory activity. The drug is powerfully hallucinatory, although, interestingly, people report that the hallucinations are recognised as not being real, and (probably because of the impact on the serotonin system) leads to a range of psychological effects; disorientation, lethargy, giddiness, euphoria, joy and even depression. Psilocybin (in the form of mushrooms) has also been used in sacred rituals for many thousands of years and has been associated many times with powerfully transformational experiences.

I find it interesting (as I write this book) partly because of the range of different perspectives on its possible utility in psychological health care. There's an interesting confluence of ideas. People from a mystical, spiritual, even shamanic, background point to the common use of psilocybin in spiritual or healing rituals in many cultures over many millennia. For me, this seems to be close to the common observed phenomena of psilocybin (presumably through a neurochemical process) intensifying emotions, encouraging deeply introspective and emotion recollection of past events and even common reports that the individual's sense of self is changed; people report no longer recognising the boundaries between themselves and other people or even objects. This intrigues my psychiatric colleagues: particularly (I suspect) the direct physiological effects; the affinity of psilocybin for serotonin receptors, the effect on neuroplasticity and the possible anti-inflammatory effects.

Psilocybin may well help people who are depressed. The striking, unusual, meaningful, significant, experiences that people report do seem to have life-changing consequences. Psychoactive chemicals may well enhance the impact of either, on the one hand, spiritually significant rites of passage or, on the other hand, psychotherapy. My personal view is that high-quality psychological therapy is likely to prove an additional necessary component to change; the chemical alone will not 'cure' depression or even, alone, be 'the answer'. Therapy is sadly only moderately effective at best, and the addition of a spiritually significant chemically assisted 'trip' might be helpful in generating new possibilities of thought, especially if that 'trip' is associated with deeper introspection, emotion recollection of past events, and a temporarily changed sense of self.

Some of the most interesting work on psychedelic drugs links the ideas of perceptual control theory and its therapeutic development, the 'method of levels' pioneered by my colleague Dr. Sara Tai and referred to in Chapter 4 of this book. Rather than assume that the drugs 'correct' some form of pathology, or even ameliorate some understandable deficit, even one induced by unbearable circumstances, it may well be the case that such extraordinary, psychedelic, experiences may affect our moods, behaviour and motivation by allowing us to gain new perspective on the conflicts that, if unresolved, hold us back. In such a scenario, a combination of novel experiences, and the ability to explore the implications for 'how we have learned to control our responses to such internal conflicts, may well be a powerful combination.

The evidence that psilocybin can help people who are depressed is still speculative at best, although it's worth evaluating anything that might be helpful. The way to do this is through a carefully constructed (carefully constructed because the issues are so complex) randomised, controlled, trial. But what intrigues me, now, is the range of different explanations put forward for WHY it might be helpful if it IS helpful. Some neuroscientists prefer a directly pharmacological mechanism, but it interests me that very well-respected scientists can differ quite fundamentally as to what those mechanisms could be. Some think that depression is a consequence of an inflammatory process, and psilocybin is helpful as an anti-inflammatory agent. Others appear to regard depression as a symptom of a fundamental pathology or dysfunction in the serotonin system and point to psilocybin's affinity for serotonin receptors. For them, psilocybin is discussed somewhat akin to a conventional antidepressant medication, and some have recommended low-dose psilocybin could be taken on a regular basis as a treatment for depression. Other people have discussed psilocybin use in a one-off dose (an approach that more closely resembles ritual uses), but have described this in chemical terms, even suggesting that the 'trip' resulting from chemical binding to serotonin receptors results in the brain 'settling down' into a new, non-depressed, state. But other colleagues (including psychiatrists) take a different approach. They look to the fact that psilocybin and other psychedelic drugs have been reported to lead to new psychological understandings and personal insights. For many of these colleagues, the chemical effects of the psychedelic drugs lead to psychological changes otherwise impossible. Still others, closer to my own views, point to the fact that any life-changing event will lead to profound changes to how we understand ourselves, other people and think about the future. This happens all the time; when we meet a new partner, meet a hero, win a personal battle, etc. In this picture, a chemically induced 'trip' is a major life event, but it's the event (not the chemical) that makes the difference.

I find all that fascinating. But I was also perplexed by the fact that the organisers of the event I mentioned earlier billed it as; '...*a great discussion about whether psychedelics are a possible cure for depression...*'. Which is fine, except I find the concept of 'cure' difficult to accept. To be fair, another message said '...*we have all been affected by depression at some point in our lives. Are magic mushrooms the answer?*' And I find 'answer' a better metaphor for the possible role of psychoactive drugs, especially the psychedelics, than 'cure'.

Drugs are Drugs

It makes sense to see psychiatric medication in the same light as a vast number of chemicals that can affect our emotions, behaviour and thoughts. Sometimes that might be helpful, but often it isn't. But in my judgement, we would all be much better off if we were to reduce our reliance on medication to address emotional distress. Medication should be used sparingly and on the basis of what is needed in a particular situation, for example, to help someone to sleep or to manage the distress of hearing voices. We should not look to medication to 'cure' or even 'manage' non-existent underlying 'illnesses'.

In practical terms, we should aim for a massive reduction in the level of psychiatric prescription. There should be many fewer prescriptions, at lower doses, for much shorter periods. This is a 'drug-based' approach in contrast to the more common 'disease-based' approach. We would do better if we were to respond to people's specific symptoms, rather than make the mistake that we're treating illnesses that can be identified by diagnosis. We need to listen to the person's own experiences indicating which drugs have helped in the past and how they are finding those currently prescribed and use what they say to guide our prescribing. Perhaps most importantly, we should only use psychiatric medication in the very short-term (i.e. for a matter of days) in the vast majority of cases.

The Prevalence of Prescription

In 2012, there was a landmark debate in the UK House of Commons. Several MPs took the opportunity to speak movingly of their own psychological problems and to call for radical new approaches in our thinking. Charles Walker MP used the debate to discuss his own battles with persistent obsessive thoughts. Like many other people in his situation, he discussed the most common form of help offered to people; medication: '...*Let us look at these, more startling statistics. In 2009, the NHS issued 39.1 million prescriptions for anti-depressants – there was a big jump during the financial crisis, towards the end of the last decade. That figure represented a 95% increase on the decade, from the 20.2 million prescriptions issued in 1998. Were all of those 40 million prescriptions necessary? Of course they were not...*'.[1]

The statistics are frightening and getting worse. According to data released by our National Health Service,[2] the number of antidepressant prescriptions dispensed in England exceeded 70 million in 2018. It means that over 7 million people received one or more prescriptions. That's 16% of the adult population of England. The rates are twice as high in women as in men and track social disadvantage; a clear indication that this represents medication for social, not biological, issues. The UK trend is replicated across the developed world, with a doubling in the number of antidepressants over the past 10 years.[3] According to the US National Center for Health Statistics, in 2011, 11% of Americans aged 12 and over were taking antidepressants.

With fewer than 60 million people of working age in the UK, these are astonishing numbers (even if we accept that very many of these prescriptions are never given to pharmacists, much of the actual medication is never taken, and each prescription may be for only a couple of weeks' supply of medication). And it's also the wrong kind of help. Back in 2012, Charles Walker MP expressed this clearly: '...*We can talk about medical solutions to mental health problems, and of course medicine has a part to play. In reality, however, society has the biggest part to play. This is society's problem....*' I agree. His fellow Member of Parliament, James Morris MP, made a similar point: '*...we must also examine whether our approach to tackling the problem is fit and appropriate for the 21ˢᵗ century. Our approach to mental illness over a number of decades has been based on what I would call the psychiatric model. The model has medicalised mental illness and treated it as something to be dealt with using drug-based therapies...*'

Charles Walker and James Morris are correct. These are serious problems. But they are serious social problems that should be addressed with social solutions. This level of prescription also comes at an astonishing cost. It has been estimated[4] that we spend around £800 million per year in the UK on psychiatric drugs. The prescription of antidepressant medication alone costs the UK National Health Service over £200 million per year. We spend £44 million on stimulants and other drugs prescribed to children for the 'treatment' of 'ADHD' or 'Attention Deficit Hyperactivity Disorder'. I agree with Charles Walker that a very large proportion (at least) of this spending is probably wasted. Although some people find medication helpful, we need to balance the positive effects of taking medication, which are almost certainly short-lived in most instances, against their adverse effects.

A Pill to take away your Sadness

Although I have a good working knowledge of the evidence base for the effectiveness of pharmacological interventions, I rely on the expertise of my colleagues with more specialist skills, experience, knowledge and qualifications. This is an important point; I am not advocating that we can do away with the specialist knowledge of medical practitioners. I rely on this knowledge and both praise and prize those who possess it. One such expert is Dr. Joanna Moncrieff, to whom I turn for systematic and intelligent reviews of the literature. In her books *The Myth of the Chemical Cure* and *The Bitterest Pills*,[5] and online,[6] Moncrieff considers the extent to which psychiatric drugs are effective in helping people and discusses the related issue of whether they are 'treating illnesses' in any meaningful sense.

Antidepressants are prescribed very frequently, and so it seems likely that at least some people think they 'work'. And, at least in the UK and most other post-industrial democracies, we approve the use of medication through complicated processes that involve expert panels making recommendations on the basis of systematic reviews of published scientific evidence. These processes lead to clinical guidelines such as those issued by the National Institute for Health and Care Excellence or NICE. These guidelines, and therefore the systematic reviews on which they are based, conclude that antidepressants 'work'. In Joanna Moncrieff's words: *'the general feeling seems to be that although they are being overused and may have some unpleasant side-effects, they certainly "work", at least in some people'*. So, do they 'work'? Do 'antidepressants' change our moods? Do they raise our levels of motivation, reduce the frequency or impact of negative thoughts?

Perhaps it's first worth pointing out that a huge range of chemicals affects our perceptions, moods and thoughts. Although it has caused problems throughout recorded history (there have been religious prohibitions on intoxication for millennia), very few people manage to avoid ever ingesting psychoactive substances. In most cultures, all around the world, people drink alcohol, chew khat, smoke nicotine-delivering cigarettes, and drink coffee... all of which have well-recognised effects on brain chemistry (as well as, in the case of caffeine, on the digestive system). Laws and social rules differ across the world, but there are enormous markets for illegal drugs; cannabis, ecstasy, heroin, cocaine, LSD, etc. The presence of the rules themselves indicates both the market demands for the substances and their chemical power. I don't advocate taking such street or recreational drugs (although I'm not very keen on legal prohibition and the so-called war on drugs has probably done more harm than good). Many chemicals—foods, illegal and legal drugs—change our thoughts, perceptions and moods. All drugs—recreational street drugs, commonplace drugs such as alcohol and caffeine, and doctor-prescribed medication—follow the basic laws of biochemistry. Once again, there is no 'abnormal biochemistry', just biochemistry. The medication prescribed in response to mental distress is specifically chosen, and often engineered, to alter our mood. It is no surprise at all to find that 'antidepressants', 'antipsychotics' or other psychiatric drugs affect our mood or thinking. That's completely different from thinking that 'antidepressants' specifically target underlying biological abnormalities responsible for an illness.

The conventional way to test the effectiveness of medication and other therapies is to conduct 'randomised controlled trials' or RCTs. I've been involved in several. Clinical recommendations, such as NICE guidelines, are typically based on systematic reviews of many such RCTs. Systematic reviews of RCTs into the effectiveness of antidepressants[7] suggest that, on average, people taking antidepressants see their scores on a mood rating scale improve a little more than do people who are taking a placebo or nothing. The difference in improvement, the degree to which antidepressants outperform placebos, is enough to establish beyond statistical chance that the medication has some kind of effect. It's worth saying that this degree of change is typically about the same as that offered by psychological therapies such as cognitive behavioural therapy (CBT). Typically, both the people given the antidepressants (or CBT) and the people given the placebo see their low mood lift over time. There are many reasons for this, including the fact that people typically seek help when their mood is at its lowest, and therefore their mood is likely to improve over time.

The benefits of antidepressant medication are small (and some people believe they act only as complex 'active' placebos; the physical side effects of the medication convincing people that they must be doing some good), and it's important to understand what these benefits might mean in practice. All these caveats apply equally to trials of psychological therapies, but what counts as 'effective' in the language of such clinical trials may not be quite what we expect in the real world. First, it usually only means that the degree to which antidepressants outperform the placebo is 'statistically significant'. That is, the difference is unlikely to be due to chance. That doesn't mean it's necessarily a large difference; 'statistically significant' does not mean 'big'. Moreover, many scientists and academics are concerned[8] that pharmaceutical companies and researchers routinely fail to publish negative results, meaning that only the positive results see the light of day.

In nearly all such trials, outcome is assessed on the basis of scores on questionnaire measures of low mood. In many senses, that's reasonable. Problems such as low mood lie on continua; some of us feel desperately low, some of us are quite miserable, others are broadly happy. It is therefore better to measure the degree of our low mood than to ask whether we are or are not experiencing 'depression'. Randomised controlled trials are powerful ways of discovering differences between two groups, but while there might be an average difference between the groups, there is usually still a very great deal of overlap. In a typical clinical trial of an antidepressant reporting positive findings, it is possible for there to be a difference between two groups (for instance, those people taking antidepressants compared to those taking placebos) of only two points on a questionnaire with a maximum score of 54. And the questionnaires used to assess low mood typically evaluate quite a wide range of problems. People will be asked about their mood, their motivation, their ability to enjoy life, their sleeping, their appetite, and their self-esteem. Although any improvement in scores is good, improvements of two or three points on these scales could well reflect improved motivation, better sleep or better appetite rather than an improvement in mood itself. These are effects that could well be related to medication; it's relatively easy to see how medication could increase our motivation, our appetite or improve our sleep. All these chemical effects are well-known, but they don't necessarily represent a 'cure' for 'depression'.

Some time ago. I was involved in a small study that looked at the effects of different clothing on our emotions.[9] It was a pretty straightforward study; we asked people to put on outfits they liked and also ones they didn't and assessed their moods; using the same kinds of questionnaires used in measuring the outcome of trials of antidepressants. Unsurprisingly, the participants felt better—happier and more confident—wearing outfits that they preferred. Unsurprisingly, these differences weren't huge... but they were about the size of the differences usually reported for antidepressants in clinical trials. When we hear good news, our mood lifts a little. When we receive a compliment, our mood lifts a little. When we wear clothes we like, our mood lifts a little. When I have a cup of coffee, I feel my mood lift a little. And when we take antidepressants, on average, our mood appears to lift... a little.

Are Antidepressants Really 'Antidepressants', or Merely Drugs?

Moncrieff points out several problems with a 'disease model' of drug action; the assumption (on the basis of their name, perhaps) that psychiatric medication offers 'cures' for 'illnesses'. Hers is a point of view that I find very persuasive. I have no doubt that 'depression' exists as a phenomenon. But I don't believe it is right to suggest that depression therefore exists as an illness. There are very many understandable reasons why we can become demoralised, unhappy and pessimistic. We can, very obviously, become depressed. We have a clear moral imperative to offer help when we see that someone else is depressed. But that isn't the same thing as saying that there exists an 'illness' called 'depression' or 'clinical depression' ('clinical depression' is a term which, if it means anything, means either 'depression that we see in a clinic' or 'depression that is serious enough to warrant professional help', and we should just say that) which requires a 'treatment'.

Antidepressants are chemicals that affect the functioning of the brain. Older antidepressants tended to be rather sedating; in other words, they made people feel tired and slowed down. This was rather unpleasant, and often dangerous. Some can, still, make people drowsy or lethargic. But some more modern antidepressants have been chosen or designed to affect our moods, but to avoid these sedating effects. They can sometimes induce a sense of indifference, which for some people helpfully takes the edge off their feelings of despair, but which others find unpleasant or even distressing. They can have other effects such as sexual dysfunction or feelings of agitation.

These are, just as with recreational drugs, the chemical effects of the medication on the functioning of the brain. Some people may find the effects helpful. If someone is feeling lethargic, a drug that improves their alertness may be positive. Many people experience unpleasant intrusive thoughts and sometimes ruminate on their problems. In that case, a sense of emotional detachment, brought about by a psychiatric drug, may be helpful. People who are depressed, especially if they are also anxious, may find that a reduction in anxiety and a slight sedative effect is calming and helps sleep. All these recognisable and understandable effects of drugs, whether prescribed or recreational, may be negative or positive. These effects may well be seen on rating scales designed to assess the severity of a depressed mood. But it is difficult to argue that these medication-induced changes in emotional states represent 'cures' or even 'treatment'. They are real; but they are what they are; the understandable effects of psychoactive chemicals.

There is no evidence that these chemicals are correcting any underlying biological mechanism. There is a danger that we are being subtly misled about the effects of medication. Messages of various kinds—in the publicity of pharmaceutical companies, in the pronouncements of senior academics, in public information campaigns by Government—often give us the impression that the medication is putting right some underlying abnormality, whereas it would be much more honest to outline the general psychoactive and physical effects of the medication. Then we could weigh up any possible benefits against possible adverse effects and decide for ourselves whether or not these effects might be useful. There are many chemicals that affect our emotions, perceptions, thought and behaviour. We swallow or smoke these chemicals for understandable reasons, and the chemicals—the drugs—have a range of effects, both good and bad. That's a long way short of a 'treatment' for an 'illness'.

The possible positive effects of psychiatric medication unfortunately also come with a cost. Antidepressant drugs have unpleasant adverse effects. Some of the newer 'selective serotonin reuptake inhibitors' or SSRIs can lead to sexual dysfunction and loss of libido. There have been distressing reports of people having intrusive suicidal thoughts when taking antidepressant medication, and some researchers believe that antidepressants are associated with an increased risk of suicide, especially in young people. This may be related to the tendency for antidepressants to make people more motivated and impulsive, which might be beneficial in some ways but also somewhat risky in someone who is depressed. Many people also report having severe and prolonged withdrawal reactions (for further discussion of all these problems, see Jo Moncrieff's 'The Myth of the Chemical Cure'[10]).

Representatives of pharmaceutical companies, and some psychiatrists, repeatedly emphasise that antidepressants 'aren't addictive'. People are naturally worried about the addictive power of cigarettes, street drugs and some older forms of psychiatric medication such as benzodiazepines (Valium). It's reassuring for people contemplating taking prescribed antidepressants to be told that they 'aren't addictive'. It does seem odd, and a strange use of language, however. Addiction is surprisingly difficult to define, but best refers to a person's dependence on a substance (in this case medication) to be able to function relatively normally. It's quite common to hear representatives of pharmaceutical companies comment that 'antidepressants aren't addictive', but then qualify this by saying 'but people can experience a recurrence of their depressive symptoms (often misinterpreted as 'relapse') when they stop taking the drugs'. Which sounds very similar to needing the drugs to function normally. Indeed, that seems to be the main selling point of the medication!

My reading of the available research tells me that antidepressant medication might be slightly better than a placebo at raising people's mood. That's not in itself something to be rejected out of hand; depression is a phenomenon that ruins (and sometimes ends) lives. The positive effects aren't dramatic, and they don't appear to represent a 'cure'. Researchers haven't been able to identify any abnormalities in the biological pathways that are targeted by the antidepressants, and in that context, the discovery of some chemicals that alter brain chemistry to make people feel a little better is hardly ground-breaking science. And the positive effects certainly come with some rather unpleasant side effects.

If you believe the 'patient information sheet' for SSRI medication (the formal information provided by the manufacturers of Selective Serotonin Reuptake Inhibitors),[11] then you'll believe not only that '...*people who are depressed or have obsessive-compulsive disorder or bulimia nervosa have lower levels of serotonin than others...*'; a statement that is highly questionable if not downright untrue, but also that; '...*it is not fully understood how ... SSRIs work but they may help by increasing the level of serotonin in the brain...*'

Unfortunately, however, the brain is more complex than this. While SSRI drugs do indeed inhibit the reuptake of serotonin, the brain responds by rapidly 'down-regulating' serotonin production[12]; reducing the brain's synthesis of serotonin. That's a real problem (for the pharmaceutical industry), as it begins to suggest that, far from 'increasing levels of serotonin in the brain', SSRIs might actually reduce them. One of the consequences is that, if you then discontinue taking an SSRI, the levels of serotonin will be low (because production has been down-regulated) but the SSRI, having been stopped, is no longer inhibiting re-uptake, meaning that the little available serotonin is more readily reabsorbed. The consequence can be a rather nasty 'discontinuation syndrome'.[13]

Weirdly, or at least confusingly, drugs that enhance the reuptake of serotonin—SSREs, selective serotonin reuptake enhancers—are used as antidepressant drugs (and as treatment for other conditions). The conclusions seem to be; serotonin is associated with depression, but we don't know how or why. Drugs that inhibit the reuptake of serotonin are prescribed to help people who are depressed, but the best guess is not that they work (if they do indeed 'work') by increasing levels of serotonin in the brain. Drugs that enhance the reuptake of serotonin are also prescribed to help people who are depressed, which rather implies that, again if they are at all helpful, complex homeostatic processes involving the production, detection and reuptake of serotonin are affected in ways that we just don't understand. This is a long way from the confident (and lucrative) messages of the pharmaceutical companies. Perhaps, as Paul Andrews, an assistant professor of Psychology, Neuroscience & Behaviour at McMaster University, concluded, after examining homeostatic processes in serotonin metabolism[14]; '*It's time we rethink what we are doing. … We are taking people who are suffering from the most common forms of depression, and instead of helping them, it appears we are putting an obstacle in their path to recovery*'. Paul Andrews' conclusion is that most forms of depression, though painful, are natural and ultimately beneficial adaptations to stress.

Pills to Take Away Your Madness

The benefits of taking antidepressants seem underwhelming when weighed against their costs. A slightly different argument applies to long-term use of so-called antipsychotic medication. There are some benefits for people in acute distress, and with particular problems, from taking antipsychotic drugs. But taken longer term, these drugs have serious, life-changing and adverse effects. These include a condition that resembles Parkinson's disease—with shaking, muscular rigidity and problems with walking and movement—and even reduced brain size in people who have been taking 'antipsychotic' medication for a long time. Because they affect various physical systems, such as our heart, liver and kidneys, as well as our brains, and because one of the common adverse effects of antipsychotic medication is a significant gain in weight, these drugs can have a significant impact on our health.

Dr. Joanna Moncrieff reports on her blog the story of a woman who was very distressed by frightening psychotic experiences.[15] The woman was scared that she had an electronic gadget implanted in her body, and that she was being watched and manipulated by malignant forces. Psychotic experiences like this are surprisingly common and very distressing for those of us involved. Moncrieff reported how, as we might expect, the young woman began taking an antipsychotic drug. Moncrieff reports that as the dose was gradually increased the young woman; '...became increasingly quiet, subdued, emotionless, expressionless and physically sluggish'. Moncrieff contrasted the conventional medical consensus that the young woman was 'better' with her own perspective; that the young woman's life; '...seemed empty and lifeless...although admittedly less distressed'.

This sums up both my own experience of observing people taking antipsychotic drugs and the scientific evidence (although not the traditional medical consensus). These powerful drugs are effective at helping people calm down and can sometimes reduce distress, but can hardly be considered cures. They have very clear effects on people, and those effects can be helpful. But they don't target biological abnormalities specific to psychosis and don't return people to 'normal'. They just have the kinds of effects that psychoactive drugs are recognised to have.

I understand that antipsychotic drugs can be very helpful for many people. In acute emergencies, antipsychotic medication can be enormously helpful and even life-saving. Decisions about medication are, or certainly should be, individual issues. Blanket advice one way or another would be foolish. But it does appear that antipsychotic medication can be helpful in suppressing acute psychotic symptoms. And it's important to recognise that many people experience highly distressing psychotic phenomena for years, either on an ongoing or a recurrent basis. Again, that means that for some of us, as Jo Moncrieff puts it: '...life on long-term drug treatment, even with all its drawbacks, might be preferable to life without it'.

There is a great deal of debate about the changes that have taken place in inpatient psychiatric care over the past six decades, and particularly about the reasons for the dramatic reduction in the number of people resident in psychiatric hospitals. The most widely accepted opinion is that the development of chlorpromazine (an early antipsychotic) in the 1950s allowed, for the first time, many thousands of people to achieve some form of relief from their distress. It's clear that many people in the early decades of the twentieth century, and before, could spend many years of their lives in extreme distress. It would be stupid and cruel to deny people effective help. But a different line of argument suggests that the reduction in society's reliance on residential hospital care was the result of profound changes both in society and in nursing practices, not because of the medication.

We also need to be clear what the effects of these drugs are, and whether they are actually 'cures' or even 'antipsychotics'. That is, do they target an underlying biological abnormality, return a person to a state of normality and substantially ameliorate the problems? We might also add: do they prevent relapse? It seems clear, and seems to have been clear back in the 1950s, that antipsychotic drugs such as chlorpromazine numb people's emotions or make otherwise stressful events seem less stressful. They can reduce emotional distress (so can, I repeat, be a good thing), but might not quite be the same thing as reducing psychosis. People who are convinced that others mean them harm (with 'paranoid delusions', in psychiatric language), and who are very frightened that they are in imminent danger, will often find their fears much less preoccupying and distressing if they take chlorpromazine.[16] That sounds a lot like the effects of opioid street drugs like heroin. It might be helpful; it doesn't sound like a cure.

A study of the recent history of psychiatry also shows us how the ways in which medication has been used, and discussed, have changed over time. Initially, psychiatrists appeared to use drugs pragmatically to help reduce distress and agitation and acknowledged their direct effects (some psychiatrists quite overtly described them as damaging the brain). Over time, however, psychiatrists began to think about (or, at least, talk about) the drugs as 'treatments' for underlying conditions. The narrative around the drugs shifted from being described as practical short-term solutions to long-term or prophylactic (preventative) remedies. Currently, clinical guidelines recommend long-term treatment with antipsychotic medication for people who have been given the diagnosis of 'schizophrenia'.[17] Those recommendations parallel the growing (but relatively recent) assumption that the antipsychotic drugs are sophisticated treatments, specifically designed to correct a known underlying biological abnormality that causes their problems.

'Antipsychotic' medication may be helpful for some people, especially in the short-term and if they are very distressed. It seems much less clear that antipsychotic medication prevents relapse. This, again, needs to be considered very carefully. Some of us have long-term problems, and may therefore find that medication (or, indeed, anything else) which helps to lessen our distress is something we wish to continue to use. But that isn't quite the basis on which antipsychotic medication is often recommended, namely that it prevents a 'relapse'; a return of the psychotic experiences. That seems a much more debatable assertion.

The use of antipsychotic medication on a long-term basis (daily or even injected as a 'depot') is so ubiquitous that it is difficult to find comparisons between groups of people who experience similar problem but who have, and have not, taken the drugs for long periods of time. These comparisons are also difficult because the medications are very powerful, so powerful, in fact, that when people stop taking their drugs (especially without expert medical advice), they often experience profound and distressing withdrawal effects, which can either resemble or induce the return of their previous psychotic experiences. However, the emerging evidence, summarised in books by Richard Bentall, Robert Whitaker and Jo Moncrieff,[18] strongly suggests that, for most of us, the long-term benefits of antipsychotic medication are significantly outweighed by their profound adverse effects. And it looks very much as if the levels of psychosis, and 'relapse' rates, are no higher in people who have previously had psychotic experiences, but who live medication-free lives than in people who take antipsychotic medication on a long-term basis. In other words, these drugs don't appear to prevent relapse. And, because these drugs have very profound side effects, those people who take the medication on a long-term basis often experience significant physical health problems (including, significantly, weight gain), as well as emotional blunting, sedation and suppression of creativity and imagination. Many wise and intelligent psychiatrists therefore conclude, as Joanna Moncrieff has done, that; '...*these are not innocuous drugs, and people should be given the opportunity to see if they can manage without them, both during an acute psychotic episode and after recovery from one'* and that; '*…if you reduce people's antipsychotics in a gradual and supported manner, people are better off in the long-term. Some will manage to stop their antipsychotics completely and do well, and overall people will not suffer higher levels of symptoms or relapses than if they had stayed on their original level of medication'.*

It is worth pointing out that many of these concerns also apply to medication used to 'treat' so-called bipolar disorder. People experience episodes of depression, and some people experience episodes of mania (feeling very agitated or 'high', sometimes leading to actions you later regret such as running up large bills) or hypomania (the same but with a lesser intensity and duration). Let's leave aside for a moment the issue of whether this diagnosis is valid or helpful, except to say that it adds nothing to label a history of manic or hypomanic episodes 'bipolar disorder'.[19] Manic episodes can be distressing and dangerous, and people who experience a manic episode once are highly likely to experience another one. We should respond with all we can reasonably do to help. Antipsychotic medication can be helpful as an immediate or emergency response, but there is much less evidence for the effectiveness of the two medications that are most commonly used to prevent 'relapse'. Because recurrent episodes of mania and depression can be disabling, there is real pressure to prescribe drugs that can be effective not only in an acute episode, but as prophylaxis, that is, to reduce the likelihood of future episodes. Lithium (a so-called mood stabiliser) is the most commonly used medication, but long-term antipsychotics are also commonly prescribed. Here, too, there are major doubts as to their effectiveness.[20] As with other mental health problems, there is precious little evidence that the medication is targeting any recognised underlying biological abnormalities or pathologies.

So Why Do We Take Them?

An editorial in the *British Medical Journal* in 2013[21] discussed the worrying proliferation of psychiatric prescription in stark terms; '*don't keep taking the tablets'.* But the situation is getting worse. Why are these prescriptions so common?

One partial explanation may be a massive level of over-diagnosis. Criteria for most mental health diagnoses are loose and vague and include a range of common and normal experiences. Worse, even these loose criteria are misused in practice; it has been suggested that only 38% of people whom clinicians diagnose with 'depression' would actually meet standard diagnostic criteria.[22] I have some problems with this analysis; I don't regard depression as a valid illness, and it is simply wrong to use such disease metaphors for normal human responses to difficult circumstances. Nevertheless, it is clear that very many people are receiving these damaging labels, and, therefore, receiving prescriptions for what are regarded (advertised, perhaps) as treatments for these non-existent illnesses.

The international pharmaceutical companies are directly guilty, too. Massive and well-funded marketing efforts are employed to sell drugs to prescribing physicians or (where the nation's legislation foolishly permits it to happen) direct to the consumer. In his excellent book *Cracked: Why Psychiatry Is Doing More Harm Than Good*,[23] James Davies describes the effort that pharmaceutical companies expend and the lengths to which they go in order to convince people to buy their products. These range from excessive promotion of positive findings through to the frankly immoral and deliberate hiding of negative ones. This is important; if industry-sponsored drug trials with negative findings (in other words, where the drugs are not shown to be successful) are not published, the only journal articles that are available for review are the positive ones. The drugs therefore appear much more effective than they really are. Researchers are also implicated. Some appear to be very well rewarded for promoting drugs companies' products. Between 2000 and 2007, the psychiatrist Professor Charles Nemeroff received $2.8 million (personally) from drugs companies while supposedly acting as an impartial scientist overseeing trials of the drugs manufactured by the companies paying him. Similarly, Dr. Joseph Biederman was dubbed the 'King of Ritalin' after receiving $1.6 million in consultancy fees from pharmaceutical companies.

But the most important marketing technique is simply to argue that our distress represents symptoms of an 'illness'. Because while understandable distress that follows the loss of a loved one triggers empathy, a listening ear and practical help, the diagnosis of a 'major depressive episode' is likely to lead to a prescription for antidepressant medication. And that represents profit.

The mouthwash, Listerine, was originally developed as a surgical antiseptic. Its main active ingredients are essential oils and alcohol. After serving as a surgical antiseptic, Listerine was subsequently sold as a floor-cleaning product and (slightly bizarrely) as a cure for gonorrhoea. The product only became highly profitable, however, in the 1920s, when it was marketed as a cure for 'halitosis'. We all know that people can occasionally have bad breath. And it makes commercial sense to offer products that can render us marginally less repellent. The genius of the Listerine marketing strategy was to develop the quasi-medical concept of halitosis; a problem for which Listerine was the solution. This was done quite deliberately; Listerine was not marketed as a product that could sweeten your breath (such products already existed, and Listerine wouldn't have had a market advantage), but as a specific cure for halitosis.

Similarly, we occasionally experience low mood; often in response to negative life events. But 'depression' is an illness that (so the logic goes) requires the prescription of antidepressant medication. People occasionally have very distressing psychotic experiences; often in response to childhood trauma. But 'schizophrenia' is an illness that (so the argument goes) requires the prescription of antipsychotic medication. Manic episodes are a major threat to our wellbeing, and it would be very sensible both to consider what medication might be helpful when they occur, and also to learn how to identify the early warning signs of episodes and help to avoid them. But 'bipolar disorder' is an illness that (so the argument goes) requires the prescription of prophylactic medication. Children occasionally have problems paying attention in class. But 'Attention Deficit Hyperactivity Disorder' or 'ADHD' is an illness (so the logic goes) that requires the prescription of stimulants such as Ritalin.

A good example of this phenomenon (a tactic that I do not approve of, of course) is the history of Wellbutrin, a brand name for the drug bupropion. Bupropion appears to affect the central nervous system by interacting with dopamine receptors. It is considered moderately dangerous in overdose, when it leads to hallucinations, delusions, vomiting, aggressive behaviour and seizures, and has been associated with deaths. The side effects are, genuinely, too numerous to list here. On the (perhaps) more positive front, bupropion has been recommended as an appropriate treatment for (there's a list): smoking cessation, 'seasonal affective disorder', 'attention deficit hyperactivity disorder' or 'ADHD', sexual dysfunction, obesity (or more properly, appetite suppression) and inflammatory bowel disease. It is quite widely used as an antidepressant. So far, Wellbutrin or bupropion looks much like any other psychiatric drug; it affects our central nervous systems, but can't in all honesty be said to be a specific treatment for a specific illness by targeting a specific biological pathology. In this context, Wellbutrin is particularly interesting because it looks very much like a product in need of an illness for which it can be classed as the treatment. And the recent decision to remove bereavement as an exclusion criterion for the diagnosis of depression may offer that opportunity. That is, there have been hints that some psychiatrists are attempting to demonstrate that Wellbutrin is an effective treatment for depression associated with bereavement.[24] This is extraordinary… find a drug that struggles to find a market, re-label a normal human response to a sad but commonplace event as a symptom of an 'illness', and then prescribe the product as a treatment for that 'illness'.

Drugs Are Drugs

Dr. Joanna Moncrieff has argued: '*Using psychoactive substances to cope with negative emotions is a longstanding human response, but also one that is fraught with difficulty. Although drug-induced effects may bring temporary relief, they may also hamper people from finding more lasting solutions to their problems. If people do want to go down this route, however, there seems no reason to restrict the repertoire to drugs currently called "antidepressants". This raises all sorts of thorny questions, of course, about why some psychoactive drugs are legal and others illegal, about what sort of drug use society approves of and what it doesn't, and why the legal dispensation of many drugs is restricted to doctors*'.[25] There are many different chemicals that we ingest to alter their mood, perceptions or thought processes. There is also institutionalised hypocrisy. At one extreme, we have strict laws controlling the possession, sale and use of recreational street drugs, even a 'war' on drugs. At the other extreme, clinicians can use the Mental Health Act (or similar laws in other jurisdictions) to compel patients to adhere to treatment plans; which almost invariably mean prescriptions for medication. The law, and public attitudes, surrounding the use of chemicals to change your perceptions and mood seem to indicate that it is simultaneously both illegal and compulsory.

Different drugs work differently. Psychiatric medication and street drugs can stimulate the production or release of neurotransmitters, can block the reuptake of those neurotransmitters or can bond directly to the receptors for specific neurotransmitters. The drugs can be specific (focussing on one neurotransmitter) or much more broad spectrum in their effects. The time they take to work and then wear off can differ. They may also differ in the ways in which they stimulate the brain to respond; by producing more or less of the neurotransmitters, altering the sensitivity of neurotransmitter receptors, affecting the number of synapses (connections between nerve cells) or stimulating the growth of new dendritic connections.

The drugs—street recreational drugs or prescribed drugs—are all different. That could, at a stretch, justify an argument that some chemical formulations may be less harmful, and more closely tailored to the chemical effects that are desired than others. It could certainly mean that some drugs are more addictive than others; crack cocaine is notoriously addictive, partly because of the speed of action. Some psychoactive chemicals encourage further use because they have euphoric or other pleasurable effects, some because they reduce unpleasant emotions, and others simply because stopping taking them have negative consequences; withdrawal effects. It means that we should choose our drugs with care. But a drug is merely a chemical that affects the functioning of the brain, for good or ill. Both Ritalin, prescribed for children who have difficulty maintaining their attention in school, and ketamine, a veterinary tranquiliser, are stimulant drugs related to amphetamine. When people take amphetamine (an illegal recreational drug) they find it easier to concentrate, stay awake and work.

That is true for all of us, not just children who have received the label of 'ADHD'. I'm not advocating the use of recreational amphetamines; but then again, I'm not advocating the prescription of stimulants to children with the diagnosis of 'ADHD'. Ketamine is a 'prescription only drug' in the UK, which means it is illegal to possess ketamine without a prescription. Ketamine is also illegal in many other countries. At the same time, ketamine is widely used as an antidepressant. It is claimed that ketamine can have an antidepressant effect within two hours... presumably the reason for its popularity as a recreational drug.

All such drugs, legal and illegal, have powerful effects on our brains. It is difficult to make coherent distinctions between 'recreational' and 'prescription' drugs. We should all, always, exercise great care and caution over the choice whether or not to ingest such powerful chemicals. I can see some arguments in favour of the use of chemicals such as MDMA or psilocybin as adjuncts to therapy; I see that as a potentially worthwhile development that builds on millennia of the human use of mind-altering drugs in spiritual or symbolic rites of passage. Many of us use mood-altering drugs, most commonly caffeine and alcohol, on a regular basis. We need to understand the differences between the different drugs. We should probably take expert medical advice, from professionals who know their subject well. But we shouldn't buy into the marketing myth that some chemicals are 'cures' for well-defined 'illnesses'.

Side Effects, Withdrawal and Addiction

All psychoactive drugs have side effects. It would be almost impossible to imagine how a drug aimed at altering the functioning of our neurotransmitters wouldn't have a pattern of adverse consequences. If we were ever to find clear biological pathologies underlying any of the kinds of problems that fall under the broad rubric of 'mental health', then we might be able to find a direct and 'clean' biological treatment. But we are a long way away from that position. First, such 'clean' treatments don't exist in conventional physical medicine either. It's not uncommon for experiences such as depression to be compared to diabetes.

Type I diabetes results from a basic inability to produce sufficient insulin, which controls blood glucose. It is usually treated with insulin injections.... which have side effects, including swelling of the arms and legs, more general weight gain, low blood sugar (hypoglycaemia) or skin reactions at the site of the injection. Even targeted medical treatments have side effects, and psychiatric treatments are far from targeted.

This book is not a pharmaceutical handbook, but it is worth pointing out quite how serious the side effects of psychiatric medication can be, presumably because of the fundamental role of the neurotransmitters that are the chemical targets of the medication. So, for instance, selective serotonin reuptake inhibitors (antidepressant medication) are associated with: feeling agitated, shaky or anxious, feeling and being sick, indigestion and stomach aches, diarrhoea or constipation, loss of appetite, dizziness, not sleeping well (insomnia), or feeling very sleepy, headaches, low sex drive, difficulties achieving orgasm during sex or masturbation, in men, difficulties obtaining or maintaining an erection (erectile dysfunction). More old-fashioned, 'tricyclic' antidepressants are associated with: dry mouth, slight blurring of vision, constipation, problems passing urine, drowsiness, dizziness, weight gain, excessive sweating (especially at night), and heart palpitations or a fast heartbeat (tachycardia). In the UK, the NHS warns that people can develop type II diabetes, perhaps directly or via the weight gain that some people using antidepressants experience. The NHS also warns of that a very few people experience '*suicidal thoughts ... when they first take antidepressants*'. Young people under 25 seem particularly at risk. Antipsychotic medication is similarly prone to nasty side effects. Again, the UK's NHS website lists: shaking, trembling, muscle twitches, muscle spasms, drowsiness, weight gain, blurred vision, constipation, lack of sex drive and dry mouth.

One problematic feature of psychiatric medication is that people experience distressing consequences when they stop taking the medication. To use just one example, if we take an SSRI (a selective serotonin re-uptake inhibitor) then the biological sequence is something like this. First, the re-uptake of serotonin is inhibited, leaving more serotonin available (and which may have a positive impact on mood). But, then, the body's restorative mechanisms mean that we tend to 'down-regulate' one of the main serotonin receptors (these receptors become less reactive to serotonin, perhaps because there's more serotonin available). But… then again, there is some evidence that, when these receptors are down-regulated, the serotoninergic neurons actually become more active and release more serotonin at their targets!

These chain reactions are incredibly complex and mean that it is difficult to say, with certainty, how antidepressant medication might work. But they also mean that antidepressant medication has been known to induce withdrawal reactions in a large proportion of users for a long time. That's because, when we stop taking the drugs, this complex set of neurochemical interactions is reversed. For some people, such reactions may be mild, not last very long, and can relatively easily be managed. For other people, even if they withdraw from the medication very slowly, these reactions are severe, long-lasting and can make normal functioning impossible. Typical withdrawal reactions include increased anxiety, flu-like symptoms, insomnia, nausea, imbalance, sensory disturbances, and hyperarousal, dizziness, electric shock-like sensations called 'brain zaps', diarrhoea, headaches, muscle spasms and tremors, agitation, hallucinations, confusion, malaise, sweating and irritability.[26]

Pill Shaming

The legitimate concerns of many people working in mental health lead them to warn about both the side effects of medication and the adverse consequences of withdrawal. These expressions of concern occasionally lead to a defensive response; both by professionals, and by people who feel strongly that their lives have been positively transformed by medication.

On the 12th November 2018, the BBC posted online a short video on 'pill shaming'.[27] It had been prepared with the help of the Royal College of Psychiatrists and featured a young woman talking about how her family, friends and some strangers had her feel ashamed and implied that she had been made to feel ashamed of taking antidepressant medication. The young woman commented on how friends and acquaintances had told her that she should 'try harder to make herself better', others said she was '*weak for taking the pills*' or asked '*why not just eat better?*' or other supposedly helpful but actually rather trivialising and insulting comments. As my friend and colleague, James Davies[28] commented, this was the first time that we saw a clear definition of a term that has been used quite widely on social media; '*pill shaming*'. At least in the BBC film, this was defined as the act of disparaging or shaming people for either taking or wanting to take antidepressants (e.g. calling them weak, asking them to try harder, etc.).

What was interesting about the BBC film was that it went further. While the explicit definition of pill shaming: the act of making others '*feel guilty for taking medication for their mental health*' was used, the definition, or rather the issues covered by the term, seemed to slip. I agree with James Davies; 'pill shaming', when defined as 'the act of making others feel guilty for taking medication for their mental health' is both wrong and indeed does happen. But, as James says, this unpleasant behaviour is not just restricted to taking pills. Discriminatory attitudes concerning mental health sadly pervade our society. People are bullied for all sorts of reasons. As I was writing this chapter, there was a newspaper article about the proposal to offer mindfulness interventions for schoolchildren. '*SNOWFLAKE KIDS GET LESSONS IN CHILLING*' shouted the headline (with the uppercase letters in the original).[29] People are 'shamed' not only for taking 'pills', but for expressing any form of understandable human emotion and for seeking (or being offered) any kind of help. And, as Davies said '*In short, whenever someone is shamed for simply trying to help themselves (especially if they believe the intervention works) we should call that behaviour out*'.

If anyone is being shamed for finding antidepressant medication helpful, then that is reprehensible. But there is also a risk that such claims of 'pill-shaming' are being used to derail discussions about the pros and cons of psychiatric drugs and to misrepresent, dismiss or discourage legitimate criticism of medication. It seems that, often, the word has been used in several rather questionable ways; either to claim the moral high-ground, to shift or derail the conversation, or as a kind of ad hominem attack; an attempt to associate important criticism with subtle or not so subtle abuse. Those who claim 'pill shaming' often seem to be explicitly mislabelling legitimate critique (which is usually a cool, scientific, weighing of the benefits against harms) as discriminatory, or more subtly implying that any legitimate evidence-based criticism of the drugs inevitably fuels or leads to pill shaming by others.

Psychiatric medication has potential benefits as well as clear harms. Antidepressants may bring some minor benefit, for some people, on average, over a short period.[30] Quite understandably, however, given that the drugs are designed to have a long-term effect and seem to lead to a consequential sequence of changes in neurotransmitter receptor biology that can take a considerable time to reverse, antidepressant drugs are imperfect at best, and have a well-evidenced pattern of nasty withdrawal effects. That discussion should mirror similar discussions of the benefits and harms of other medication, such as statins.[31] It should be respectful and follow the evidence. Probably because mental health naturally touches on issues such as motivation, optimism, and—quintessentially—our thoughts about ourselves, other people the future and the world, our discussions can sometimes inappropriately descend into moralistic judgements. We'd be much better off if we were to stick to the facts.

Stop Pushing the Drugs…and Offer Real Alternatives

We would all be better off if we were much more cautious and more sparing in our use of psychiatric drugs. In practical terms, we should aim for a significant reduction in the level of psychiatric prescription. We may all be healthier if there were many fewer prescriptions, at lower doses, for much shorter periods. We need to respond to people's symptoms, rather than make the mistake that we're treating illnesses that can be identified by diagnosis. We could listen to the people's own experiences of how medication has and hasn't worked for them, or how it's working for them now, and use that as the basis of our prescribing. Perhaps most importantly, in the vast majority of cases we should use psychiatric medication in the very short-term only.

This more pragmatic approach should also see any use of psychiatric medication as part of a 'psychobiosocial model', where we at least attempt to understand why a person is distressed and how medication could act as a short-term adjunct to other forms of psychosocial care.

This echoes Moncrieff's 'drug-centred, not disease-centred' model; moving away from the myth that ingesting these chemicals in some sense 'cures' 'illnesses'. That would result, in practice, in a substantial reduction in the use of medication. We would see fewer prescriptions, for lower doses of medication, taken over shorter periods. If I were forced to make some practical recommendations, I'd suggest that we should aim immediately to reverse the doubling of prescriptions that has happened over the past decade; that is, halve the number of new psychiatric prescriptions as soon as is practical. If we were able to reduce the number of prescriptions to no more than 10% of their current levels, we would save the UK around £720 million per year in the costs of the drugs. It would also save many thousands, even, millions, of us from the harm these drugs do to our bodies.

That would mean, even require, profound changes to the role of psychiatrists. At present, most psychiatrists spend a great deal of their time 'diagnosing' 'mental disorders' and prescribing medication. The vision for the future that I'm presenting here includes an important role for medical expertise, but it equally suggests that medical colleagues need to adopt a different and more integrated role. If we were to accept a 'psychobiosocial' model for mental health care and agree that medical advice concerning the use of psychiatric medication should be based on a pragmatic or 'drug-based' model, then it follows that community psychological health teams would have a different relationship with medication and with the medical practitioners who have expertise in its use.

Accepting a 'drug-based' approach to the prescription of psychiatric medication would not only see a substantial reduction in prescription, a focus on symptomatic relief rather than 'cure', and short-term rather than prophylactic prescription, but it would also see a shift of responsibility from secondary care psychiatrists based on so-called secondary care mental health units to medical practitioners (usually GPs or family doctors) working in community teams. If psychiatric drugs were in fact highly specialist treatments that target discrete, diagnosable, illnesses, then it would be appropriate to assume that most people who use mental health services would require referral to secondary care, hospital-based, clinics. But if we regard psychiatric medication as a potentially useful, although sometimes problematic, part of the care plan for those of us struggling to cope with the stresses and pressures of normal life, it would make more sense for the drugs to be managed by GPs within primary care as part of an overall 'psychobiosocial' care plan.

Psychiatric medication, the professional involvement of psychiatrists (and, to be clear, all other forms of mental health care, including the work of clinical psychologists) should be coordinated through community-based psychological health and wellbeing teams. These teams should not only adopt a psychosocial ethos, but be managed as part of local authority social services. Most of the medical aspects of this care in relation to both mental and physical health would best be delivered by GPs and nurses attached to those community teams, rather than via the medical services of hospitals and (in the UK) NHS Trusts.

A model whereby GPs provide support to community-based psychological health and wellbeing teams would mean additional responsibilities. But if there were to be a very marked reduction in the use of medication and commensurate rationalisation of the numbers of hospital-based psychiatrists, such pressures would easily be managed. Indeed, increased investment in primary care should be broadly welcomed.

There are several visionary (and very successful) services that have already adopted these kinds of approaches. Describing a model service for people with very complex problems which occasionally attract the label of 'personality disorder', Marsha Linehan introduced the idea of 'pharmacotherapists'. Her service uses medical colleagues as occasional consultants to be drawn on when decisions need to be made about one small part of a wider care plan, specifically the use of medication.[32] We can see this, too, in how London's Drayton Park Crisis House[33] uses its allied GP service for pragmatic prescriptions. And these are not trivial examples; the women who use the Drayton Park Crisis House are going through serious psychological health crises which would warrant hospital admission were the crisis house not available. In the UK, Tony Morrison (Professor of Clinical Psychology at the University of Manchester) and colleagues have recently shown that psychological therapies can be helpful for people with distressing psychotic experiences without the need to use any antipsychotic medication at all.[34] The Soteria Project, initiated in San Jose, California, USA by the psychiatrist Loren Mosher, is a community-based alternative to traditional psychiatry services based on the Soteria model and philosophy (in Sweden, Finland, Germany, Switzerland and Hungary as well as the USA[35]) employ primarily non-medical staff and emphasise the autonomy and human rights of residents and rely on very minimal use of antipsychotic medication. In Norway, new legislation has recently required all mental health units to allocate some provision specifically for people who do not wish to take medication, but who nevertheless require residential care.[36] Work is also underway in the UK to help people who have experienced manic or hypomanic episodes identify the early warning signs of a return of a manic episode and make plans accordingly.[37] Often, those plans involve medication (short-term medication can be effective in the early stages of a manic episode), but this is a very different prospect to the long-term, prophylactic, prescription of traditional psychiatry.

Notes

1. Hansard, the record of the UK Parliament, is available online. This particular debate is at: http://www.publications.parliament.uk/pa/cm201213/cmhansrd/cm120614/debtext/120614-0003.htm.
2. https://www.bbc.co.uk/news/health-47740396.
3. Michael McCarthy, "Antidepressant use has doubled in rich nations in past 10 years," *British Medical Journal* (2013): f7261. https://doi.org/10.1136/bmj.f7261.
4. Stephen Ilyas and Joanna Moncrieff, "Trends in prescriptions and costs of drugs for mental disorders in England, 1998–2010," *The British Journal of Psychiatry* 200, no. 5 (2012): 393–398. http://bjp.rcpsych.org/content/200/5/393.long.
5. Joanna Moncrieff, *The myth of the chemical cure* (London: Palgrave Macmillan, 2008); and Joanna Moncrieff, *The bitterest pills: The troubling story of antipsychotic drugs* (London: Palgrave Macmillan, 2013).

6. http://joannamoncrieff.com/2013/11/27/why-theres-no-such-thing-as-an-antidepressant/.

7. Joanna Moncrieff and Irving Kirsch, "Efficacy of antidepressants in adults," *British Medical Journal* 331, no. 7509 (2005): 155–157. https://doi.org/10.1136/bmj.331.7509.155.

8. http://www.badscience.net.

9. Wendy Moody, Peter Kinderman, and Pammi Sinha, "An exploratory study: Relationships between trying on clothing, mood, emotion, personality and clothing preference," *Journal of Fashion Marketing and Management: An International Journal* 14, no. 1 (2010): 161–179. http://www.emeraldinsight.com/journals.htm?articleid=1840473.

10. Joanna Moncrieff, *The myth of the chemical cure* (London: Palgrave Macmillan, 2008).

11. Many (perhaps all) of the patient information leaflets can be found online. The leaflet for Prozac can be found here: https://www.medicines.org.uk/emc/files/pil.3768.pdf.

12. See, for example: https://www.sciencedaily.com/releases/2015/02/150217114119.htm.

13. James Davies and John Read, "A systematic review into the incidence, severity and duration of antidepressant withdrawal effects: Are guidelines evidence-based?" *Addictive Behaviors* (2018). https://www.sciencedirect.com/science/article/abs/pii/S0306460318308347?via%3Dihub.

14. https://www.sciencedaily.com/releases/2015/02/150217114119.htm.

15. http://joannamoncrieff.com/2013/12/09/long-term-antipsychotics-making-sense-of-the-evidence/.

16. Pierre Deniker, "Experimental neurological syndromes and the new drug therapies in psychiatry," *Comprehensive Psychiatry* 1, no. 2 (1960): 92–102.

17. National Clinical Guideline Number 178. Psychosis and Schizophrenia in Adults: Treatment and Management. issued: February 2014, last modified: March 2014. London: National Institute for Health & Care Excellence. https://www.nice.org.uk/guidance/cg178.

18. See: Richard P. Bentall, *Doctoring the mind: Why psychiatric treatments fail* (London: Allen Lane. 2009); Robert Whitaker, *Anatomy of an epidemic: Magic bullets, psychiatric drugs, and the astonishing rise of mental illness in America* (New York: Random House, 2010); and Joanna Moncrieff, *The bitterest pills: The troubling story of antipsychotic drugs* (London: Palgrave Macmillan, 2013).

19. Steven H. Jones, Fiona Lobban, Anne Cooke et al., *Understanding bipolar disorder: Why some people experience extreme mood states and what can help* (Leicester: British Psychological Society, 2010). https://www1.bps.org.uk/system/files/Public%20files/cat-653.pdf.

20. http://joannamoncrieff.com/2013/12/09/long-term-antipsychotics-making-sense-of-the-evidence/.

21. British Medical Journal, "Don't keep taking the tablets," *British Medical Journal* 347 (2013). https://www.bmj.com/content/347/bmj.f7438.

22. Christopher Dowrick and Allen Frances, "Medicalising unhappiness: New classification of depression risks more patients being put on drug treatment from which they will not benefit," *British Medical Journal* 347 (2013): f7140. https://doi.org/10.1136/bmj.f7140.

23. See previous footnotes: James Davies, *Cracked: Why psychiatry is doing more harm than good* (London: Icon Press, 2013).

24. Sidney Zisook, Stephen R. Shuchter, Paola Pedrelli, Jeremy Sable, and Simona C. Deaciuc, "Bupropion sustained release for bereavement: Results of an open trial," *The Journal of Clinical Psychiatry* 62, no. 4 (2001): 227–230. http://www.ncbi.nlm.nih.gov/pubmed/11379835.

25. https://joannamoncrieff.com/tag/placebo-effect/.

26. See note 13.

27. https://www.bbc.com/news/av/health-46212595/medication-for-mental-health-call-to-end-pill-shaming.

28. http://cepuk.org/2018/11/20/dr-james-davies-lets-clear-pill-shaming/.

29. https://www.dailystar.co.uk/our-paper/2018-12-07.

30. Andrea Cipriani, Toshi A. Furukawa, Georgia Salanti, Anna Chaimani, Lauren Z. Atkinson, Yusuke Ogawa, Stefan Leucht, et al., "Comparative efficacy and acceptability of 21 antidepressant drugs for the acute treatment of adults with major depressive disorder: A systematic review and network meta-analysis," *Focus* 16, no. 4 (2018): 420–429. https://www.sciencedirect.com/science/article/pii/S0140673617328027.

31. Fiona Godlee, "Adverse effects of statins," *The Lancet* (2014): g3306. https://www.bmj.com/content/348/bmj.g3306/rr/702257.

32. Marcia M. Linehan, *Combining pharmacotherapy with psychotherapy for substance abusers with borderline personality disorder: Strategies for enhancing compliance. NIDA research monograph series: Integrating behavioral therapies with medications in the treatment of drug dependence* (Rockville, MD: National Institute of Health, 1995), 129–142.

33. https://www.candi.nhs.uk/services/drayton-park-womens-crisis-house-and-resource-centre.

34. Anthony P. Morrison, Douglas Turkington, Melissa Pyle, Helen Spencer, Alison Brabban, Graham Dunn, Tom Christodoulides, et al., "Cognitive therapy for people with schizophrenia spectrum disorders not taking antipsychotic drugs: A single-blind randomised controlled trial," *The Lancet* 383, no. 9926 (2014): 1395–1403. https://doi.org/10.1016/s0140-6736(13)62246-1.

35. See: http://www.soterianetwork.org.uk.

36. https://www.madinamerica.com/2017/03/the-door-to-a-revolution-in-psychiatry-cracks-open/.

37. See, for example, the work at the Spectrum Centre at the University of Lancaster in the UK: www.lancaster.ac.uk/shm/research/spectrum/.

10

Residential Care: Hotels not Hospitals

When we are in crisis, we may need residential care, but this does not need to be seen as a medical issue. Hospitals could therefore be replaced with residential units designed and managed from a psychosocial perspective. The best model for such a design may well be a 4* hotel rather than a clinic or hospital ward. The staff on such units may well include medical, psychiatric, experts as important and valued colleagues, but medical professionals could more effectively act as consultants to the team, rather than being seen as having sapiential authority over the team.

In 2014, my book *A Prescription for Psychiatry*[1] included a brief account of a woman who had been admitted to an inpatient psychiatric ward under a section of the Mental Health Act as a consequence of her self-harm. I reported, five years ago, how this young woman was under constant observation. Nurses were under instruction to accompany her everywhere, whether receiving medical care for her wounds (when, incidentally, the nurse told her that she was '*just there to observe, not to talk to you*') or, on one occasion, on a visit to her friend's house. On returning from the visit, personal pictures were removed from the young woman's room. The rationale was that she was being punished for 'bad behaviour' with by their removal and her 'good behaviour' would be rewarded with

P. Kinderman, *A Manifesto for Mental Health*,
https://doi.org/10.1007/978-3-030-24386-9_10

their return. This is callous and illogical. The young woman was detained in a psychiatric hospital—considered 'ill', considered insane and believed unable to control her own behaviour. And yet, hypocritically, she was also apparently believed to be merely wilful and able to bring her behaviour back under control (and within acceptable bounds) by sheer force of will, reinforced and shaped by the application of contingencies of reward and punishment. Or, perhaps more likely, this was merely a return to the kinds of punitive treatment felt necessary in earlier time to subdue the animal-like and regressed insane patients. The details of this young woman's treatment would bear out a rather more unpleasant interpretation. As well as the incident with the pictures, this pattern of punishment was repeated—punishment for behaviour that was simultaneously regarded as 'symptoms of an illness'—with the removal of her laptop computer or (apparently malevolently) moving her bed away from the wall of her bedroom (where she felt safe) into the centre of the room.

Five years after the publication of *A Prescription for Psychiatry*, the young woman is still detained in hospital. A second-opinion report (written by an eminent professor of psychiatry and recommending substantial changes in the care offered) has been ignored, and she remains both detained and closely observed. Most recently, she has been told that it would be impossible for her brother and father to visit her and equally inappropriate for her to meet them away from the hospital… because she would only be able to leave the ward if escorted by a nurse, and staffing levels mean that nobody would be available. Most tellingly—most irritatingly and frighteningly—the clinicians in charge of her care appear not only to be able to predict that she would be unsafe to leave the ward without escort and that the staffing levels would be inadequate… five months before the planned meeting. It's very difficult to see this only as an issue of clinical care, and it's also a human rights issue.

Care or Coercion?

Human rights challenges are particularly clear when we examine the use of coercion and the use of the Mental Health Act. Mental health care is unusual within healthcare specialities in the use of coercion. Whereas decisions in routine medical care are predicated on the basis of 'informed consent', this principle is far from universal in mental health care. A common argument is that coercion is necessary because people 'lack insight', but my experience is that the real reason is different. While people are undoubtedly suffering and in need of help, the 'care' and 'treatment' on offer are often not what people want or need. Often, what is offered is so unpleasant or feared that we need to coerce people into accepting it. In the UK, in the year from 2015 to 2016 (the latest period for which statistics are available) people were 'Sectioned' under the Mental Health Act on 63,622 occasions, with around 20,000 people in psychiatric hospitals against their will at any one time.[2] International comparisons are complex (partly because people can be subject to involuntary treatment either while physically detained in hospital, or be subject to various forms of compulsory treatment orders in community settings), but the numbers worldwide are likely to be disturbing at best.

As the statistics indicate, people with a wide range of problems can find ourselves caught up in coercive practices.[3] There is clear evidence of widespread disregard of the normal clinical emphasis on informed consent.[4] For example, it is relatively common, at least in the UK, to offer people a choice: 'either come into hospital voluntarily, or we'll "Section" you'. This is coercive at best. If I am told that I'll be detained against my will if I don't agree, my agreement is hardly anything other than under duress. It may or may not be technically illegal in the UK at present. Contemptibly (and I am personally both entirely opposed to this state of affairs and campaigning to change the law), the UK Mental Health Act not only applies once we are unable to make decisions for ourselves. European and international law theoretically protects our rights to make autonomous decisions (and have them honoured), but this has not impacted on the authorities' powers to compel us to accept mental health care even when we disagree. Once detained in hospital, shamefully, we are often exposed to coercion, force and even violence. The use of physical force is frequent.

Autonomy

Coercion, choice and autonomy are ignored or brushed aside. Medication as routinely used as a control technique. Sometimes it's very subtle, intimately associated with the medical ethos and 'disease-model', and justified as necessary to save lives or prevent suffering. But a moment's thought can reveal the heartlessness involved.

I was once asked to write a commentary for a book chapter describing clinical dilemmas on an inpatient psychiatric ward. The idea was to have a book consisting of a chapter describing an ethical or clinical dilemma and then a brief commentary. The case example that I was sent involved a woman who was very distressed and agitated. She was described as experiencing a 'manic episode'. As I read the description, the story became both very clear and rather disturbing. The clinical dilemma was written from the perspective of persuading her to take medication. While nursing or medical staff were sitting with her and talking with her about her various (admittedly rather incoherent) concerns, she was described as being relatively calm. Whenever the subject of medication was raised, or if the nurses suggested that they might have to leave, she would become very distressed. The account ended with a rather heartfelt description of how the staff felt that they had no option but to force medication on her, a very distressing experience. I remember being struck by the contrast between the medical approach—the principled feeling that the client needed to receive the medicine that would help her—and my own feeling that, since she seemed to be comforted by having a professional sitting with her and listening, then that should continue, for hours if necessary, until sleep offered respite. The contrast in assumptions was striking.

But there are more insidious threats to our fundamental rights. And at least some of these are inherent to the system. A few months ago, the campaigner Alison Cameron tweeted a photograph of the private (i.e. profit-making) psychiatric hospital to which she had been admitted. In her words, it was: '*[a s]hocking place. This cage was where v unwell patients were put for "fresh air"*'.[5] The facility isn't that unusual. In many establishments, the managers have been put in the position of making compromises—between the regulations that forbid smoking, and the need to offer residents some access to the outside world, and the perceived need for security. It looks very much as if the establishment has been built to a very non-specific architectural plan, with no particular design considerations to balance those competing needs. And, like many such establishments, built on the cheap with only afterthought consideration of the residents' requirements, the facilities for people to go outside for a smoke or for a breath of fresh air are best described as a *'cage'*.

If we have problems so serious that we need to be admitted to a secure psychiatric hospital, presumably because there are fears that we might wish to take our own lives, what we need is an environment that gives us hope and optimism, reminds us that we are valued and loved, makes us feel good and is even (perish the thought) a little luxurious and pampered. But instead... we get a shabby cage.

It goes deeper than that. On a personal trip to Australia, I was fortunate enough to visit a mental health facility in a rural hospital, on the edge of the 'bush'. It was a secure facility, but actually very attractive. It was light, airy and well-designed. But it was also quintessentially medical. It was a hospital ward, and its design resembled every other medical unit. It reminded me of a small piece of work I did in my first job after qualifying as a clinical psychologist. I had been asked by my boss to offer a psychological perspective on the construction of a new residential mental health unit. The hospital in which we worked was expanding and modernising, and a new mental health unit was included in the plan. When I visited the manager responsible for commissioning the development and liaising with the architects, I found that the hospital manager was briefing the architects using a standard NHS document offering guidance on the design of hospital wards. Although very helpful, it merely assumed that beds on hospital psychiatric wards naturally required all the paraphernalia of general hospital wards caring for people with serious physical health conditions. To the authors of this guidance, a ward was a ward, and a hospital bed was a bed. To be fair, I didn't check at the Australian facility whether the beds were supplied with an alarm button for the nurses, a vacuum attachment, oxygen and other pipes and devices. But the point is... the symbolism and message being sent are still those of illness. The 'cage' tells you that you're dangerous and undervalued, the 'ward' tells you that you're ill, that there's something fundamentally wrong with you.

When people are in crisis, residential care may be needed, but this does not need to be seen as a medical issue. Since a 'disease model' is inappropriate, it is also inappropriate to care for people in hospital wards; a different model of care is needed. As with other services, residential units could be based on a psychosocial model. Residential social workers or nurses who have retrained in a psychosocial approach (and possibly with a more appropriate professional title) are likely to be best placed to lead such units.

The need for compulsory detention would be much reduced within this new approach. In those instances where compulsory detention was necessary, decisions would be based on the risks that individuals are thought to pose to themselves and others, together with their capacity to make decisions about their own care. This approach is already the basis for the law in Scotland. The law in England and Wales permits the 'responsible clinician' (the person who is legally responsible for someone's care, traditionally a psychiatrist) to be a psychologist, nurse or social worker. This should be routine. When we reject a 'disease model' of care and adopt a 'human-centred' model, the law relating to psychological health could change significantly. There would be different criteria governing to whom the law applies, different ways of assuring that people are offered care that is (in the words of the current law) 'least restrictive', with a psychosocial focus, new roles for new professions and a greater focus on social justice and judicial oversight.

In previous roles, I have contributed to a number of reviews of the mental health legislation (as well as having professional experience of working with people detained under the Mental Health Act). I draw on that experience, and a comprehensive review of the relevant literature, to explore what a non-pathologising, capacity-based approach to mental health legislation would look like and how it would change life for people in receipt of mental health services.

Services planned on the basis of a psychosocial model would offer a very radical alternative. Instead of seeing care for people with mental health problems as a specialist branch of medicine, with links to social care, we would see such support as essential part of social provision, with specialist input from our medical colleagues. In such a world, people would default to a psychosocial explanatory model, and the disease model of mental disorder would be redundant. That would lead to more empathy, more compassion and more understanding of people's needs both by professionals and wider society.[6] It would give people more of a sense of agency, a belief in their ability to help themselves. People's problems would be understood as just that; problems, and diagnoses would be largely replaced by formulations. For people in extreme distress, places of safety would still be needed to replace the niche filled at present by inpatient wards. However, these should be seen as places of safety, not medical treatment units, and should therefore be led by lay people, people who have themselves used mental health services, social workers or possibly psychologists, rather than doctors or nurses, and physically designed as homely, welcoming, houses rather than 'wards'. On those units, our medical, psychiatric colleagues would still play a valuable role, but would act as consultants to the care team on specifically medical issues, not necessarily leaders of those teams. The ethos of care on such units would be based on recovery, not treatment or cure, and be firmly based on a psychosocial formulation of the problems facing each service user. Good quality, humane, care and taking seriously the person's own views about their difficulties and needs rather than insisting that they see themselves as 'ill' and accept medication, would minimise the need for compulsion. When compulsion is needed, however, the legal criteria should be based on the principle that people should only be subject to coercion when they are unable to make the relevant decisions for themselves, a capacity-based approach.

For most of us, though, mental health care is already community-based. In the vision of care proposed here, reconfiguring services as psychosocial rather than medical would transform care. Links to other community-based services such as primary care (GP) and public health services are strong and should remain so. Interestingly, public health services are already based in local authorities. Their ethos would shift from medical to psychosocial and shift from medical dominance to a model whereby medical colleagues offer consultancy on primarily medical issues (e.g. the prescription of drugs) to those psychosocial teams.

If we were in crisis, what would we consider to be a 'place of safety'? What would we want in such circumstances? We can be clear about what isn't needed. Most people in acute distress are not 'ill' and do not need to be in 'hospital'. I am aware that this is a challenging thing to say. But I mean precisely what I say. As I made clear earlier in this book, 'illness' and 'diagnosis' are inappropriate metaphors for understanding emotional distress. When problems are serious or acute, people can certainly need help, and occasionally medication can be useful. But they aren't 'ill', and there is no good reason to suppose that a 'hospital' is the most appropriate place of safety. Instead, people deserve to be offered a high-quality, welcoming, supportive and calm environment in which to recover and receive the help they need.

Physical Health

People with psychological health problems often have major physical health problems too. Admission to a psychiatric hospital offers an opportunity to help clients access the physical health care that they need. But, in practice, people at present find it difficult to access such help, despite being an in- or outpatient in a 'hospital'. The conclusion has to be that hospital care is failing even in that respect.

In the UK, both the Royal College of Psychiatrists and the Department of Health have expressed serious concerns over the physical health of, and physical health care provided to, people in residential psychiatric care. There are two issues here: the identification of relevant medical conditions at admission, especially medical conditions that might help explain a person's problems, and ongoing physical health care of residents. It is important to understand and then address any medical conditions that might affect our mental health. In truth, however, these are rare. Despite the assertions of the pharmaceutical companies, the emotional and social problems labelled as 'mental health problems' are primarily just that social and psychological issues. Although we cannot separate our physical from our psychological health, that is simply not the same as assuming that mental health problems are 'illnesses' and that they should be treated as such.

People rarely come to the doors of psychiatric wards without first having contact with a number of health and social care staff. The majority of people admitted to hospital are already known to the services, whose needs and care plans are understood, but whose social circumstances are such that, at least occasionally, they need additional support. Many people are in acute crises, and access services through Accident and Emergency departments, following calls to the ambulance

services or via the police. In such circumstances, it is indeed important
that people have their primary medical needs assessed. About ten years
ago, I worked as a clinical psychologist on a 'psychiatric intensive care
unit'. One Monday morning, we held our usual 'ward round' (and,
yes, of course, we definitely need to change that terminology) and were
updated on a young man who had been admitted over the weekend.
The psychiatric registrar reported (rather proudly) that the young man
had been brought into the unit late on Friday afternoon by an ambulance crew after his friends had reported that he had been acting very
oddly in a Gestalt therapy session—he began speaking incoherently and
defecated in public. Understandably, his behaviour led to an immediate emergency call and, because he was extremely uncooperative with
the paramedics, an admission directly to the nearest secure psychiatric
inpatient unit. Our registrar colleague reported that, over the weekend,
she and the nursing staff had observed some worrying signs: incoher-
ence in speech that sounded more like delirium than 'thought disorder',
intermittent visual hallucinations (of tiny human beings) interspersed
with much more calm and reasonable periods. The registrar employed
her excellent medical skills and referred the man to a neurology clinic.
A scan revealed a bleed from a ruptured aneurism in the frontal lobes
of his brain. By the time we arrived on Monday morning for the 'ward
round', the young man had already had surgery. Remarkably, by that
time he was back to his normal self, coherent and calm. When we met
to discuss his experiences, and to tell him that an acute psychiatric ward
was the wrong place for him, he was one of the most content residents
on the ward.

It is probably correct that: '…an acute psychiatric ward was probably the wrong place for him…'. But that tells us something remarkable.
These kinds of medical emergencies are very rare. It is hugely important
that they are spotted and addressed. I should make it clear: in any residential psychological health unit based on a psychosocial ethos, medical
advice would be vital. But when such medical emergencies are discovered, it turns out that psychiatric units are exactly the wrong place for
people concerned: they need, as in this example, medical or neurological care. Any sensible plans for residential units should ensure that such
medical support is easily available if needed. But it is also important to

note how rare examples like this are in reality. The majority of people admitted to psychiatric units are either already well known to ward staff, including the doctors, or have reached the doors of an inpatient unit following a string of contacts with services. In all contacts with GPs, with outpatient psychiatrists, with psychologists, social workers and community psychiatric nurses, at Accident and Emergency departments, with the police and with paramedics attached to ambulance services, it is important that staff are able to identify and refer to medical colleagues anyone who needs their help.

We need to be able to identify and respond to critical medical emergencies. Any changes to the design and management of residential, or inpatient, provision must address this issue. But this is only a small element of the present psychiatric inpatient system. In truth, such medical emergencies are rare. And high-quality medical care can be provided in a range of settings. Indeed, there are good reasons to believe that different arrangements may be beneficial.

In our current system, the physical health of residents in inpatient psychiatric wards is a matter of concern. In 2012, the Royal College of Psychiatrists and the Healthcare Quality Improvement Partnership reviewed the 'in-patient' care offered to people who had received a diagnosis of 'schizophrenia'.[7] Part of their report addressed physical healthcare needs and the extent to which services met the specific requirements of the NICE clinical guidelines. The NICE clinical guideline for the care of people with a diagnosis of 'schizophrenia' sets out eight indicators against which physical health should be monitored. These include: body mass index (BMI), blood levels of glucose and lipids (total cholesterol and other fats), blood pressure, smoking habits, alcohol and other substance use, blood levels of the hormone prolactin (where relevant) and a history of cardiovascular disease, diabetes, hypertension or hyperlipidaemia in members of the service user's family. All of these can be addressed quite simply through a brief interview and a blood test; I was recently offered precisely this service from my GP, a 'men's health check'.

Unfortunately, the 2012 audit revealed some rather worrying statistics. Monitoring of BMI, blood glucose and lipid levels and blood pressure was only offered to 50% of people (even those who had been in the service a long time). In some 90% of cases, substance use, alcohol use or smoking status were recorded, but prolactin levels had been recorded for only about 10% of cases. In only 29% of cases were the most important 'cardiometabolic risk parameters' recorded. In other words, these crucial health checks were only infrequently offered.

Members of the public who use mental health services need high-quality medical care for their physical health needs. Unfortunately, our current service structures may not allow psychiatric colleagues to provide it. A 2009 report from the Royal College of Psychiatrists[8] concludes that '...*there is a growing body of evidence that many psychiatrists lack the skills required to provide for the general healthcare of people with mental health problems. This situation may have arisen for good reason – psychiatrists have sought to specialise in mental health matters, regarding physical healthcare as the province of other clinicians*'. My point is that the present system is failing even to live up to the requirements of a biomedical approach to mental health care. Once again, we need something different.

Social Breakdown

When I worked in a psychiatric intensive care unit, one client was a middle-aged man whose primary problem at the time of admission was hearing distressing voices ('auditory hallucinations', in medical language). He had received, inevitably, a diagnosis of 'schizophrenia' several years earlier and had (more or less) adhered to a prescription for 'anti-psychotic' medication ever since. When we met to discuss his case, a lesser clinician may have responded to ongoing auditory hallucinations by increasing (dangerously) the man's prescription. Luckily, the psychiatrist with whom I worked was better than that. For a while, we discussed possible ways that we might be able to help the man to overcome or eliminate the voices. But then...it occurred to us. This man had lived with his voices for many years. He struggled, and he needed help of various kinds, but for many years, he had lived successfully on his own while hearing those voices. More recently, something had gone wrong, his self-care had deteriorated, and his problems had escalated.

There were reasons for this deterioration, but that's not my point here. My point is that he had found a way of living successfully despite quite distressing auditory hallucinations, but a deterioration in his social circumstances had led to a crisis requiring an emergency response. It struck us all in the 'ward round' that a reasonable outcome in the short-term would be for him to be able to return to his apartment and able to live his life in a manner of his choosing, with appropriate support, despite hearing voices. It would be lovely to see him free of them, but his ability to live independently was clearly not dependent on their absence. With that realisation, our care plan changed; instead of trying to remove the voices, instead of assuming that his discharge from hospital would be dependent upon successful reduction in the hallucinations, we aimed to help him return to an ability to live independently.

There are many different reasons that people end up in hospital. For a close relative of mine, the trigger for a serious 'relapse' was the withdrawal of benefits. The UK government has recently initiated a change to the 'Employment and Support Allowance' paid to people unable to work. To receive these payments, claimants have to pass a 'work capability assessment', a short medical test carried out by a private contractor. Many, including my relative, 'fail' this test…and the consequences can be serious. In his case, the resulting anxiety led to a deterioration in his psychological health. My point is that it is life events and circumstances that lead people into crisis, and into the need for care. We know, clearly and unambiguously, that people get into difficulty because of such things as loved ones becoming ill or dying, bullying and abuse, major life events, redundancy and unemployment, financial difficulties and debt, marital problems and loneliness.

When our lives come crashing down around us, when we lose hope or lose touch with reality, we need support. Sometimes, we need a place to stay, a 'place of safety'. We should commission those services that might actually address real-world problems: social services, debt counselling, housing advice, benefits advice, employment support, training and educational opportunities, occupational and psychological therapies and physical health care. But none of that means that we need to offer a place in a 'hospital'. We have examples of what is possible from other areas of social and personal care. Care for people with learning disabilities is often delivered in residential units that are predicated on social rather than medical ideas. Residential care for older adults offers a wide range of specialist services in non-medical settings, and hospices are frequently designed and organised in deliberately non-medical ways. There are government plans for more home-based and non-hospital care.[9] Innovative psychological health and social services already operate residential crisis units away from traditional hospital sites yet welcoming people in acute distress and in need of immediate support.

Where Would I Go in a Crisis?

It would not be an appropriate use of taxpayers' money to offer all users of psychological health services a Maldives chalet by the shores of the Indian Ocean, but I do think it's reasonable to consider what we would look for in a decent hotel. People who are stressed, confused, hopeless and low in self-esteem need to be offered accommodation that is high-quality, welcoming, supportive and calm and where they can receive the help they need. In many ways, like a well-staffed 4-star hotel, rather than an emergency medical facility.

I do not doubt that everybody involved in crisis care aspires to offer high-quality and physically attractive accommodation. But, within a medical, 'disease-model' ethos, the main function of an inpatient ward is to keep someone safe while their underlying 'illness' is diagnosed and treated. Other aspects matter less: the atmosphere, the furnishings, the possibility of privacy, the 'messages' that the physical surroundings give about people's worth and status and even staff attitudes. In a 'health' service, there is always a danger that design considerations will follow from medical ways of thinking. People entering residential, inpatient care are often at their most desperate. Few, if any, will feel good about themselves. How must it feel to walk through 'air-lock' style security doors to enter the ward, to be faced with noisy, crowded, functional rooms with institutional, clinical, utilitarian, often shabby fixtures and fittings? But, on the other hand, what could it do for someone to find themselves in an environment which is calm, welcoming, comfortable, elegant and well designed?

The history of mental health services reveals something curious, however. Throughout history, moral considerations have impinged on the otherwise practical, scientific or medical ways of thinking. Perhaps this isn't too surprising. Our psychological health and wellbeing are intimately related to the framework of understanding that we have about ourselves, other people, the world and the future. They relate to who we are and why we do what we do, the meaning and purpose of our behaviour and why our lives have turned out as they have. Most importantly, ideas about mental health are invoked to explain why people behave in ways which are frowned upon socially. Moral and even religious perspectives have been important concomitants of understanding, care and treatment. This has meant that people with mental health problems have variously been seen as sinners, morally 'lost', animalistic or diseased. And quite barbaric 'treatments' have been used—chairs that spin people around until they are sick, cold baths, insulin 'shock therapy', electric shock therapy, restraint of various kinds and the use of a wide range of sedating drugs. Punitive 'treatment' seems (unconsciously I hope) to have been designed to shock or even punish people—maybe they even have the gall to complain that they have been abused.

Which all means that many people will feel a historical shudder when I propose offering people the equivalent of 4-star hotel accommodation. We have, I fear, a vestige of these blaming, stigmatising, discriminatory attitudes, an unspoken desire to punish people or to shock them into sanity. My own profession of psychology has been complicit here, not only in looking for people's so-called deficits, but also in helping design interventions based on 'negative reinforcement' or 'aversive stimuli'. There may be those who object to using taxpayers' money to providing hotel standard accommodation to people who are variously 'unemployed', 'on benefits', 'drug-users', 'mentally-ill'.... A simple reading of the media headlines of recent years tends to suggest that as a society we have some rather unpleasant views about how we should treat people. It is uncontroversial to suggest that general hospitals should aspire to offer the amenities of a 4-star hotel (e.g. that a hospice for people with terminal illnesses should be comfortable, elegant, calm and well appointed). Any difference in attitude reflects long-standing stigma and discrimination against those of us who admit to emotional distress. Therefore, yes, we should aspire to high-quality residential care and confront the discriminatory attitudes that argue against this.

Having worked in acute mental health units for most of my professional life, I am well aware that safety and security are important. Most mental health professionals are very keen to preserve their clients' personal, family and home lives and to maintain people's mental health without resorting to residential care. Therefore, especially these days, admission to residential mental health care tends to be reserved for people in acute crisis. It is an unfortunate fact that, therefore, many people in such establishments are either very vulnerable or pose a degree of risk to themselves. We need to keep people safe. For example, since some people are likely to be experiencing suicidal feelings, it is important to reduce the risk of suicide by hanging. And one of the best ways to do that is by removing ligature points (things that people could use to harm themselves).[10] I am also very aware that people, when frustrated, confused, angry and hurt, occasionally pose a real risk to others.

So residential units for people in crisis need to be secure. That costs money, in design and in staffing. And while good design might cost little, part of the lamentable quality of psychiatric units at present may be due to cost savings. But it is entirely possible to design well and maintain security. Part of my job has involved visiting junior civil servants and, very occasionally, government ministers, in Whitehall. Their offices are elegant, occasionally impressive…and always very secure. When we design for civil servants and politicians, we manage to combine attractive environments with excellent security. It clearly isn't impossible. There are undoubted challenges in designing high-quality, secure, residential units. But I cannot conclude that a medical ethos adds anything positive to the experience of residential care. Ultimately, a reliance on chemical restraints is a bad thing.

Notes

1. Kinderman, P. (2014). A prescription for psychiatry: Why we need a whole new approach to mental health and wellbeing. Springer.

2. https://www.theguardian.com/society/2018/jan/23/nhs-patients-having-to-be-sectioned-to-get-help-says-regulator.

3. https://www.cqc.org.uk/sites/default/files/documents/cqc_mental-health_2012_13_07_update.pdf.

4. https://www.madinamerica.com/2018/03/patients-overlooked-compulsory-treatment/.

5. https://twitter.com/allyc375/status/854220687489323008.

6. See, again: Sheila Mehta and Amerigo Farina, "Is being 'sick' really better? Effect of the disease view of mental disorder on stigma," *Journal of Social and Clinical Psychology* 16, no. 4 (1997): 405–419; and John Read and Niki Harré, "The role of biological and genetic causal beliefs in the stigmatisation of 'mental patients'," *Journal of Mental Health* 10, no. 2 (2001): 223–235. https://doi.org/10.1080/09638230123129.

7. https://www.rcpsych.ac.uk/improving-care/ccqi/national-clinical-audits/national-clinical-audit-of-psychosis/national-audit-schizophrenia.

8. http://www.rcpsych.ac.uk/files/pdfversion/op67.pdf.

9. https://www.england.nhs.uk/wp-content/uploads/2016/02/Mental-Health-Taskforce-FYFV-final.pdf.

10. Isabelle M. Hunt, Kirsten Windfuhr, Jenny Shaw, Louis Appleby, and Nav Kapur, "Ligature points and ligature types used by psychiatric inpatients who die by hanging," *Crisis: The Journal of Crisis Intervention and Suicide Prevention* 33 (2012): 87–94. http://www.ncbi.nlm.nih.gov/pubmed/22343063.

11

The Mental Health Act

When, regrettably, the powers of the Mental Health Act are needed, any deci-sions taken by mental healthcare professionals need to first place human rights at the centre of decision-making. The law should respect our rights to make decisions for ourselves unless we are unable to do that, and then should be based on the risks that we pose to ourselves and others, rather than whether or not we are considered 'mentally ill'. We should aim to reduce the use of com-pulsory powers and provide for much greater judicial oversight within the use of mental health legislation. Once again, psychosocial, rather than biomedi-cal, principles should guide our decisions.

I have spent my career divided between clinical and academic work. Much of my work has been focussed on inpatient settings and with peo-ple who have quite severe and disabling problems. After qualifying, I divided my working week between inpatient, hospital-based, psychiatric ward and an outpatient clinic. When I conducted my Ph.D., I spent a great deal of my time interviewing people who were resident on inpa-tient psychiatric wards. In my academic career, I have been responsible for randomised, controlled trials of CBT for people with serious men-tal health problems: this again frequently brought me into contact with people staying in hospital. And throughout my career I have continued

© The Author(s) 2019
P. Kinderman, *A Manifesto for Mental Health*,
https://doi.org/10.1007/978-3-030-24386-9_11

to work with people with serious problems, who are often frequently admitted to hospital. But I have to confess that I had not visited a psychiatric ward for several months until recently, when one of my clients was briefly admitted to hospital. And I was shocked by her experience.

The details of my client's mental health problems are not relevant here, but, like many people who are admitted to psychiatric hospitals, she had been experiencing problems for a number of years. From time to time, the challenges of caring for her became too much for her parents, and (occasionally following the intervention of the police) she spent a few days in hospital. It is significant for the narrative of this book that there has never been a dramatic change in the care offered during her admissions—no new diagnosis, no new or insightful formulation, no change in prescription. The main reason for her admission is to provide some respite for her parents. So, this particular admission was not unusual. In truth, my client welcomed it. Her anxieties were such that admission to hospital represented 'safety' for her.

On visiting her in hospital, my first impression was poor. I had expected to walk in, to be greeted by a nurse or other healthcare worker and, within the sensible parameters of visiting regulations, spend time with the person I had come to visit. I had expected the environment to be inappropriately medical, but I expected clinical cleanliness and tidiness. Instead, I was confronted by a peculiar 'air-lock' style arrangement—I entered through a conventional automatic, sliding, door, but had to wait until that door had closed, and locked, behind me. Then a security guard—not a receptionist—asked me my business. I said I was a friend of a patient (the guard asked for her name) and was asked to give my name before being issued with a visitor's badge and the second automatic door was opened. I was already uncomfortable; my client was a voluntary patient; she had not been detained under the Mental Health Act and was therefore—in theory at least—entirely free to come and go as she wished. That right should extend to her visitors. I can see why psychiatric units need to consider security, but the immediate impression was unpleasant. The theme was immediately one of risk, dangerousness and threat. Certainly not one of calm. I made my way to the ward, and, once through the main doors, there was no immediate sense of control or coercion. I met my client in a general activity room, but there was an odd, institutional feel. The unit was busy, even crowded.

There were some comfortable chairs, but they were upholstered in a plasticised, waterproof, material; the kind you find on the chairs in an Accident and Emergency waiting area. In any case, the only space that my client and I could find was sitting in upright chairs at a table which doubled as a dining unit. There were artworks on the walls, but there were also boards for posters, information leaflets and health-related messages. Those of us who work in, or visit, psychiatric wards will recognise this picture. I have a different vision.

Too Much Coercion?

In February 2013, my colleague (and former Ph.D. supervisor), Professor Richard Bentall, wrote a short article for the *Guardian* newspaper on the subject of coercion in mental health services. It is worth reading in full and coincides closely with my own views.[1] It is also worth reading a commentary on Richard's article by Dina Poursanidou, a member of the Asylum Collective and someone who can speak from personal experience.[2] In his article, Richard makes reference to the fact that coercion is increasing in mental health services. He points out that coercion is 'routine', with many people who are in hospital on a 'voluntary' basis nevertheless detained in all but name, with it being made clear to them that, if they don't agree to the care that is being offered, they will be detained and forced anyway. Richard points out how important a sense of autonomy—the right to make choices—is for all of us, and therefore how coercion and the denial of rights are traumatic. Given that many people using mental health services have already been subjected to physical and sexual abuse, bullying and other kinds of victimisation, further coercion may be particularly traumatic. As Dina comments, the ward to which she was compulsorily admitted became '...*the ultimate symbol of an oppressive, terrifying, non-therapeutic and unsafe space in my psyche, a space that I came to hate and despise vehemently... the ultimate symbol of a deeply traumatising experience....*' It had come '...*to symbolise the culmination of my mental distress for me – a place where I was deprived of my liberty, where I was treated as somebody with diminished capacity and insight....*' Dina comments how involuntary detention '...*was a source of profound feelings of humiliation and shame, as well as a source of a deep sense of failure, unfairness/injustice and stigmatisation – all acutely disempowering emotions...it was an immensely scarring experience whereby the very core of my existence was deeply shaken and all my certainties collapsed – something that I experienced as a brutal assault on my identity'.* Richard Bentall argues that many of the arguments in favour of compulsion are flawed. People are not always (as is often implied) irrational in rejecting care, the medication that is almost always the first choice for clinicians is not always beneficial, and such care often does not have positive long-term outcomes.

Dina is more powerful, commenting that her experience was one of a '*...complete lack of therapeutic care on the ward'.* Her comments about what happened in reality are worth reading. Bentall concludes that '*... sometimes, coercion is difficult to avoid. But if coercion is a necessary evil it is still an evil and mental health services need to find ways of resorting to it less. This will require a change of culture and, perhaps, for some mental health professionals to consider alternative careers. In the long term, the solution to the problem of coercion in psychiatry is to design services that patients find helpful and actually want to use'.*

I agree. That is precisely the thrust of this book. But if coercion—even very occasionally—is a necessary evil, how might we best frame and use the law?

Do we need the Law at all?

One radical proposal is that the law should be silent about our psychological health. For those of a radical, liberal, tradition who take a psychosocial view of psychological health issues, there is no need to consider specific legislation permitting compulsion. If someone is distressed, their argument goes; they should be able to choose for themselves whether to accept psychiatric (or any other form of) care. In this view, a person has every right to reject the advice of doctors that they should, for example, take medication or come into hospital. In this view, we have no right to compel people to undergo psychiatric care.

Few people accept this argument entirely. We have always been vulnerable to great distress, confusion and hopelessness. Each year about 6000 people in the UK and 800,000 across the world take their own lives. I mentioned earlier how around 1000 more people killed themselves in the years between 2008 and 2010 than would have been expected, and that this has been associated with the economic recession. I do not regard these people as suffering from 'disorders', but equally I cannot accept that our proper response should be to offer people in huge distress, and not in their usual or 'right' frame of mind, the promise that services are there if they want them and then merely leave them to make their own decisions. Frequently, we are unable to make rational decisions.

The Mental Health Act

In England and Wales, compulsory care for people with mental health problems is overseen by the Mental Health Act 2007. The Mental Health Act states that it is intended to provide for; '... *the reception, care and treatment of mentally disordered patients, the management of their property and other related matters*' where '"*mental disorder" means any disorder or disability of the mind*'. This circular language ('mental disorder means a disorder of the mind') is common in legal circles, and I find it frustrating. The Act has many sections (the origin of the term 'to be sectioned' meaning to be detained in hospital under the provisions of the legislation), but central to most people's experiences are Sections 2 and 3.

Section 2 of the Mental Health Act (as amended) allows for a person to be admitted to hospital—whether or not they consent—for assessment for up to 28 days. The legal procedure is that an 'approved mental health professional' or the person's 'nearest relative' (both of these are legal terms, which are largely self-explanatory, the exact legal details can be found online[3]) can apply for admission via the normal referral routes of the health services. Any admission must be authorised by two doctors, who must both agree that: '...*the patient is suffering from a mental disorder of a nature or degree that warrants detention in hospital for assessment; and that the patient ought to be detained for his or her own health or safety, or the protection of others...*'. In an emergency, a person can be detained for up to 72 hours, if one doctor has confirmed that '...*the detention is of "urgent necessity..."*' and that '...*waiting for a second doctor to approve the detention...would cause an "undesirable delay"*'. In addition, as mentioned earlier, police officers have the authority to take people to a 'place of safety' if they appear to be suffering from a mental disorder, in order that they be assessed by a doctor and an approved mental health professional.

Section 3 of the Act is very similar, except that it permits detention in hospital for up to six months, and for the purposes of treatment as well as assessment. In the words of the Act, '... *detention can last for up to six months after two doctors have confirmed that the patient is suffering from mental disorder of a nature or degree which makes it appropriate for the patient to receive medical treatment in a hospital, the treatment is in the interests of his or her health and safety and the protection of others and appropriate treatment must be available for the patient*'. Of course, some people remain in hospital for longer than this, in some cases for years. Detention under Section 3 can be renewed for a further six months and thereafter for periods of 12 months at a time. Once in hospital, people are under the care of a 'responsible clinician', who (in most cases) will be responsible for deciding when discharge is appropriate.

A Psychosocial Perspective

The powers of the Mental Health Act are used about 50,000 times a year in England and Wales. This does not mean that 50,000 people are detained in hospital, because some people may be detained several times within a year. With very few exceptions, all professionals working in mental health services are very well aware of the serious threat to civil liberties and human rights that this entails, and the frequent trauma that ensues for the individuals involved. My colleagues (or, at least, all those whom I admire) therefore only use the Act when they believe it to be necessary and in the best interests of their clients. For me, this means two things. First: while there is very widespread acceptance that we should try to reduce the number of people subject to compulsion under mental health legislation, there is no set figure—25,000 or 10,000, say—that is agreed to be the 'correct' figure. Second: the driving force behind our use of compulsion in mental health care is necessity; the idea that some people need urgent help, and that we cannot, in conscience, abandon them. Nevertheless, significant revisions of the UK's mental health legislation are required. These can learn from, and possibly inform, other jurisdictions' approaches.

The present UK Mental Health Act is, like many other national variants, a very odd piece of legislation. In any normal state of affairs, it would be illegal—a form of unlawful imprisonment—to require someone to stay in hospital if they wished to leave, and equally illegal—a form of assault—to force a person to take medication if they did not consent. These things are not illegal if performed under the auspices of the Mental Health Act and if the required conditions are met. I hinted earlier at Section 136 powers, which enable a police officer to take someone whom they believe to be 'mentally disordered' from a public place to a 'place of safety'. Interestingly, if the person is in a private place, the Act (in Section 135) requires a police officer first to obtain a warrant from a magistrate (junior judge). And that contrast illustrates how the Mental Health Act is a permissive Act; it permits people to do things that would otherwise be illegal or require a warrant.

And the things it permits are serious. If deployed incorrectly, use of mental health legislation could lead to serious breaches of human rights. Article 3 of the European Convention on Human Rights (and therefore of the UK Human Rights Act 1998) states that 'no one shall be subjected to torture or to inhuman or degrading treatment or punishment'. Many of us would argue that much of current mental health care is perceived by a very large number of people to be degrading and inhumane. Article 5 states that *everyone has the right to liberty and security of person. No one shall be deprived of his liberty save in the following cases and in accordance with a procedure prescribed by law...*' One of these 'cases' concerns; '... *the lawful detention of... persons of unsound mind...*'. The term 'of unsound mind' is not defined in the Human Rights Act, but case law has referred to people with 'real illnesses'.[4] Not only do I believe that there are no such things as 'real mental illnesses', I believe the notion is irrelevant. If we were to accept, for the point of argument, that a 'real mental illness' was to be defined as 'meeting the criteria for a recognised mental illness as defined by one of the major diagnostic manuals', clearly this would not render a person liable to detention and treatment under mental health legislation; caffeine dependence and trichotillomania (hair pulling) are 'recognised mental disorders' in those manuals, and nobody would suggest the Mental Health Act could be used in such cases.

Under what circumstances should we be permitted to override a person's right to liberty, to be able to choose for themselves where they reside and whether or not to accept professional advice? Article 8 of the European Convention on Human Rights affirms that 'everyone has the right to respect for his private and family life, his home and his correspondence' and 'there shall be no interference by a public authority with the exercise of this right except such as is in accordance with the law and is necessary in a democratic society in the interests of national security, public safety or the economic well-being of the country, for the prevention of disorder or crime, for the protection of health or morals, or for the protection of the rights and freedoms of others'. Article 8 therefore is also of key importance in the context of compulsory mental health care. It provides for compulsion in the case of necessity.

55 Steps Towards Autonomy

The movie '55 Steps' opens with a harrowing scene of a woman screaming as she is manhandled, forcibly injected with sedatives and locked in seclusion on a psychiatric ward.

'55 Steps' stars Helena Bonham Carter as Eleanor Riese and Hilary Swank as her lawyer, Colette Hughes. Written by Mark Rosin, directed by Bille August, and released this year, the film documents Eleanor's ground-breaking 1987 Californian court case, establishing that people have a right to the exercise of informed consent. That statement would be commonplace in all fields of medicine… except psychiatry, but until Ms Riese was obliged to go to court to enforce her rights, Californians admitted to hospital, and who were capable of weighing up the medication's benefits and risks, had no right to refuse, and no right to be consulted.

The movie follows Eleanor's case from the harrowing opening scene, though the long-winded and tiresome legal process, to her success… and then her early death as a result of the medication she had been forced to take. This wasn't an easy struggle; the movie ends with a funeral, and the title refers to fact that Eleanor struggles to keep walking up the 55 steps to the courtroom for repeated hearings after she loses her first claim.

'55 Steps' is a film about abusive and coercive mental health care, it's a film about an important court case, it's a film about the adverse effects of psychiatric medication and about the contentious nature of informed consent. As the (real) court case developed, the *New York Times* reported on the discussions. In their words: '*A panel of the State Court of Appeal has ruled that... patients could not be forced to take the medication unless a judge determined that they were incapable of making an informed decision about their medical care*'. Well, of course, you might say. Unless unable to make an informed decision, a citizen's autonomous wishes should be sovereign. But Eleanor's case is so important because that simple and apparently obvious conclusion was opposed by the medical, psychiatric, establishment at the time.

Eleanor Riese's case hinged on a number of arguments; her First Amendment right to freedom of expression, because her medical notes clearly stated that she had been medicated for being 'sarcastic', her right to autonomous decision-making, but also the adverse effects of the medication being administered; particularly tardive dyskinesia (a particularly nasty, often permanent, side effect of antipsychotic drugs where the muscles of the face and body make involuntary jerky or twisting movements). The psychiatric establishment at the time was, at best, equivocal on this issue. In 1980 (a few years before the '55 Steps' court case), the American Psychiatric Association published the findings of a 'taskforce' on the issue of tardive dyskinesia, a common side effect of so-called anti-psychotic medication. Included within that report was a survey of psychiatrists on the issue of informed consent. In other words, whether they thought people had a right to be told about such adverse effects. It was striking that 58%—a majority, but hardly a sweeping majority—believed that '*good medical practice required such discussions*' but only 11% believed that it was appropriate for such discussions to involve written agreement.

It's extraordinary that Eleanor Riese's case was fought out in my lifetime. The forcible and even violent usurping of our rights to determine our own health care, our own psychological health, the physical sanctity of our bodies and the conceptual sanctity of our autonomy should have been outlawed years ago. But, right now in 2018, in the UK, Eleanor's victory is unfulfilled. When discussing tardive dyskinesia, the charity MIND comment that: '*... awareness of tardive dyskinesia has improved over the years, but unfortunately doctors don't always remember to tell people about this risk when they prescribe antipsychotics*'. Eleanor's campaign for informed consent clearly has a long way to go; we can't exercise informed consent without a discussion of risks.

It seems extraordinary that we could have contemplated withholding citizens' rights to informed consent about such powerful, dangerous, and potentially damaging drugs. But there is also another extraordinary element to this case, and indeed to the UK's Mental Health Act (at least as it applies in England and Wales). In 1987, Ms Riese won the right for all citizens of California to exercise informed consent '... *unless a judge determined that they were incapable of making an informed decision about their medical care*'. But, explicitly, this ruling applied to people who were '... involuntarily committed...' Unfortunately, Eleanor's lawyers did not secure a ruling that meant that the process of involuntary detention itself could only be used if a person was '... *incapable of making an informed decision about their medical care*'. And that's still the case in England and Wales. In England and Wales, despite Eleanor's victory, we can still detain people against their will and, by definition, override their capacity to give or withhold informed consent. The struggle, clearly, continues.

Autonomy and Capacity

In my opinion, it is right that the criteria include the requirement to the effect that 'the person is experiencing psychological health problems of a nature or degree which makes it appropriate for them to be admitted to a residential care establishment'. It is also appropriate to include a criterion to the effect that 'it is necessary for the person's health or safety or for the protection of other persons that they should be admitted to a residential care establishment'. These essentially reflect key criteria already in the Mental Health Act of England and Wales. They reflect the serious and compassionate judgement shown by colleagues as they implement the Act. But the English and Welsh Act does not include a further vital criterion. It does not include any reference to the person's ability to make decisions for themselves.

In a psychological approach, a concept such as 'of unsound mind' would only make sense if a person were unable to make valid decisions for themselves. This, vital, extra criterion is absent from the English and Welsh Mental Health Act. Scotland, famously, is a separate nation, with a separate legal system. In Scotland, the Mental Health (Care and Treatment) (Scotland) Act, 2003,[5] includes a criterion; '… *that because of the mental disorder the patient's ability to make decisions about the provision of such medical treatment is significantly impaired*'. In Canada, the relevant criteria include that '…*the person is unable to understand and to make an informed decision regarding his or her need for treatment, care or supervision as a result of the mental disorder*'.

Were English and Welsh law to adopt this criterion, it would draw mental health legislation much closer to the UK's Mental Capacity Act. The Mental Capacity Act is designed to protect people who may permanently or temporarily not be able ('lack capacity') to make some decisions for themselves. The Act covers issues such as 'Enduring Power of Attorney' and is designed to deal with important decisions relating to an individual's property, financial affairs, and health and social care. It also applies to everyday decisions, such as personal care, what to wear and what to eat. It sets out tests for such decision-making capacity and sets out how people may make decisions for people in those circumstances; bearing in mind the legal responsibility to ensure that any decision made on their behalf is made in their best interests. There are obvious points of similarity between the Mental Capacity Act and proposed revisions to the Mental Health Act.

Until recently, compulsory mental health care was very largely restricted to inpatient hospital settings. But discharge has always been a matter of concern. In the UK, clinicians had been in the practice of occasionally offering people 'long leave'; retaining the element of compulsion because the individual was officially 'detained in hospital' but discharged 'on leave'. This practice was ruled unlawful, and in 2007 the UK government introduced 'community treatment orders'. These allow people to be discharged from hospital, but they are required to adhere to a care plan drawn up by their 'responsible clinician'. I have little faith in the benefits of long-term medication, and I passionately support the principle of autonomy for people able to exercise it. But equally I don't think that people are 'ill', and I don't believe in the concept of 'hospital care' in this context. Many mental health problems are not only serious but also longstanding or recurrent. If someone requires ongoing help, it may be a 'least restrictive alternative' to supervise people in their own homes. I do think, therefore, that there are circumstances where it might be reasonable to see psychological health legislation outside a hospital setting. Indeed, rather controversially, my colleague Dr. Sara Tai and I argued this in a paper published in 2008.[6] Community treatment orders are highly controversial. Many people feel that they are entirely unwarranted intrusions into a person's private life. Many people feel that they are merely legal tools to enable compulsion to be continued even after hospital discharge. There are conflicting views on their effectiveness.[7] My view is that we should be guided by both principles (in this case, particularly, fundamental rights) and science. If the evidence is that community treatment orders help to reduce coercion and unnecessary intrusion into our private and family lives that would generally support their use. If, on the other hand, there is evidence that people are inappropriately subjected to coercion (for instance, people being placed on community treatment orders when they do not meet the legal criteria) or if there is evidence that they do more harm than good, then we should change our policy. But it should always be the case that the same principles—necessity and lack of capacity—should guide the use of such legislation. We should only be subject to community treatment orders, or hospital detention, if we are no longer able to exercise consent. In such circumstances, but only in such circumstances, it is reasonable to consider the least restrictive ways in which our best interests can be protected. There should be much greater judicial oversight.

Warrants

In my opinion, a further change to the law is also required. The deprivation of rights and liberties represented by the use of mental health legislation is serious. Although it is reasonable—even necessary—that we care for someone if they are temporarily or permanently unable to exercise rational autonomy, it is important that we have proper judicial oversight over this process. Other intrusions into peoples' rights and liberties are governed by the strict application of warrants, only under exceptional circumstances do we tolerate a 'permissive' approach, merely allowing authorities to override our rights. We (at least in the UK) require a judicial warrant to arrest someone (an 'arrest warrant') or to search someone's house (a 'search warrant'). These aren't particularly difficult to obtain; a police officer makes an application to a duty magistrate, presents evidence that the necessary criteria are met, and the process is sanctioned. Importantly, sanctioned under legal authority. All applications of mental health legislation (in England and Wales, the Mental Health Act) should be sanctioned by warrant. That would, necessarily, put a hurdle in the process of 'sectioning'. That is right and proper. It is simply appropriate that such a serious legal, as well as clinical, decision should be legally sanctioned. And any pressure to reduce the level of compulsion in mental health care should be welcomed. Most importantly, it is right that evidence that someone meets the criteria for the legislation to be applied. This should include the criterion that they are not able to exercise their own decision-making autonomy at that point. It should also be presented to a neutral, judicial, authority before action is taken.

In my opinion, it is only right for us to use the savage powers of mental health legislation when a magistrate or judge has issued a warrant; after first being persuaded both that detention is necessary for the person's health or safety or that of others, and also that the person is unable at that point to make an informed decision regarding their care. This would certainly not mean that a person in great and acute distress (and, perhaps, causing a public disturbance) would be left without help while complex bureaucratic processes are pursued to obtain a warrant. It is important to balance a desire for judicial oversight with a need for urgent action to assist people in distress. As with arrest or search warrants in the criminal justice system, it is perfectly possible to legislate for a reasonable balance in these issues. The various sections of the UK's Mental Health Act already include provisions for immediate response to acute need, with subsequent actions required within 72 hours. What would differ if there were proper judicial review is that, within 72 hours, a warrant would be required from the courts. This is different from the present system that merely requires compliance with the provisions of the legislation without specific judicial oversight.

As a minor historical note, as I was writing this book, I was offered access to Liverpool City Council's historical archive. This includes paperwork relating to admission to local 'Asylums' dating from 1851 (and a lot more besides). It's noteworthy that, in 1851, the procedure was that a properly credentialed 'surgeon' presented evidence to a Justice of the Peace (a local judge) who issued the order of admission to the asylum on the basis of the evidence provided. In other words, we appear to have reduced the level of judicial oversight needed before our rights can be overturned.

Psychologists and Compulsion

Until recently, psychologists have not been directly involved in imposing compulsory mental health care. In England and Wales, the amendments to the Mental Health Act in 2007 brought a significant change in the form of the new role of 'responsible clinician'. The 'responsible clinician' replaces the old role of 'responsible medical officer' and is the person responsible for a person's care while detained under the Mental Health Act. Clinical Psychologists as well as psychiatrists can now be 'responsible clinicians'. This is a profound change in our potential role within mental health care (although it will apply to those of us who adopt this responsibility). Indeed, the psychologist David Smail has said: '... *what makes [psychologists] different from other professions in the field is...[that we]...can't lock them up; we can't drug them or stun them with electricity; we can't take their children away from them. The only power we have is the power of persuasion and this... more or less forces us into an attitude of respect towards our clients*'.[8] This relationship between clinical psychologists and their clients could be threatened by compulsion. But what makes psychologists different from other professions is not only a historical absence of formal power but also a markedly different framework of knowledge and skills. The argument made in this book is that a different, new psychosocial model of care is required. Although I am well aware of the potential dangers, I am also of the opinion that this different approach to care planning should be available to people in the most acute need. In time, it should be routine for the 'responsible clinician' to be a psychologist or social worker.

Notes

1. http://www.guardian.co.uk/commentisfree/2013/feb/01/mental-health-services-coercion.
2. http://www.asylumonline.net/too-much-coercion-in-mental-health-services-by-richard-bentall/.
3. The Act can be read here: http://www.legislation.gov.uk/ukpga/2007/12/contents but it is quite complex and legalistic. The Wikipedia page is, therefore, helpful: http://en.wikipedia.org/wiki/Mental_Health_Act_2007.
4. The specific case involved (Winterwerp v. The Netherlands [Article 50]—6301/73 [1981] ECHR 7 [27 November 1981]) is discussed in: Michael L. Perlin, Heather Ellis Cucolo, and Alison Lynch, *Mental disability law: Cases and materials* (Durham, NC: Carolina Academic Press, 2017).
5. The Scottish Act can be found here: http://www.legislation.gov.uk/asp/2003/13/contents.
6. Peter Kinderman and Sara Tai, "Psychological models of mental disorder, human rights, and compulsory mental health care in the community," *International Journal of Law and Psychiatry* 31, no. 6 (2008): 479–486.
7. Susham Gupta, Elvan U. Akyuz, Toby Baldwin, and David Curtis, "Community treatment orders in England: Review of usage from national data," *British Journal of Psychiatry Bulletin* 42, no. 3 (2018): 119–122. https://europepmc.org/articles/PMC6048733/.
8. David Smail, "Putting our mouths where our money is," *Clinical Psychology Forum* (1993) 61: 11–14.

12

Working Practices

Services must be equipped to address the full range of people's social, personal and psychological as well as medical needs. Teams should be multidisciplinary, democratic and aligned to a psychosocial model. This would involve a greater reliance on psychological therapies and suggests that many nursing and medical colleagues should consider retraining. This model also implies a new role for consultant psychiatrists: as expert colleagues, but with leadership of multidisciplinary teams determined by the skills and personal qualities of the individual members of the team. In a psychosocial model of psychological health and wellbeing, there would be no assumption that medical psychiatrists would retain their current authority and status.

If we had the courage to implement a genuinely psychosocial approach to service delivery, we would see increased investment in the full range of professionals able to deliver therapeutic services that address people's genuine problems and—vitally—the root causes of those problems. We would not 'diagnose' so-called illnesses, but instead identify (and record) each person's experiences (using revised versions of the established ICD and DSM phenomenological codes), and equally, we would identify (and record) relevant social and environmental causal factors (again using established ICD and DSM codes). There would be a major emphasis on

© The Author(s) 2019
P. Kinderman, *A Manifesto for Mental Health*,
https://doi.org/10.1007/978-3-030-24386-9_12

prevention. We need to address such issues as divorce, marital difficulties, unemployment, stresses at work, financial difficulties, illnesses in family members, crime (both as a victim and as a perpetrator, when caught up in the criminal justice system), assaults, bullying and childhood abuse, and we need to make sure that these are recorded in the system.

Psychological therapies have their place, because we know that the way that we make sense of and respond to events is important, and therefore, the opportunity to talk through what has happened and how it has affected us is vital. But we also need to offer more practical responses. It is perfectly reasonable to expect easy access to practical business advice. If we are anxious and depressed because our businesses are in trouble (maybe problems with cash-flow), then why not offer professional financial advice and support, rather than focus on the mental health aspects? As Anne Cooke put it: '*It's no good just mopping the floor and leaving the tap running*'.

We need to work collectively to ensure that mental health services (perhaps we should be honest, and refer to these as psychological health services) can work with the criminal justice agencies to ensure both protection and justice, investigating and preventing assaults. Because marital separation is a major source of emotional stress, we should ensure that there is sufficient support for people going through separation or marital difficulties, such as mediation services, support for single parents and practical, legal and emotional support for people in difficulty in their relationships. These sources of support should be integrated with psychological health services. This presents a challenge, because if we want such services to be a fully integrated part of a comprehensive psychological health service, rather than adjunctive social services dealing with a separate, if related, issue, we need to think carefully about the management of such services. Similarly, because unemployment is a major source of distress, we should aim for full employment and certainly do what we can to protect people from the emotional and economic impact of unemployment. Many jobs are themselves sources of stress, however. We should aim to ensure equitable and supportive employment practices, including employee relations, a living wage, decent terms and conditions and appropriate employee representation. We should use some of our massive tax revenues to offer practical support for people engaged in the economic activity of our communities.

All of this is, however, more than mere political aspiration; it is a vision for how services could operate. To illustrate how our basic assumptions could change, I recently set a very standard formulation task for my students, asking them to consider a man of working age, depressed, following some difficulties in his relationship and problems in his business. All the students were excellent, and their formulations were both evidence-based and compassionate. But, in each case, their automatic assumption was that the appropriate (or expected) response was to focus on the individual, whether or not he was depressed, the predisposing, precipitating and protective factors in the development and maintenance of that depression and whether couples therapy or CBT might help. While the students mentioned rumination, mindfulness and the benefits of exercise, none of the students discussed business support interventions. Nobody recommended help that might be available from the local Chamber of Commerce, the pressures of cash-flow, or the rateable value of small business premises, or government grants. I am a clinical psychologist, so it's reasonable to expect my particular competence to address our thinking, and behaviour, and how these can maintain our problems, but we shouldn't think that this is the only way to understand the situation. Imagine, for example, that I had set students on an Masters of Business Administration (MBA), economics or politics course a similar task. My guess, or hope, is that they, too, would recognise the human challenges, but would make much more practical plans, which might, ultimately, have a greater chance of real success. Our mental health services, as presently constituted, and the default operating assumptions of our professions tend to divert our attention away from these kinds of considerations and the more effective solutions that might follow.

Those of us working in psychological health services should be supported, as part of our normal, contracted, work, to engage with employers to address workplace stresses and offer people who are out of work practical, as well as emotional, support. Services such as Citizens Advice, debt counselling agencies and Victim Support are vital to help people in financial difficulties, victims of crime and people dealing with a range of other traumatic life events. We should ensure that any psychological health services are fully integrated with these other social services that support families and parents in difficulty. It also means working with teachers and educational psychologists in schools, and it means supporting a network of children's services. This doesn't merely mean that we should have rapid and fluid pathways for referral between separate 'mental health services' and educational services (we have those already, although they are not always as rapid and fluid as they should be). It means moving the psychological health services from the medical NHS (in the UK context) into its proper realm. Debt and money worries are serious sources of stress, so we should not only offer emotional support and counsel people in financial difficulties, we should also offer people practical help and financial advice. And this means employing professional financial advisors, not merely expecting mental health workers to pretend to have skills they do not possess. We should support people in negotiations with statutory benefits agencies to ensure people have the financial and legal support that they deserve, and we should be prepared to engage with financial systems (such as 'pay-day loan' companies) that conspire to keep people indebted. Recreational street drugs can prove a threat to people's psychological health and wellbeing, and so we should ensure that psychological health services have intimate links to services that help people who have problems with drug use. Providing these services properly, in the correct configuration, will entail significant change. Many of these issues are currently largely ignored, at least tacitly. Mental health professionals are aware of these issues and make referrals when necessary, but the services are separate, and the evidence of mental health professionals' failure to record psychosocial stressors indicates not that these are unknown, or even considered a low priority; they are considered to be the responsibility of a different part of the system, the responsibility of people outside of the health service. As a result, many such links and referrals are ill-coordinated. Apologists for the present systems will argue that all these services are currently part of the care offered to clients. They might well argue that we need to improve the services that we have, rather than press for radical change. The experiences of those of us who have passed through the system would tend to suggest otherwise.

The adoption of a 'psychosocial' model for the provision of psychological health services would have significant implications, as colleagues and I have argued for some time.[1] As I have argued throughout this book, services would be planned on the basis of need and helping people find 'real-world' solutions that work for them, rather than providing 'treatments' according to unscientific and dehumanising diagnostic categories. Where residential care is necessary, we would all benefit from completely new residential units, operating according to wholly different rules, to replace 'hospitals'. This would mean that services would fully embrace the recovery approach; people would not be 'treated' for 'illnesses', but would be helped to regain (in the words of the European Commission) '... *their intellectual and emotional potential... their roles in social, school and working life'*. In this approach, those of us who use, or have used, the services would be intimately involved in their development and management as well as in the actual provision, with 'expertise by experience' highly valued. And, perhaps speaking more professionally as a clinical psychologist, any therapies, interventions and services should, in my professional opinion, be guided by individual formulations drawn up collaboratively between the person using the service and any professionals involved.

In such an approach, there would continue to be an emphasis on specialist teams, but they would be planned and organised on the basis of psychosocial rather than medical principles. As a psychologist, I am naturally likely to argue this, but better, more effective, more humane, services would be possible if psychologists were prepared to offer consultation and clinical leadership and supported in those decisions. Medicine would remain a key profession, but with emphasis placed on a return to the key principles of applying medical expertise as it assists a multidisciplinary team in the understanding of someone's problems and offering help, rather than on an unquestioned assumption that doctors should lead clinical teams. Nurses could help build better services if they were to be supported in diversifying from attending to the medical treatments prescribed by doctors and develop increasing competencies in psychosocial interventions. Occupational therapists and social workers should play much more of a role in building and leading services of the future and thereby see their roles develop and strengthen. We should be open to new possibilities; it would be particularly valuable to employ people skilled in practical issues such as finding employment or training, managing finances and caring for children. Finally, we would all benefit from improved services if we were to see the increased and explicit employment of peer professionals, people with lived experience of psychological health problems. Personal experience of psychological health problems should be seen as a desirable characteristic in colleagues, part of the positive reasons to employ someone, rather than an exclusion criterion.

Access to and Provision of Services

Decisions about the provision of psychological health care should be based on individuals' experiences and the impact of those phenomena on their personal and social functioning, rather than diagnosis of illness. Given the huge impact of mental health problems discussed earlier, there are good arguments for a substantial increase in funding for mental health care. Nevertheless, difficult decisions have to be made about to whom and in what circumstances services should be made available. Diagnostic distinctions between 'real illnesses' and 'normal reactions' are alien to psychological models of psychological wellbeing. Instead, priorities should be based on the severity of, consequences of, and risk posed by, a person's problems.

Many of my colleagues accept unquestioningly the spurious quasi-certainties of a medical diagnostic approach, where we can expect a service if we are 'ill' and not if we aren't. Some take this further. Their faith in the diagnostic system (understandably, given their training) is such that they often firmly believe that any other approach would necessarily be a loose and vague arrangement. But the assessment of psychological difficulties can be conducted following different assumptions, assumptions that have the major advantage of 'ecological validity'; they make sense in the real world.[2] The alternatives to psychiatric diagnoses are not merely narrative accounts, subjective stories. Formulation, although a necessary part of psychological health care, is not an alternative to diagnosis, either (at least in my judgement). What we need, in my professional opinion, is a system based on the operation definition and systematic recording of real, relevant, human experiences, not assumed 'symptoms' of illusionary 'mental illnesses'. As we saw earlier, these approaches not only make sense to applied scientists, they are already imbedded (although rarely used) in the standard diagnostic frameworks.

Teams, Multidisciplinary Teams and Democratic Multidisciplinary Teams

There is widespread agreement that care should be a team-based activity, but perhaps less agreement on what this means in practice. When we are referred to psychological health services, whether seeing an individual therapist, attending alternative day services or admitted to residential care, we should expect to have their full range of relevant needs assessed and then addressed by an appropriate range of properly qualified specialists. As I have made clear throughout this book, the range of needs; social, psychological and medical (in different proportions for different people) means that the team requires a range of specialists working together.

Looking to the future, my vision—my manifesto—is for greater breadth and integration in psychological health care. That means explicitly aiming to address a broader spectrum of problems and integrating the skills needed to address them. We should therefore aim for a broader, yet more integrated, team of professionals with diverse skills. Our role is to help people solve problems and resolve the understandable psychological consequences, not merely 'treat' illnesses'. This approach implies that medical colleagues will still clearly remain valuable members of the team, but they would best be thought of as consultants *to* the team rather than having sapiential authority *over* it.

I apologise for introducing the word 'sapiential'. It was new to me, too, until a few years ago. I was first made aware of this interesting word when I was involved in the discussions surrounding the New Ways of Working report.[3] One of our tasks was to look at both the shared, generic, and the 'specific and distinctive' contributions that each profession makes to a multidisciplinary team. We received a draft document from the working party looking at the distinctive contribution of the consultant psychiatrist. To begin with, the document acknowledged that: '...*a well functioning multi-disciplinary team requires leadership from several individuals with different levels of expertise in different areas – leading on what each knows best...*'. I agree. But the (draft) commentary continued, immediately, to argue that: '...*such is the clinical primacy of the consultant in dealing with treatment resistant, acute, severe or dangerous clinical situations that require the broadest possible approach covering all physical, legal, psychological, and social aspects, as well as analysing and making explicit the value and ethical aspects of choices or decisions to be made. It is more sapiential than hierarchical leadership. This will become much clearer with the shift from delegated to distributed responsibility for patients in community mental health teams. It will be up to the autonomous professional to decide when to seek advice or case review with a consultant. And every time that happens it will give meaning to the clinical primacy of the consultant with whom the "buck stops" in given situations'.*

I'm sorry for such a lengthy quote, but it is important (and quite shocking, really). In other words, multidisciplinary teams need to employ people with a range of skills (by definition), but the consultant psychiatrist should always be in charge. Deconstructing the language used is important. 'Clinical primacy of the consultant' is a phrase that implies a medical professional should be in charge, directly contradicting the immediately preceding statement: '*... individuals with... expertise in different areas – leading on what each knows best...*'. It's impossible for both statements simultaneously to be true. This point becomes even clearer when the text suggests that: '*...the autonomous professional...*' should '*... seek advice or case review from a consultant... with whom the "buck stops"...*'. So much for autonomy!

These comments were, as I said, in a draft document for a Department of Health report on multidisciplinary working. As a member of the working party, I had serious objections to this draft. But I was also intrigued by the use of the word sapiential. I had not come across it before and had to look it up. The dictionary definition is: '*...relating to wisdom...*'. Most dictionaries add that the word is 'from ecclesiastical Latin' and relates particularly to the wisdom of God.

I agree that: 'a well functioning multidisciplinary team requires leadership from several individuals with different levels of expertise in different areas – leading on what each knows best'. I do not agree with the concept of 'clinical primacy', I do not agree that 'autonomous professionals' should have their decisions reviewed by a 'consultant' (that makes a mockery of 'autonomous') and I do not believe that any one profession has 'sapiential leadership'. Fortunately, I and my colleagues were able to impose common sense on the proceedings (although I confess that I asked a colleague to accompany me to the next meeting of the working party, at which this draft was to be reviewed, for moral support). This wording does not feature in the final report.

The right place for psychological health care is in the community, alongside GPs, public health physicians and social workers. There should be a network of community-based care teams, linked to social services provision and other local authority care and services, as well as to the NHS and third-sector organisations. In the UK, this is consistent with a general policy for integration of current mental health services with physical health care and social care. We've seen a major integration of GP services with wider community and social services. Importantly, we've also recently seen UK public health services transferred wholesale into local authority management. This is a highly controversial move and coincides with (perhaps even permitted) significant cuts to public health services. But it also offers a precedent and a model for similar transfer of responsibilities for psychological health care. This would see opportunities for GPs, properly trained in psychological health care, in helping to support our psychological wellbeing. It would see many more clinical psychologists, but, as with our medical colleagues, they would be working in the community, not in hospitals or 'clinics'. And, consistent with the conclusions of our 'New Ways of Working' report mentioned earlier, medical psychiatrists would be vital colleagues, but consultants to, not in charge of, those teams.

When I was writing *A Prescription for Psychiatry*, I turned to a colleague, a senior and respected psychiatrist (whom it would be unwise and unhelpful to name), to help check the validity of some points I was making. My colleague's response was helpful on the specific questions, but also took the opportunity to comment on the wider argument: '… *I think you can make a perfectly coherent argument for the total dissolution of psychiatry. In an ideal world, I don't think it would exist, or if it did, it would simply be medical professionals interested in the care of the mad alongside other professionals, much as it started out being in the asylum days of the 19th century…*'. That was, remember, a psychiatrist writing, not me. But I largely agree. Since our mental health and wellbeing are predominantly a social and psychological phenomenon, since diagnosis is unhelpful and the prescription of drugs is best reserved for a minority (and managed in a more pragmatic manner than at present), we would do well to see a much greater reliance on GPs to provide for the holistic health care of their patients.

Again, in *A Prescription for Psychiatry*, I commented that: '*In this vision, medical psychiatrists would still perhaps have roles: as specialists, as consultants to GPs and as consultants to residential units*'.

In retrospect, I can see why the addition of the word 'perhaps' may have caused offence. The phrase '... *would still have roles...*' may well have passed unchallenged. Adding *'perhaps'* appears to have been a red rag to a bull—questioning the 'sapiential authority'; and 'clinical primacy' of a socially dominant profession.

Nevertheless, I stand by my views. The scientific evidence, and the political and policy considerations that follow, argue for a major rebalancing of investment away from what is now traditional psychiatry towards a different system. Not the 'total dissolution of psychiatry', but a very significant change. And this implies change for several professions.

Psychology

For my chosen profession of clinical psychology, adopting this manifesto for change could have significant consequences. The profession of clinical psychology has its roots in mental health, and it is highly likely that addressing psychological health problems will remain the key focus of our work for the foreseeable future. Clinical psychologists are experts in psychological therapies (and, in the UK at least, must be competent in at least two forms of psychological therapy in order to retain their professional registration with the Health and Care Professions Council), so it is highly likely that we will continue to offer one-to-one therapy. But other professions are also skilled therapists, and as well as providing therapy, clinical psychologists have been calling for more socially responsible, more fully holistic, services for many years.

Most of my colleagues would welcome more engagement across all the domains of psychological wellbeing discussed earlier. We value one-to-one engagement with clients and (generally) believe that we have skills to offer in that respect. But we know that real change requires deeper engagement. For some of my clinical psychology colleagues, this does not require a wholesale rejection of what I call the 'disease-model' of mental health care. For many of my colleagues, their therapies (often CBT or cognitive behaviour therapy) are effective and helpful, and they are fully supportive of a preventative approach, addressing social determinants of conditions that are accepted as 'mental disorders'. Many colleagues are agnostic about the diagnostic debate. Many are comfortable with the tacitly pathologising (but not biologically reductionist) idea that 'thinking errors' lie behind those mental disorders. Many colleagues are critical of diagnoses. For me—as I hope I have made clear—my rejection of the 'disease-model' approach, my rejection of the notion that pathologies lie behind our difficulties (a rejection based soundly on the available evidence) and my scepticism, therefore, that either therapy or medication are anything other than 'sticking-plaster' solutions, means that I look to my own profession for deeper and more meaningful engagement.

That means seeing clinical psychologists working in occupational health and occupational psychology services, helping people reduce workplace stress, minimising the likelihood of absence due to emotional problems and maximising productivity. It means seeing clinical psychologists working with schools and teachers, helping children learn, but also helping children, teachers and parents deal more effectively with emotional issues. In the model for psychological health I am advocating, we would expect to see clinical psychologists working more closely with the physical health services, supporting patients with serious physical illnesses, helping them adjust to illness or injury, helping with rehabilitation and maximising the likelihood that people take steps towards becoming fitter and healthier. Across a wide range of community services, I want to see clinical psychologists offering their skills in sports and leisure, with charities, with local authority services... across the full breadth of the domains of wellbeing, in all areas of psychological health and across all social services.

To achieve these aims, our employers need to understand—and support—this shift. Most clinical psychologists in the UK are currently employed by NHS Trusts. It is perhaps unfortunate that our history of close links with mental health services, and our undoubted expertise in one-to-one psychological therapies, mean that clinical psychologists are often seen as valued staff if and when they see individual clients, but are less often encouraged to pursue any broader roles. We would be better able to enact the changes I am advocating, if psychological health services as a whole, including clinical psychologists, were managed in local authority settings.

A wider focus, beyond 'mental health', or, worse 'mental illness', and instead addressing psychological wellbeing, would mean looking at the links between 'clinical' psychology and the other applied psychologist groups. I would welcome the integration of clinical psychologists' interest in psychological health with occupational psychologists' interest in employment, educational psychologists' interest in education, health psychologists, forensic psychologists and so on. All these sub-groups share the overarching professional discipline as applied scientists of applying our knowledge of psychological theory to addressing social problems and improving wellbeing. That makes this is less a call for clinical psychologists as a very specific group to broaden their ambitions across all of life, but rather more a call for applied psychologists to work together to apply their skills and knowledge in a coherent manner across all these domains of psychological health and wellbeing. We should be confident, but applied psychology itself needs to reform.

Our clients—individuals, families, organisations and communities—would benefit if we were to unify our currently disparate 'brands' of applied psychology into a single profession... and we need to make that profession more genuinely fit for purpose. That means reforming our professional body, the British Psychological Society. In 2017, when I served as President of the Society, I argued that psychologists—and therefore the British Psychological Society—were experts in things that really matter to people: relationships, education and learning, health, mental health, politics, sport, crime, work, how organisations function, prejudice and intercultural understanding and more. As professionals, we have a duty to act in the best interests of our clients and to protect and promote their fundamental rights. Perhaps most importantly the British Psychological Society is a charity, and therefore, it does not primarily exist to serve itself or even its members, but the public.[4]

To embrace this responsibility, we should also look at our training. As long ago as 2002, I recommended that one way to make our profession more suited to the model of psychological health recommended here would be to be more integrated into our training.[5] I suggested that we consider training occupational, clinical, health, educational and forensic psychologists together in a generic curriculum in the first year of our three-year doctoral training, tapering to more specialist training in year three. This would ensure that each person would finish their training with the skills necessary to register as a member of each branch of applied psychology (clinical or occupational or whatever). I still think it would be a good idea if our trainee psychologists follow a pathway through training involving a much greater degree of integrated exposure to other approaches within applied psychology and the wider social context of psychological health.

Psychologists as Prescribers?

Some of my clinical psychologist colleagues have discussed the possibility of extending their professional responsibilities into the limited prescription of psychiatric drugs. There are precedents for this, both internationally (psychologists in several nations or states already have limited rights to prescribe medication) and in terms of other professions, such as nursing, whose members have had the right to prescribe medication for some time. In most cases, this is regulated as 'supplementary prescribing', whereby a medical practitioner will approve a certain list of medications which can be administered to certain patients according to a pre-approved schedule or plan. In this scenario, it has been suggested by some of my colleagues (including, as it happens, my former Ph.D. supervisor) that clinical psychologists could take on a similar role in mental health care.

In the USA, some psychologists working for the US Department of Defence were given limited prescribing privileges in a carefully monitored pilot project that began in 1988. Now, because the USA has a federal legislative system, psychologists are allowed to prescribe medication in five US states (New Mexico, Louisiana, Illinois, Iowa and Idaho), if working for the military and in the US territory of Guam. The general opinion is that these initiatives have proceeded successfully and safely. Given the relative similarities of US and UK healthcare, and the training and skills of both psychiatrists and psychologists in the two countries, it seems reasonable to think that psychologists could learn to prescribe safely in the UK if there were sufficient will and resources to make this happen.

There are some positive arguments in favour of giving psychologists prescribing privileges. Given that the NHS in the UK is currently struggling to recruit a sufficient number of young doctors to train and work in psychiatry, and because the NHS as a whole is suffering from serious funding cuts (and especially in mental health), anything that saves money might be seen as beneficial. If one profession (psychology) were to be trained in both psychological and biomedical approaches to care, this might also help speed the routes through training. It has been argued that people using mental health services might find it helpful if the same professional was responsible for both pharmacotherapy and psychological therapy. For example, a psychologist might wish to prescribe medication in the short-term to someone who is entering therapy during a crisis. It has been argued that, then, the psychologist would be in a good position to taper their client off the medication as the therapy progresses. It is important to remember that any right to prescribe medication is also a right to take a person off medication, and this may well be a good proposition in the light of the adverse effects noted earlier.

However, from my perspective, I would be very unhappy if psychologists were to begin to offer medication. As I have argued throughout this book, we, collectively, rely on medication too much, at too high doses, too much as a 'knee-jerk' reaction to problems that are not illnesses. That means, as Jo Moncrieff argues, while medication may be a pragmatic response of a civilised society, these chemicals aren't 'cures' and aren't putting right underlying pathologies. These mistakes have not happened because there is something particularly wicked, venal, stupid or unimaginative about my psychiatrist colleagues. I don't think they would magically disappear if psychologists, rather than psychiatrists, were to be in charge of the prescription pad.

It has been argued that psychologists should be prepared to hold the reins of psychiatric medication, so they can limit use, and that the 'pragmatic' approach fits better with a psychologist's remit. It has been argued that psychologist could help their clients withdraw from medication. The 'prescription privileges' argument also plays well to psychologists in their (occasional) desire to have authority in clinical teams; it's argued that, with these rights, psychologists could either negotiate with colleagues on equal terms, or even render them redundant. I disagree and even worry about the opposite effect that psychologists who have the capacity to prescribe medication might spend less time delivering psychological therapies. Indeed, as one of the proponents of psychologist prescribing has himself said: '...*the biggest risk of allowing psychologists to prescribe might well be the weakening of the only NHS workforce that is specifically dedicated to the promotion of psychological approaches*'. My worry is that, just as the medical profession has gravitated towards the use of prescription, a supposedly effective, cheap, readily-available, understandable (but inappropriate) quasi-solution to social problems, we would too.

Instead, psychologists would be perfectly placed to lead teams which include people with specialist knowledge that we do not, because of our training and education, possess (just as we possess specialist skills and knowledge that they do not have). My view is that we should not incorporate the role of other professions within our skill set, we should, instead, employ them under our direct (and authoritative) leadership. My view is that, if the technical knowledge relevant to medication prescription or de-prescription is needed, we should bring on board people with those skills to supplement our team, as and when we need those skills.

Social Work

Social factors are the most important in the origin of our psychological problems, and this places a priority on social interventions. It logically follows that the most appropriate professionals to coordinate psychological health services may well be social workers. My argument throughout this book has been that our emotional distress is largely determined by our social circumstances, the events that happen to us, and how we have learned to appraise and respond to those events. It makes sense, then, to see psychological health services as integral to the social services delivered (in the UK) by local authorities. As I will set out in more detail in the next chapter, not only do I envisage a much more 'social' ethos to those psychological health services, I also believe that our mental health—psychological health—services would be most effective, most humane and most accessible, if they were managed within wider social services and indeed organised and managed through local authority structures. Meaningful recovery, defined in the European Commission terms of social, psychological or occupational functioning, is influenced as much by social class, opportunities for employment and economic and social policy as by 'successful' treatment of what we currently incorrectly think of as psychiatric illnesses.[6] Social workers are currently the only mental health workers with specific and comprehensive education and training in the application of social science to practical effect in individuals' lives.[7]

The training of social workers, like psychologists, psychiatrists and nurses, covers a wide range of theoretical perspectives and skills. The distinctive contribution of social workers, perhaps especially in promoting social inclusion, means they are vital in organising and commissioning care packages beyond the health systems. I value this, but we could go further. Like other professions (psychology, nursing), I would like to see many more social workers leading teams. I would prefer to see a dominant social ethos to mental health (at present, 'psychological health' in the future) services. I would therefore prefer to see a medical ethos and the distinctive medical skills of my colleagues contributing to a multi-disciplinary team managed, organised, and led, by social workers.

Psychological health services, and those of us who use such services, may also benefit from greater use of the slightly more direct and therapeutic role offered by 'social pedagogues' elsewhere in the EU.[8] Social pedagogues are members of a profession which is widely recognised in many countries but relatively unknown in the UK. Social pedagogy is a profession with a particular focus on early years education, but which can be useful with any age group. Not unlike occupational therapists, social pedagogues deploy a wide range of academic disciplines (sociology, psychology, education, philosophy, the medical sciences and social work) to help us develop our skills and self confidence in dealing with emotions and relationships.

Psychiatry

In the vision for multidisciplinary psychological health services that I am proposing, psychiatrists (medically qualified doctors specialising in psychiatry) will continue to have an important role. Paradoxically, rather than recommending that my medical colleagues become some form of ersatz psychotherapists (aping the role of colleagues who are trained, skilled and qualified in psychological therapies), or attempting to usurp the role of social workers (attempting to observe and analyse the impact of social and environmental factors on our wellbeing), medical practitioners should use their education, skills and training to focus on medical health care and on the specifically biological aspects of mental health.

There is no reason to deviate from the basic principles of the 'New Ways of Working' approach that a multidisciplinary team should be made up from colleagues with complementary skills. I have great respect for the medical skills of my colleagues and recognise that I don't possess such skills myself. Equally, the eight years of specialist education, experience and training that led to my qualification as a clinical psychologist also give me some specialist skills. It would be foolish to build teams where there is total duplication of skills, even if that were possible. On the other hand, even though I believe that a social model of psychological health (as opposed to a 'disease model') is fundamentally correct, and even though I repudiate the diagnostic approach and wish to see a radical reduction in the use of medication, I am nevertheless of the view that there remains a vital role for medical colleagues in the multidisciplinary psychological health teams of the future.

At one rather tense meeting, I was once informed by a very senior psychiatrist that, as well as the (enormously comprehensive and taxing) curriculum of physical medicine, he and his medical colleagues had studied both sociology and psychology during their training. I presume, but didn't bother asking, that he meant the odd lecture as part of his medical studies, rather than anything more comprehensive. He asserted, therefore, that he was able to do the job of both social workers and clinical psychologists, but they, because they hadn't studied medicine, couldn't do his. A colleague (another psychiatrist, but someone I consider a friend) actually physically restrained me with a firm hand on my shoulder.

Instead of attempting to do everybody else's job (poorly), there would be massive benefits for members of the public who use psychological health services if medically qualified members of the team were to retain a specific focus on the application of medical knowledge. Although family doctors or GPs would be the most appropriate medical practitioner for most people, psychiatrists have key roles. These would, in the model of care that I am proposing, include identifying those very rare cases where a person's apparent psychological problems have a physical cause, as in the example of the young man with an aneurysm mentioned earlier. Although such cases are extremely rare, it is important to provide this service. More importantly, because it is much more common, we know that the physical health of people with serious psychological problems can be badly affected. It follows that medical, as well as nursing, colleagues are vital, not so much to address the psychological issues, but to address primary physical health concerns. I have made it clear how important, and equally how inadequate such physical health care is in the current configuration of services… bizarrely, since our mental health care system is too medicalised, it simultaneously neglects the medical welfare of patients. Such physical health care requires close liaison with community-based, primary care healthcare systems (in the UK, the GPs who offer our comprehensive first point of care and family doctor services), another good reason to prefer a primary care rather than secondary care focus.

Finally, psychiatrists have a role in the prescription of psychiatric drugs. I really don't need to repeat that I would wish to see a sharply reduced reliance on such medication. I have also discussed how the evidence points to how social, rather than biological, factors have a dominant role in the origins of psychological problems. Nevertheless, it will always remain important that psychological health services have access to competent medical professionals to assess the possible contribution of biological factors and to prescribe drugs (if people want to take them). Psychiatrists would therefore remain a crucial component of care, although, in the vision that I am setting out here, their role might change a little.

Nursing

Paralleling the profound changes in the use of medical staff that would follow if we were to adopt the kind of psychosocial model for psychological health services outlined here, we could imagine significant changes to the role of nurses. In most countries, certainly in the UK, mental health nurses form the backbone of services, acting as front-line carers, and are the most common staff group offering 24 hours a day, 7 days a week care. There are over 45,000 mental health nurses in the UK, more than the number of psychiatrists and clinical psychologists combined. Mental health nurses work in all areas of mental health services and frequently act as care coordinators. For many people, nurses are the only direct care providers, although their role is increasingly being taken over by unqualified 'support workers'.

My vision for psychosocial care offers new opportunities for mental health nurses. My proposals involve a very substantial shift from a medical to a psychosocial approach. That means a greater application of social and psychosocial solutions and less reliance on medical interventions. Nurses do much more than support the use of medication and do more than act as functional adjuncts of doctors, and it is those more autonomous professional competencies, especially in psychosocial interventions that I would wish to develop. In essence, I would like to see a profound shift in nurses' professional activity to mirror the paradigmatic shift in psychological health services from a medical, disease-model, approach to a psychosocial ethos.

We can already see this shift within the profession, especially in the UK and the USA. Basic nursing training, for mental health nurses, now emphasises psychosocial perspectives and interventions. In the UK and USA, nurses practise forms of structured psychological therapy such as CBT regularly. Indeed, the UK's 'IAPT' programme, the government-backed policy of increasing substantially the number of people able to access psychological therapies, relies heavily on nurses and other mental health professionals (and, largely, not qualified clinical psychologists), who are offered additional training in those psychological therapies and an improved role. Incidentally, part of the IAPT programme involves learning lessons from the early days of developing CBT for people with more serious psychological problems. We were able to train psychiatrists and nurses in the basic principles of CBT, and that they were (in most cases) able to practice competently. But it proved difficult to implement widespread CBT in practice, because the working style of mental health nurses in traditional roles tended not to support the regular scheduled appointments needed for such therapy. Reforms of the system, as well as additional skills, are needed. So, my observation is that my nursing colleagues are actively developing their skills as psychosocial practitioners.

We could even consider changing the name of mental health nurses to reflect a new emphasis. The 'nurse' role and title stem from physical health care, from medicine and appear slightly inappropriate in a psychosocial service. The name and role of the nurse also, wrongly, imply a subservience to medicine. Although undoubtedly to be controversial, renaming 'mental health nurses' might be a very powerful way to signal change in the system. Of course, it would be for my colleagues to choose and define their own identity, but a possibility would be something like 'psychosocial therapist'. I also have at least one anecdotal reason to believe that at least some senior nurses would welcome the kind of transformational change I am recommending.

When people in my line of work attend meetings to discuss policy issues, we often stay overnight (usually in very cheap, wholly unappealing, hotel chains). On one occasion, I was having an evening meal (again, I should stress, the least glamorous option available) with two senior colleagues, an employee of the government Department of Health and the then representative in our discussions from the mental health nurses' section of the UK's Royal College of Nursing. We were chatting, developing our ideas a little more fluidly in an informal setting, and I expressed some views along these lines. My nursing colleague simply said: '*I've been saying that myself for years*'.

The model of psychological health services I am proposing would also support the development of the autonomy and independence of nurses in a 'consultant' role, as well as strongly supporting the development of nurses' competencies in psychological aspects of care and in psychological interventions. In recent years, the role of the mental health nurse has already evolved in this direction, but there is a convincing argument for a substantial change in the nature and profile of the nursing role. The training of 'nurses' should reflect the science of psychological health and should therefore emphasise psychosocial, not medical approaches and interventions.

Occupational Therapy

Meaningful and purposeful activity is an important element of all forms of psychological health care, in both community settings and residential care. Earlier in this book, I quoted a short extract from a letter I had received from a man describing his experiences on a psychiatric inpatient ward. This is not at all what residential units should be like. My correspondent's experience may be unusual, and it may reflect a practice that is dying out. I hope that's true. But in any case, I would like to imagine a world in which a day spent in a residential unit would involve practical steps towards psychological health in the form of physical exercise, a trip to a gym or to a swimming pool, perhaps, and but also other valuable, purposeful, activity during the day; activity that is therapeutic is geared towards the 'five ways to well-being' and is meaningful to each person.

We tend to stress physical activity and exercise. There is very good evidence that physical exercise is excellent for our psychological health. But I would want more. If I were a resident of a psychological health unit, I would want access to exercise, but also access to books writing materials, the Internet, music (both to listen to, and to create), art (again, both beautiful artworks, and more than the institutional murals so common in clinic environments, and creative activities), nature, learning (history, geography, science), discussion, dance… Given the very circumstances that very understandably lead people to develop psychological problems, I'd also expect access to training, financial advice, legal and business advice, self-defence training… All this would require investment, but I simply don't think that it's too much to ask for.

This kind of thinking, which is inherent to the model of psychological health I'm advocating, could see greater opportunities for colleagues working in occupational therapy. And, rather than being mere distraction while in residential care, such therapy may have far-reaching implications. While we must protect people from unreasonable expectations (particularly from right-wing politicians who seem to believe that people who have benefitted from the structures of society are owed something by the most vulnerable and poor), there is plenty of evidence that meaningful, valued, freely chosen, employment is valuable in promoting recovery for those of us who have experienced psychological problems.[9] Unsurprisingly, however, those of us who have had such problems often face major challenges in the employment market.[10] Occupational therapy aims to address 'the nature, balance, pattern and context of occupations and activities in the lives of individuals, family groups and communities'[11] but, like nurses and indeed psychiatrists, occupational therapists are now also rapidly developing skills in psychological therapies. Like social workers, occupational therapists also have a particular focus on issues of social inclusion. Occupational therapy, then, should be central to any psychological health service along the lines advocated here.

Is This Really a Change?

Many of my colleagues, especially from conservative professions, might point out that these changes are happening already. It is certainly true that, over recent years, a number of government initiatives have supported psychosocial approaches, have emphasised patient-centred services and have supported a 'recovery' approach. The UK government's IAPT ('*Improving Access to Psychological Therapies*') programme has seen over £1bn ring-fenced investment in psychological and psychosocial therapies. Policies such as the 'New Ways of Working' discussions have repeatedly stressed the importance of multidisciplinary teams and of a biopsychosocial model underpinning care. Most importantly critics who might argue that my manifesto is redundant would point to the many policies recommending the inclusion of such services as debt counselling, drugs services, court diversion schemes and the creative arts of various kinds in the 'landscape of care'. Mental health services are now, they would argue, working: 'more closely with grass-roots voluntary agencies and self-help groups, including offering helping-the-helpers support, or taking responsibility ourselves for training and supervising community members'.[12]

I agree. All these are positive. But failing to challenge the 'disease model' of mental health, even positive evolutionary changes can leave intact the basic, damaging, idea that currently drives our mental health services, namely that psychological and emotional difficulties are merely symptoms of an underlying physical 'mental illness' or brain disease. For many of my colleagues who promote a more humane approach, half-hearted claims to be addressing social issues usually boil down to suggesting that they, themselves, will continue to offer a medical specialism, but *somebody else* needs to add a dose of social perspective. This simply threatens to perpetuate the status quo. Real change—a paradigm shift—will come when we move beyond the idea that psychological health issues are essentially medical problems with social aspects (like any other illnesses) and acknowledge that what we are talking about are essentially social and psychological problems. Radical change is needed to ensure that the management, leadership and practices of services reflect this.

Notes

1. Peter Kinderman, William Sellwood, and Sara Tai, "Policy implications of a psychological model of mental disorder," *Journal of Mental Health* 17, no. 1 (2008): 93–103. https://doi.org/10.1080/09638230701530226.

2. Anne Cooke, *Understanding psychosis and schizophrenia: Why people sometimes hear voices, believe things that others find strange, or appear out of touch with reality... and what can help* (Leicester: British Psychological Society, 2017). Available from: www.understandingpsychosis.net.

3. National Institute for Mental Health in England, *Guidance on new ways of working for psychiatrists in a multidisciplinary and multi-agency context* (London: National Institute of Mental Health in England, 2004).

4. My Presidential Address to the British Psychological Society can be found here: https://thepsychologist.bps.org.uk/volume-30/june-2017/psychology-action-not-thinking-about-oneself.

5. Peter Kinderman, "The future of clinical psychology training," *Clinical Psychology* 8 (2002): 6–10.
6. Richard Warner, *Recovery from schizophrenia: Psychiatry and political economy* (New York: Routledge, 2013).
7. Care Services Improvement Partnership and National Institute for Mental Health in England, *The social work contribution to mental health services—The future direction* (London: Care Services Improvement Partnership and National Institute for Mental Health in England, 2006).
8. See, for example: http://www.rywu.org.uk/wp-content/uploads/2010/05/Social-Pedagogy-Report.pdf as well as Jacob Kornbeck, "Reflections on the exportability of social pedagogy and its possible limits," *Social Work in Europe* 9, no. 2 (2002): 37–49 and Stewart Asquith, Chris L. Clark, and Lorraine Waterhouse, *The role of the social worker in the 21st century: A literature review* (Edinburgh: Scottish Executive Education Department, 2005). http://www.scotland.gov.uk/Resource/Doc/47121/0020821.pdf.
9. Jed Boardman, Bob Grove, Rachel Perkins, and Geoff Shepherd, "Work and employment for people with psychiatric disabilities," *The British Journal of Psychiatry* 182, no. 6 (2003): 467–468.
10. Peter Huxley and Graham Thornicroft, "Social inclusion, social quality and mental illness," *The British Journal of Psychiatry* 182, no. 4 (2003): 289–290 and Office of the Deputy Prime Minister, *Mental health and social exclusion: Social exclusion unit report* (London: Cabinet Office, 2004).
11. National Institute for Mental Health in England, *Guidance on new ways of working for psychiatrists in a multi-disciplinary and multi-agency context* (London: National Institute of Mental Health in England, 2004).
12. Alison Hauenstein Swan, "Lessons I learned in war zones," *Clinical Psychology* 46 (2005): 6–9.

13

The Social and Political Prerequisites for Genuine Psychological Health and Wellbeing

Our psychological health and wellbeing are largely dependent on our social circumstances. To promote genuine psychological health and wellbeing, we need to protect and promote universal human rights, as enshrined in the United Nations' Universal Declaration of Human Rights. Because experiences of neglect, rejection and abuse are hugely important in the genesis of many problems, we need to redouble our efforts to protect children from emotional, physical or sexual abuse and neglect. Equally, we must protect both adults and children from bullying and discrimination: whether that is racism, homophobia or discrimination based on sexuality, gender, disability or 'mental health' or any other characteristic. We can all do more to combat discrimination and promote a more tolerant and accepting society. More generally, if we are serious about preventing psychological health problems from developing and about promoting genuine psychological well-being, we must work collectively to create a more humane society: to reduce or eliminate poverty, especially childhood poverty, and to reduce financial and social inequality. We need to work harder to promote peace, social justice and equity and ensure that citizens are properly fed, housed and educated and living in a sustainable natural ecosystem. We need to promote social mobility and social inclusion, encourage actions aimed at the common or collective good (for instance through practical support of local charitable activities) and reduce both corruption and materialistic greed. In a fair society, in a society that protects our psychological health

© The Author(s) 2019
P. Kinderman, *A Manifesto for Mental Health*,
https://doi.org/10.1007/978-3-030-24386-9_13

and wellbeing, we would ensure that everyone had a meaningful job or role in society and we would eliminate unhealthy organisational cultures at work.

Dainius Pūras, the UN Special Rapporteur, emphasised: '*the preconditions of poor mental health, such as violence, disempowerment, social exclusion and isolation and the breakdown of communities, systemic socioeconomic disadvantage and harmful conditions at work and in schools......* *There exists an almost universal commitment to pay for hospitals, beds and medications instead of building a society in which everyone can thrive...*'. When speaking in public about these issues, I frequently asked questions (or more properly, challenged) along the lines of '*I agree with you, Peter, but how do we actually achieve change?*'. The answer lies not in the winning or losing of arguments between academics and professionals, but instead in the success of citizens' ability to assert their fundamental human rights and demand choice in a range of evidence-based, humane, effective services.

Maladjusted ... to Injustice

In 1967, Martin Luther King Jr. spoke to the American Psychological Association about links between racism, unemployment and living conditions. Now, we can see continuing economic crisis and the impact of policies of austerity, right-wing populism and nationalism. And these are not just economic or political matters; they are crucial psychological issues too. Quite literally, these are matters of life and death. Between 2008 and 2010, immediately following the most recent economic crisis (not yet the self-inflicted economic wounds of Brexit), there were 1000 more suicides in England and Wales than would be expected on purely historical trends, and many of those deaths can be attributed to rising unemployment.

Psychologists, whose professional role is the promotion of wellbeing and the prevention of distress, have a duty to speak out about those social, economic and political circumstances that impact on our clients and the general public and to bring such evidence to politicians and policy makers. For example, it's clear that unemployment and exploitative employment practices (such as zero-hours contracts, insecure jobs, the 'gig economy') are damaging to our wellbeing regardless of our age, gender, level of education, ethnicity or the part of the country in which we live. The longer someone remains unemployed, the worse the effect, and people do not adapt to unemployment. Their wellbeing is permanently reduced. In contrast, finding a decent job leads to higher wellbeing.

Martin Luther King said: '*There are some things in our society, some things in our world, to which we should never be adjusted*'.[1] Another Nobel Prize winner, Albert Camus (distinctive in that he occupied himself during the Nazi occupation of France editing the clandestine newspaper of the Resistance), wrote in his private notebook in May 1937: '*Psychology is action, not thinking about oneself*'.[2]

Psychology is about the things that really matter, relationships, optimism, a sense of meaning and purpose and personal agency. These are the core of wellbeing: a key element of government policy. Similarly, philosophical concepts like fairness, respect, identity, equity, dignity and autonomy underpin our fundamental human rights and have clear links to psychology. Indeed, we have to avoid the trap of 'psychologising' issues, focussing all our attention on individual psychology, on what happens inside, rather than outside, people's heads. I am and remain a proud clinical psychologist. I am very proud of the work that my colleagues (including nurses, psychiatrists and others) do to address the psychological wellbeing of individuals. How we make sense of the world is vitally important and something that we can influence. But we learn to make sense of the world because of what happens to us.

We grow up influenced by our social circumstances, our peers at school and our position in the world. If we grow up in circumstances of abuse, poverty, racism, discrimination, neo-liberal exploitation and the denial of our rights, we will grow up devoid of that sense of meaning and purpose, that sense of agency and optimism that is so vital to psychological wellbeing. That's why we need to keep talking to our political leaders about the psychology of mental health and wellbeing. It's also why it's vital to remember that the fundamental building blocks of society are, indeed, fundamental. All human beings need our fundamental rights; we need a sound economy and an equitable economy. We need protection and a secure start in life. We need education and decent employment, and we need protection and care when things are difficult and when we grow old. These fundamentals aren't additional to or alternative to psychology; they shape our psychology.

Psychology is action. And as Martin Luther King said: '...*there are some things in our society, some things in our world, to which we...must always be maladjusted if we are to be people of good will. We must never adjust ourselves to racial discrimination and racial segregation. We must never adjust ourselves to religious bigotry. We must never adjust ourselves to economic conditions that take necessities from the many to give luxuries to the few. We must never adjust ourselves to the madness of militarism, and the self-defeating effects of physical violence. ... There comes a time when one must take a stand that is neither safe, nor politic, nor popular. But one must take it because it is right*'.

Psychologists and Human Rights

Applied and community psychologists are deeply concerned with human rights issues. Many of the clients of applied psychologists suffer or have suffered as a result of human rights abuses; the everyday practice of applied psychologists is frequently subject to the provisions of the UN and European Conventions on Human Rights, institutionalised in the UK through the Human Rights Act 1998, and psychologists have a distinctive perspective on human rights.[3]

Psychologists are closely involved in understanding and caring for people whose human rights have been infringed and work with such bodies as the Medical Foundation for Victims of Torture and Amnesty International. Psychologists work every day with people receiving mental health care under compulsion, as well as with people who cannot care for or make decisions for themselves. Psychologists work in the Prison Service and in the Immigration Service, as well as in education and in social services. In mental health services, psychologists work with some of the most socially excluded and discriminated against sectors of the society, with people who have been abused and assaulted, victims of domestic violence and rape, as well as with the perpetrators of such abuse. The related issues of human rights and the provision of high-quality public services are therefore of everyday professional importance.

Abraham Maslow argued that a variety of human needs (from basic physiological needs such as food, water and sleep, through needs such as safety and security to higher social needs such as love, self-esteem and respect from others) must be met before we can achieve our full potential in life. But such basic human needs are expressed and negotiated in social relationships. At a time when we had a more left-wing government, the then Lord Falconer, The Lord Chancellor, said: '*The big human rights questions ... they turn on views about what is necessary in a democratic society. They are about balancing one person's interests against another ... values we can all share, and practical respect for each other's dignity*'.[4] This reflects the idea that human rights are less legal obligations and more like the codifications of how we collectively understand our relationships and obligations to each other.

The UK Human Rights Act 1998 incorporates the provisions of the European Convention on Human Rights (ECHR) into UK law, and human rights law affects the practice of psychologists in many ways. Article 3 of the UK's Human Rights Act states that: '*no one shall be subjected to torture or to inhuman or degrading treatment or punishment*'. This is, surprisingly, little used in mental health care, despite the fact that a very great deal of such mental health care is degrading and inhumane.

Article 5 of the Human Rights Act states that: '*everyone has the right to liberty and security of person. No one shall be deprived of his liberty save in the following cases and in accordance with a procedure prescribed by law...*'. Clause (e) addresses '*the lawful detention of ... persons of unsound mind ...*', etc. This Article has quite wide applicability and is of key importance in the context of compulsory mental health care. It explicitly allows for exemptions in the case of persons 'of unsound mind'. This term is not defined in the Human Rights. The implication of the psychological approach I have advanced in this book is that people are of 'unsound mind' if they are unable to make valid decisions for themselves. In England and Wales, both psychologists and psychiatrists have argued that mental health legislation should be based on the principle of autonomy, perhaps (as I have argued) in the wording of the Mental Health (Care and Treatment) (Scotland) Act (2003): '*that because of the mental disorder the patient's ability to make decisions about the provision of such medical treatment is significantly impaired*'.

Article 14 of the Human Rights Act 1998 states that: '*the enjoyment of the rights and freedoms … shall be secured without discrimination on any ground such as sex, race, colour, language, religion, political or other opinion, national or social origin, association with a national minority, property, birth or other status*'. The Human Rights Act sets out positive obligations for public bodies. Services (including the work of psychological health services) must be offered in non-discriminatory ways. Because psychology addresses our shared societal consensus of how personal needs and desires are negotiated in social relationships, psychologists should be assertive in advocating the application of psychological evidence to such policies.

Psychologists for Social Change

I am not the only psychologist to hold similar views. The rather wonderful group 'Psychologists for Social Change'[5] established by Professor Sally Zlotowitz shares my aims. In May 2018, Annabel Head and Jessica Bond published an article in the Independent newspaper arguing that: '*we need to address the socioeconomic causes of mental health issues if we really want to tackle the problem*'.

Head and Bond praise the fact that mental health and psychological wellbeing are now securely on the political agenda. Increased awareness of psychological health issues and the willingness to discuss them put pressure on policymakers to fulfil their promise to put as much proportionate investment into psychological health as is committed to physical health.[6] But, if we want to make a real difference, we need to raise awareness not only of the issues of mental health and psychological wellbeing, but also about the root causes of psychological distress. This means understanding our society and the communities in which we live and how their social, political and economic forces affect our wellbeing.

As Head and Bond point out (as I have been saying), there is robust evidence for the role that social, economic and environmental factors play in psychological health. It is an uncomfortable fact psychological distress (and the labels of 'mental disorders' that some of our colleagues like to use) is a sign of and consequences of inequity. Poor people and more socially disadvantaged people are more likely to suffer than those of us more fortunate.[7] Hardly surprising, disadvantage is associated with misery. All the evidence is, in fact, strikingly unsurprising when presented in ordinary language. Poor people are more likely to be depressed and anxious[8]… but then poverty is depressing and frightening. Those of us in debt[9] and in unpleasant jobs (for instance zero-hours contracts or jobs in which we have little control over what we do)[10] are more likely to be depressed and anxious… because it's depressing and frightening to be in debt, and because it's soul-destroying to work like a dog for meagre rewards. When we lose our jobs, we are likely to become depressed and even contemplate suicide[11]…. but who wouldn't be depressed in this world if we lost our meaning and purpose in life at the same time as losing the means for financial security? If we go to bed each night and wake up each morning in inadequate accommodation[12] or live in a neighbourhood blighted by crime and violence[13]… well, it's obvious enough if we ask the question: 'would you feel happy, optimistic and safe, living in a dangerous neighbourhood?'.

In truth, it's not rocket science. But we need actually to do something about it. I'm a practising clinical psychologist, and I want to use my professional skills to help anyone who's depressed or anxious. But I am concerned that personal therapy, while necessary and in that sense therefore welcome, can be a sticking plaster, an ambulance at the bottom of the cliff when we could be erecting a fence. As Head and Bond put it: *'People may feel insecure, less in control of their lives or even unsafe…. If someone feeling like this went to their GP or to a mental health service, their response to these life experiences may be interpreted as "symptoms" of a mental health problem…. Antidepressants or CBT to cope with anxiety may or may not be offered and may or may not temporarily help the individual. But it is not going to change their situation or prevent others from ending up in the same place… It is a person's brain that is the problem and not these wider factors. This individualisation of psychological distress not only puts the onus for recovery squarely on the individual's shoulders, but it shifts the focus away from the societal, cultural and political factors which contribute to people being in these positions in the first place'.*

These comments echo my views and those of Dr. Dainius Pūras. We can understand why individual professionals and health services might wish to offer therapeutic help; the help is needed and it's our job. We might also understand why politicians might like it this way; it's hard (and expensive) to tackle poverty, inequality, poor housing and deprivation and much easier to express admiration for heroic doctors and nurses. But psychological health is, obviously and essentially, a political issue.

Some politicians recognise this. Recently, the UK Parliament's Education and Health and Social Care Select Committees joined forces to examine child and adolescent mental health policies. Their report[14] found that the government *'lacks any ambition and fails to consider how to prevent child and adolescent mental ill health in the first place'*. This is unacceptable… but at least the Select Committee were asking the right questions and pointing out the unacceptability of the responses.

More recently, Luciana Berger, MP for the part of Liverpool in which I work, commented on how she would wish to see *'a revolution on mental health'*.[15] Her argument echoed, again, that of Dainius Pūras (and me): *'… we need a revolution in mental health, moving away from crisis toward prevention and early intervention; from mental illness to mental health'*. Luciana was clear: *'"Revolution" suggests a complete overthrow of the old order and a new system to replace it; I choose this word quite deliberately. We need a wholly new approach to mental health, of which counselling and psychotherapy should be a central part … Societies which are more equal and more prosperous enjoy better mental health and wellbeing. For this reason, if no other, social justice should run through our social and economic policies like a golden thread'*. I agree.

Unfortunately, we still have a long way to go. In 2018, a different United Nations Special Rapporteur visited the UK. Philip Alston, UN Special Rapporteur on Extreme Poverty and Human Rights, reported on the suffering that has been inflicted through the callous approach to austerity taken by the government since 2009 and the relationship between poverty, inequality and mental health difficulties.[16] Alston noted that, in the world's fifth largest economy, there was *'… immense growth in foodbanks and the queues waiting outside them, the people sleeping rough in the streets, the growth of homelessness, the sense of deep despair that leads even the Government to appoint a Minister for suicide prevention and civil society to report in depth on unheard of levels of loneliness and isolation. And local authorities, especially in England, which perform vital roles in providing a real social safety net have been gutted by a series of government policies. Libraries have closed in record numbers, community and youth centers have been shrunk and underfunded, public spaces and buildings including parks and recreation centers have been sold off.... The results? 14 million people, a fifth of the population, live in poverty....For almost one in every two children to be poor in twenty-first century Britain is not just a disgrace, but a social calamity and an economic disaster, all rolled into one... great misery has also been inflicted unnecessarily, especially on the working poor, on single mothers struggling against mighty odds, on people with disabilities who are already marginalized, and on millions of children who are being locked into a cycle of poverty from which most will have great difficulty escaping...'.* Professor Alston commented how the UK government's approach to benefits was '*... punitive, mean-spirited, and often callous ...'*. The Lancet, the UK's leading medical journal,[17] particularly highlighted Professor Alston's conclusion that in the UK, '*... poverty is a political choice. Austerity could easily have spared the poor, if the political will had existed to do so...'*. Of course, as Luciana Berger says, '*...social justice should run through our social and economic policies like a golden thread...'*. We're not there yet.

Social Agents in a Social Model

In a vision of psychological health care, we would act primarily as social agents in a social model of care. The best system for organising and delivering this care would therefore be through the social services of the local authorities. In the UK, this would see what is now considered part of the National Health Service (NHS), the health care system, becoming part of the local authority social services provision. In other countries, the systems for provision are slightly different, but the basic separation of social and medical care is commonplace. The transfer of responsibilities that I am suggesting may, in fact, be somewhat easier in other countries than in the UK, because city and regional authorities often have responsibilities for health care, which in the UK is organised on a quasi-national basis.

A concrete (literally) example is the city in which I work, Liverpool in North West England. I would like to see Liverpool City Council take over responsibility for the strategic direction, management and delivery of psychological health care for the city. In this vision, all the psychological health care—the services that are now delivered through health services structures such as NHS Trusts—would be managed and delivered by local authorities. This would see psychiatry and associated professions organised and managed alongside existing social services and the public health colleagues who have already been brought under local authority management. Of course, at present, much of our mental health care is already delivered in community settings. But it remains part of, and organised by, the NHS. And residential care in particular remains dominated by hospital-based inpatient psychiatric wards. A more appropriate model would be for psychological health to be based entirely within local social services. That would mean seeing local authorities assuming management of the whole system, including residential services. This would lead to inpatient wards being reconfigured as residential units along social, not medical, lines. This would be a fundamental change.

From the top down, and from the bottom up, mental health care is currently predicated on a medical model. In the UK, the most influential single individual is the Medical Director of the National Commissioning Board. Mental health care is currently part of the medical infrastructure, which in the UK is the NHS. The government's Department of Health provides funding and significant strategic direction, but more detailed decision-making is deferred to the 'arms-length' National Commissioning Board, the Medical Director of the Board and the 25 National Clinical Directors. These clinical leaders provide expert advice and research on conditions and services, ranging from obesity and diabetes to emergency preparedness and critical care. This is all positive and necessary. But it does mean that mental health care falls under the directorship of a clinical director within this very medicalised structure and system. This 'clinical primacy' is also seen further down the system. NHS Trusts (the UK's core delivery organisations) have 'medical directors' to lead and guide services. While as individuals and as a group, medical directors, and the national clinical directors, perform a valuable service, any service run in and by a healthcare system will reflect the ethos and dominant methodologies of that system. This profoundly affects every aspect of our mental healthcare system. Indeed, even the term 'mental health care' conveys this medical dominance, psychological health or psychological wellbeing may be much more appropriate phrases.

In my experience, working as a clinical psychologist and as a researcher and educator, there are important consequences of this medical dominance. Decision-making within organisations is often dominated by the specific role occupied by psychiatrists. While individually often excellent, this nevertheless reflects only one particular perspective in the hierarchy of the organisations. On a clinical level, key decisions are often made by consultant psychiatrists, with multi-disciplinary team meetings only convened in order to discuss how those decisions should be implemented, rather than actually to make decisions. And those multi-disciplinary meetings are usually strongly influenced by a biomedical perspective. It's also significant that, if the consultant psychiatrist is absent, then frequently the meetings are postponed or automatically led by a more junior psychiatrist rather than a more senior non-medical member of the team.

Those of us struggling emotionally and psychologically need care to be organised very differently. Instead of an inappropriate medical service, treating presumed (but non-existent) 'illnesses', we need a new, psychosocial, approach. We need a network of community-based care teams, linked to social services and other local authority provision, as well as to the NHS and third-sector organisations. As I said at the very beginning of this book, I'm an optimist. And, fortunately, I see this as the direction of travel nationally, if not internationally. In the UK, there is policy backing to integrate mental health care, physical health care and social care. There has been a major integration of GP services with wider community and social services, and, importantly, we've seen UK public health services transferred wholesale into local authority management. This should continue, especially in terms of psychological health care.

Ideally, psychological health would be a local authority-managed, social and community resource, not a medical, hospital-based service. This does not mean dispensing with psychiatric colleagues nor denying their importance. Contrary to some responses on social media (usually by colleagues who haven't in fact read my work), I am not an 'anti-psychiatrist'. Psychiatrists' contribution would remain substantial and important.

But I see my psychiatry colleagues as consultants *to*, not automatically in charge *of* those local teams. I have used, before, the analogy of the medical advisor to Manchester United Football Club. Proper medical care and advice are undoubtedly vital to such a physical, high value organisation. It would be hugely risky if a multi-million-pound, international organisation, based on the physical prowess of a small number of athletes, were to ignore their physical health. Medical care is an essential element of any world-leading athletics body. But Sir Alex Ferguson (or his many replacements, over the years that Manchester United have struggled following Ferguson's retirement) would never have suggested that his medical consultant had managerial authority above him. The psychiatrist would be a consultant *to* the team, not the manager *of* the team.

The NHS

In the UK, just after the Second World War, there was a revolution in a wide range of social services. Boosted by the contributions made by millions of individual citizens in the war, there was pressure for a new, more egalitarian, system. Despite leading the anti-Nazi coalition, Winston Churchill lost to a socialist Labour Party. Consequently, the NHS was founded in 1948 (established by an Act of Parliament passed in 1946, to explain a few anomalies with dates). Many people (including doctors) found the idea of a nationalised, socialised system both concerning and controversial. Initially, the British Medical Association formally opposed the idea of a NHS. But the idea of a NHS has always had enormous popular support that, through general taxation, every citizen has immediate access to a universal system of gold-standard healthcare free at the point of need. In 1946 UK politics, however, there was considerable debate as to whether the network of healthcare providers should be organised through existing local authorities that each local city or county council should manage their local hospitals and doctors in the new proposed scheme or through a new, national, structural organisation. For various reasons, it was eventually decided that the local authority solution was less attractive than the idea of a new, national, structure, and the NHS as we know, it was born.

The NHS was therefore established as a structure independent of local authorities, city mayors and town councils. But, then, there was considerable discussion over whether mental health services should be part of this system. Some commentators believed (an opinion that I would now share) that mental and physical health care services were essentially sufficiently different that mental health care should be separately organised and should fall under local authority control. Three powerful arguments led, eventually, to inclusion of mental health care within the NHS.

What may well have been wise in 1946, when local authority administration was considerably different, seems much less appropriate today. Since 1948, the network of community-based mental health services has developed and expanded. Now, we have a growing and positive relationship between community-based NHS mental health Trusts offering both traditional 'out-patient' services and residential 'in-patient' units with the extensive (if currently threatened by political decisions) social services provided by local authorities. Healthcare is an important part of our economy, but is also intimately tied to our various specialist community teams and social services. So, for example (and this is definitely not an exhaustive list), the NHS offers specialist mental health care for new mothers (often delivered by community mental health Trusts, but based out of general hospitals or maternity hospitals) and child and adolescent mental health services (CAMHS), sometimes delivered by community mental health Trusts, but occasionally by specialist children's hospitals. It offers a very wide range of services for people of working age, specialist learning disabilities services, services for people with physical disabilities, services for people with substance misuse problems, support for people returning to work, help for offenders who have psychological health problems and services for older people. There are even very specialist services for, for example, commercial sex workers, asylum seekers, military veterans and young people leaving local authority care. All these services interface with family doctors (GPs) and with similar, complementary, services offered by local authorities and third-sector organisations.

The close liaison between NHS and local authority services can be seen in what are called 'Section 75 arrangements'. Local authorities and health services have developed (relatively) effective and efficient ways of working together. These are facilitated by Section 75 of the National Health Service Act 2006 (hence the terminology) which encourages and legally enables health Trusts and local authority social services departments to pool money, delegate functions to each other and to integrate their resources and management structures. This effectively means that a nurse, a psychologist or a psychiatrist could find themselves employed by an NHS Trust, but under day-to-day management by a local authority manager and funded by local authority funds... or vice versa. This helps plan and deliver services across a wide range of areas of psychological health care, but has so far been particularly used in learning disability services, in services for children and for older people.

Collaboration between health and local authorities is further strengthened by the development of local Health and Wellbeing Boards in the UK. In 2012, the UK government introduced the Health and Social Care Act 2012,[18] which included, controversially, steps towards increasing private (commercial) provision within the NHS. But that piece of legislation also did something rather wonderful. It provided the legal basis for the establishment of Health and Wellbeing Boards in each major local authority. These Boards bring together NHS and local authority managers, as well as leaders and opinion-formers from the wider community to plan and coordinate the commission of health and wellbeing of their local population and to reduce health inequalities. These Health and Wellbeing Boards bring together clinical commissioning groups and local councils to develop a shared understanding of the health and wellbeing needs of the community, a Joint Strategic Needs Assessment (JSNA), and then agree to a joint strategy for action. Although, at present, each agency is independently responsible for its budget, the Boards enable joint commissioning and integrated services across health and social care, joined-up services between the NHS and local councils and stronger democratic legitimacy and engagement. Because local authorities are responsible for services such as housing and education and are closely linked to fire and rescue services, the police force and housing providers, there is huge potential for more integrated services.

Nobody would deny the benefits of direct medical care. But progress in improving the health and wellbeing of citizens also requires intervention at the population level. In the case of physical health care, many of the deadliest killers, heart disease, diabetes, stroke, cancer and sexually-acquired infections, need to be addressed through public health measures for maximum benefit. This is also true for psychological health. Therapy, even medication, may be helpful for some, but real improvements in the overall psychological health of the population require action at a societal level. We need to address the causes listed earlier. Because marital separation is a major source of emotional stress, we need to ensure that there is sufficient support for people going through separation or marital difficulties: mediation services, support for single parents and equitable laws concerning divorce proceedings and child custody. Because unemployment is a major source of distress, we must aim for full employment, and certainly do what we can to protect people from the emotional and economic impact of unemployment. Conversely, work-related stress is also a big issue for many people. We need to ensure equitable and supportive employment practices, including employee relations, a living wage, decent terms and conditions and appropriate employee representation. Services such as Citizens Advice (a government-funded, but independent, network of advice agencies with offices in most towns across the UK), debt counselling agencies and Victim Support are vital to help people in financial difficulties, victims of crime and people dealing with a range of other traumatic life events. Similarly, drugs advice and drugs counselling services play vital roles in maintaining the wellbeing of citizens. Psychologists and psychiatrists throughout history have realised that our experiences in childhood are fundamentally important in determining future psychological health problems, and that emotional neglect, bullying and childhood emotional, physical and sexual abuse are all powerful direct causes of psychological health problems. It is therefore vital that we, as a society, act to protect children, not merely mop up the emotional consequences later in life. This means developing coordinated services to support families and parents in difficulty. It means supporting teachers and educational psychologists in schools, and it means supporting a network of children's services. And, no matter how politically controversial it might be, we must press for social justice and in particular for a more equal society.

For all these reasons, I see local authorities as the right place for the management of psychological health care. Psychological health care will remain inappropriately dependent on a medical, disease-based, ethos so long as it is seen as another branch of medicine. I see the journey of public health from NHS management to local authority management as offering a pioneering route for the transfer of mental health care from hospital-based services to local authority control.

Psychological Health Care in an Age of (Continuing) Austerity

When, four years ago, I wrote *A Prescription for Psychiatry*, I commented that the policies of a right-wing government in the UK had put public spending under considerable pressure. Unfortunately, this has continued and got worse. Central government financial support for local authorities has continued to fall, placing communities under great strain. UK politics (driven by citizens, who have always valued their National Health Service—the NHS—very highly) has meant that government ministers have always pledged to protect the funding for the health services to ensure that they are universal and free at the point of need. Remarkably, this pledge seems not yet to have been broken. Unfortunately, however, the protection of public funding has not extended to social services (especially because these tend to be provided by local authorities, and national governments can easily shift the blame for the consequences of funding cuts). And because so many health conditions are dependent on social and community services, as we see cuts in social services, we see pressure on health services. As our living conditions worsen, all kinds of health conditions—from obesity to tuberculosis—are made worse. And, as we cut social services, it becomes increasingly difficult safely to discharge people (especially vulnerable people) from hospital. Pressures build up, and discharge back-logs grow.

It seems to be a matter of pride to some in government (again, right-wing politicians) that the UK is planning to reduce the funding for public services to a level not seen since 1948.[19] In other industrialised countries, not least the USA, a declared aim to 'shrink the state' seems popular. It is popular with extremely rich people and those in charge of large commercial enterprises, because 'shrink the state' really means 'pay less tax'. This is all a matter of concern, if not shame, for me. Policies aimed at ensuring full and comprehensive health and social services, universally available, funded by progressive taxation and free at the point of need, are both vital in order to enable the provision of appropriate services and good for society.

But local authorities are, as I write this, under enormous financial pressure. It is in this context of financial pressure that many of my colleagues have been concerned about the transfer of public health services to local authority control. Their argument is that it is much better to keep as many services as possible within the ring-fenced NHS budget than to expose them to the pressures of a shrinking local authority funding model. But, while this may be an important concern in the current UK context, it does not negate my wider argument. The temporary details of public service funding in the UK in 2018 should not prevent a larger debate about what the appropriate ethos and service model might be for psychological health and wellbeing services more generally. In my opinion, any concern about the funding of and costs of services makes the case for integrated care even more strongly.

Notes

1. Martin Luther King's speech can be read here: https://www.apa.org/monitor/features/king-challenge, and was published as: Martin Luther King, "The role of the behavioral scientist in the civil rights movement," *Journal of Social Issues* 24, no. 1 (1968): 1–12.
2. Albert Camus, *Carnets 1935–1942* (London: Hamish Hamilton, 1963). See also: https://thepsychologist.bps.org.uk/volume-30/june-2017/psychology-action-not-thinking-about-oneself.
3. Peter Kinderman, "Psychology and human rights," *Science and Public Affairs* 6, no. 10 (2004).
4. Lord Falconer's speech is referenced here: https://publications.parliament.uk/pa/jt200304/jtselect/jtrights/78/78we06.htm.

5. 'Psychologists for Social Change' can be found here: http://www.psych-change.org/.

6. Annabel Head and Jessica Bond, "We need to address the socioeconomic causes of mental health issues if we really want to tackle the problem," *The Independent*, Sunday 20 May 2018. https://www.independent.co.uk/voices/mental-health-help-how-change-awareness-causes-treat-a8357741.html.

7. Jonathan Campion, Dinesh Bhugra, Sue Bailey, and Michael Marmot, "Inequality and mental disorders: Opportunities for action," *The Lancet* 382, no. 9888 (2013): 183–184. https://www.thelancet.com/journals/lancet/article/PIIS0140-6736(13)61411-7/abstract.

8. Erik Blas and Anand Sivasankara Kurup, eds., *Equity, social determinants and public health programmes* (Geneva: World Health Organization, 2010). http://www.who.int/iris/handle/10665/44289.

9. Rachel Jenkins, Dinesh Bhugra, Paul Bebbington, Traolach Brugha, Michael Farrell, Jeremy Coid, Tom Fryers, Scott Weich, Nicola Singleton, and Howard Meltzer, "Debt, income and mental disorder in the general population," *Psychological Medicine* 38, no. 10 (2008): 1485–1493. https://www.ncbi.nlm.nih.gov/pubmed/18184442.

10. Jessica Allen, Reuben Balfour, Ruth Bell, and Michael Marmot, "Social determinants of mental health," *International Review of Psychiatry* 26, no. 4 (2014): 392–407. https://www.ncbi.nlm.nih.gov/pubmed/25137105.

11. Ben Barr, David Taylor-Robinson, Alex Scott-Samuel, Martin McKee, and David Stuckler, "Suicides associated with the 2008–10 economic recession in England: Time trend analysis," *British Medical Journal* 345 (2012): e5142. https://www.bmj.com/content/345/bmj.e5142.

12. Christine Liddell and Ciara Guiney, "Living in a cold and damp home: Frameworks for understanding impacts on mental well-being," *Public Health* 129, no. 3 (2015): 191–199. https://www.ncbi.nlm.nih.gov/pubmed/25726123.

13. Sarah J. Blizzard, Jeanne Kemppainen, and Julie Taylor, "Posttraumatic stress disorder and community violence: An update for nurse practitioners," *Journal of the American Academy of Nurse Practitioners* 21, no. 10 (2009): 535–541. https://www.ncbi.nlm.nih.gov/pubmed/19796287.

14. The Select Committee Report can be found here: https://publications.parliament.uk/pa/cm201719/cmselect/cmhealth/642/642.pdf.

15. See: http://www.lucianaberger.com/2018/12/07/we-need-a-revolution-in-mental-health/.
16. For the United Nations' press release on Philip Alston's visit, see: https://www.ohchr.org/EN/NewsEvents/Pages/DisplayNews.aspx?NewsID=23881&LangID=E.
17. The Lancet Public Health, "Poverty is a political choice," *The Lancet Public Health* 3, no. 12 (2018): e555. https://www.thelancet.com/journals/lanpub/article/PIIS2468-2667(18)30243-3/fulltext.
18. The Health and Social Care Act can be found here: http://www.legislation.gov.uk/ukpga/2012/7/contents/enacted and you can read about the controversies here: http://en.wikipedia.org/wiki/Health_and_Social_Care_Act_2012.
19. You can read about this depressing policy here: http://www.bbc.co.uk/news/business-25240202.

14

A Manifesto

If we are to continue to improve psychological health care, we need to shift from a 'disease model', which assumes that emotional distress is merely a symptom of biological illness, towards social and psychological approach to mental health and wellbeing. While all of our thoughts, behaviours and emotions emanate from the biological activity of our brains, this does not mean that psychological health problems need therefore to be regarded as brain diseases. Psychological health services would better meet our needs if they were based on the premise that our mental health and wellbeing depends on the things happen to us, how we make sense of those events and how we respond to them. The assumption or assertion that our distress is best understood merely as a symptom of diagnosable 'illnesses' is only one perspective. Rather than employing medical, pathologising, language and methods, we can and should use effective, scientific, understandable alternatives. To understand and explain our experiences, and to plan services, we need to develop co-produced 'formulations' and sharply reduce our reliance on medication. Hospitals could be replaced with residential units designed and managed from a psychosocial perspective, and psychological health legislation must respect our rights to make decisions for ourselves unless we are unable to do that and provide for much greater judicial oversight. Teams work best when they are multidisciplinary, democratic and aligned to a psychosocial model, and psychological health services could be managed as social services, alongside other social,

P. Kinderman, *A Manifesto for Mental Health*,
https://doi.org/10.1007/978-3-030-24386-9_14

community-based, services. Finally, because our psychological health and wellbeing are largely dependent on our social circumstances, we must work collectively to create a more humane society: to reduce or eliminate poverty, especially childhood poverty, and to reduce financial and social inequality. Fortunately, such a vision is—nearly—within reach.

Disagreements within the profession of psychiatry have been visible for years, largely between biological and social perspectives. But there are things upon which we agree. All professionals working in mental health are fundamentally committed to the best interests of those members of the public who use our services (that's why we argue with passion). We also (almost without exception) believe that greater investment in mental health services is needed, both as an absolute sum and as a proportion of health care. We all believe in ensuring the highest standards of care and on the importance of genuine leadership (not merely participation) by the users of services themselves. We all agree on the benefits of prevention (although some people tend also to emphasise the importance of caring for people with very serious problems) and we believe in the elimination of discrimination against people who use mental health services.

We cannot simply rest on our laurels and assume that good will protect our rights and promote high-quality services. Here, I have set out a manifesto for such a programme of reform. It's worth setting out what that might look like in reality.

A Paradigm Shift

The American physicist and philosopher Thomas Kuhn introduced the idea of a 'paradigm shift', a fundamental change in the basic concepts and experimental practices of a scientific discipline. Examples of these Kuhnian paradigm shifts in science include the transition from a Ptolemaic geocentric cosmology to a Copernican heliocentric one, germ theory rather than miasma theory of disease, Charles Darwin's speciation through natural selection, and the transition from classical Newtonian physics to quantum mechanics and Einstein's theory of relativity.

These scientific developments are paradigmatic shifts because they don't merely reflect new insights or applications within a way of seeing the world; they represent changes in the way the world is seen. In Ptolemaic geocentric cosmology, highly intelligent astronomers and mathematicians worked hard to make sense of the movements of stars and planets, but they did this from the basic assumption that the Earth was at the centre of the universe (partly because the Christian Church from time to time ordered people who disagreed to be tortured to death in public). The paradigmatic shift was the (brave) idea to challenge the basic assumption and conclude that the sun was at the centre of the solar system.

There is a similar paradigmatic shift underway in mental health. The shift from seeing those difficult or troublesome thoughts and emotions that are currently seen as 'symptoms' of 'mental illnesses' to seeing these experiences as what they are—psychological phenomena—is a radical change in perspective. We would do away with ideas of disorder and pathology and abnormality. We would stop thinking about the aetiology of 'major depressive disorder' and start thinking about what makes us depressed. Or, more radically still, what gives us a sense of meaning and purpose in life. We would stop describing the completely understandable consequences of traumatic events a 'disorder' and instead understand and describe how those events impact on our lives. And we would stop seeing our helping responses as 'treatment'. We may well treat diabetes or Dupuytren's contracture, but we don't 'treat' racism or poverty; or, to be precise, when we use the analogy, we realise that it's an analogy. Similarly, we would definitely try to prevent these kinds of problems occurring in the future, but there is absolutely no reason to believe that we have to think of these problems as 'illnesses' before we get on with the job.

These shifts in thinking are profound. In a rather poor poem in 1895, Joseph Malins contrasted prevention and treatment by imagining a building a fence to protect citizens falling from a dangerous cliff with supplying an ambulance to care for people who've fallen; '*some said, "put a fence around the edge of the cliff", some, "an ambulance down in the valley"'*. When we see mental health problems as illnesses or disorders, we naturally think of ambulances; of doctors, of illnesses, of aetiologies, of pathologies, of treatments and of cures. When we think of the ways in which human beings respond to adversity, with all our glorious variation, and all the understandable emotional and cognitive consequences, we think in terms of fences. Or, to put that less poetically, we think of social justice, of economic and political equity, of protection of the more vulnerable members of society, of the protection of children from abuse or bullying.

Thinking of depression as a phenomenon rather than an illness would bring other paradigmatic changes. The asset-based community development model is an example of a completely different—paradigmatically different—approach to building individual and community wellbeing. I'm not suggesting that this approach could, alone, replace the infrastructure of biomedical psychiatry, address the wide variety of problems swept up in the concept of 'mental health' and meet all the needs of highly distressed people at risk of harming themselves or others. But it does illustrate how differently issues are seen from different perspectives. The asset-based community development model focusses on the strengths and potentials of communities, rather than disorders within individuals. This means assessing the resources, skills and experience available in a community, and then working with the community to facilitate moving people towards action. This aims to use the assets and resources of a community as the basis for development and it aims to empower the people of the community, particularly by encouraging them to use the assets they already possess.

One significant consequence of this approach is the change in power dynamics and the role of professional expertise. Advocates of the asset-based community development approach have pithily contrasted the 'medical model' as 'to; everything is done to us and without us', the 'charity model' as 'for; everything is done for us; without us', the 'social model' as 'with; nothing for us without us', but the 'community development model' as 'by; everything is done by us, for us'. This sounds wonderful, but also somewhat threatening. As a professional (and for that matter, as a White, male, Western professional), it's easier to live with a social model (where I can convince myself that I am being democratic) and embrace the 'nothing about us without us' message, but my professional specialness is still valued. The full-hearted democratic equity of the community development model is wonderful… but threatening.

In 1973, the American Psychiatric Association voted to accept the recommendation of their scientific committee that 'homosexuality' should no longer be regarded as a mental illness. It fascinates me how most of my colleagues (now) seem so entirely to accept this point that they find it perplexing when I draw obvious parallels. This decision illustrates how so many decisions about psychiatric diagnosis depend on social judgements and values that change through history. That we could stop regarding 'homosexuality' as an illness and appreciate the wonderful variety of human sexuality is a simple illustration of how we can change our minds about things we call 'mental health' issues. We could relatively easily realise that experiences such as depression and anxiety represent less desirable aspects of what it means to be human. My colleagues don't see things in the same way. For them, the rejection of the illness label in the case of our sexuality represents progress within (not a challenge to) the dominant conceptual model. Their argument is that some things are clearly mental illnesses, but it's been decided that homosexuality isn't one of them. There is, for many of my colleagues, no inherent challenge to the idea of 'mental illness' itself.

Many of the ways in which this argument is played out are contradictory. It is pointed out, for instance, that we cannot be happy and productive when we are also depressed or anxious, justifying a label of 'disorder'. This is an argument which fits uneasily with the contention that problems such as depression and anxiety are characterised by brain abnormalities. Equally difficult to square with these arguments is the contention that 'disorder' is merely a word used to reflect useful but essentially arbitrary cut-off points on various continue. The argument here is that we look at obesity or blood lipid levels or even average intake of alcohol as issues that range across continuous dimensions, but it makes sense to define (on the basis of sound epidemiological science) working definitions of 'overweight' or 'hypercholesteremia' or to define recommended alcohol consumption levels. Similarly, the argument goes, the same applies to mental health; that to identify a 'disorder' is merely to identify a useful working definition for action.

What interests me about these arguments is that they don't tend to challenge the basic assumption that there are 'disorders', but instead argue whether or not this or that label is appropriate within that conceptual model. That is, the question isn't whether a diagnostic approach is valid, but whether it's right that homosexuality (and other phenomena) should leave or enter the diagnostic lexicon, on a variety of grounds. Those arguments aren't necessarily bad arguments. It's perfectly legitimate to argue that either individual distress or the impact on personal, social, occupational or educational functioning allows us to distinguish phenomena such as depression and anxiety from different expressions of sexuality. A distinction could be made between 'disorders' which reflect an underlying pathology and phenomena that don't. And it's not invalid to argue that we make pragmatic judgements about cut-off scores in continually varying phenomena across health care (although these might be thought of as somewhat contradictory arguments). My point is that these are all arguments that continue to accept the reality of a group of phenomena called 'disorders' or 'mental illnesses' and then attempt to justify the position of certain phenomena as either inside, or outside, that group. None of these arguments challenge the notion of the validity of that group in the first place.

This is what makes my argument a Kuhnian paradigm shift. It does not merely recapitulate pre-existing ways of looking at the topic, it challenges the underlying assumptions. This seems to be such a profound point that many of my colleagues fail to see it or understand it. When I raise the issue of sexuality and remind colleagues of the 1973 vote, the most common response is to be a little bewildered, to point out that the concepts of sexual orientation and low mood (for instance) are simply different concepts. My point isn't merely to welcome the fact that the American Psychiatric Association redrew the line in 1973, moving homosexuality from one side to the other. I do recognise that, and I welcome it. My point is that we shouldn't be drawing that line in the first place; that we would do better if we were to think about things entirely differently.

A Manifesto

If we are to continue to improve mental health care, we need to shift from a 'disease model', which assumes that emotional distress is merely a symptom of biological illness, towards social and psychological approach to mental health and wellbeing. While all of our thoughts, behaviours and emotions emanate from the biological activity of our brains, this does not mean that mental health problems need therefore to be regarded as brain diseases. Mental health services would better meet our needs if they were based on the premise that our psychological health and wellbeing depends on the things happen to us, how we make sense of those events and how we respond to them. The assumption or assertion that our distress is best understood merely as a symptom of diagnosable 'illnesses' is only one perspective. Rather than employ medical, pathologising, language and methods, we can and should use effective, scientific, understandable alternatives. To understand and explain our experiences, and to plan services, we need to develop co-produced 'formulations' and sharply reduce our reliance on medication. Hospitals could be replaced with residential units designed and managed from a psychosocial perspective, and mental health legislation must respect our rights to make decisions for ourselves unless we are unable to do that and provide for much greater judicial oversight. Teams best meet our needs when they are multidisciplinary, democratic and aligned to a psychosocial model, and psychological health services may best be managed as social services, alongside other social, community-based, services.

This is a manifesto for reform. While biomedical research is valuable, we must reject claims that overstate or misrepresent the evidence base. This means no longer treating mental health issues as predominantly caused by brain pathology, but rather embracing evidence that psychological health issues are usually responses to social and environmental factors. This change will reduce stigma, more accurately capture the nature of distress, reduce the emphasis on pathology in our mental health discourse and promote the research and implementation of more effective non-biomedical alternatives.

Psychiatric drugs are now prescribed to over 20% of the adult population. Antidepressant use has doubled over the past ten years, as has the average duration of antidepressant use. While we need to recognise the role drugs can play, we need reform of excessive as well as unnecessary long-term prescribing due to the associated harms of dependency and withdrawal. As recent research also shows that long-term use leads to worse outcomes (and can be linked with rising psychological health disability), doctors could prioritise short-term prescribing, always with a plan for coming off. Additionally, patients must be properly informed regarding potential harms as well as benefits and must no longer be misled by unsubstantiated rationales for prescribing, such as notions of brain chemical imbalances.

We must reform the essential structures of psychological health provision delivery. While psychological health care requires appropriate funding, and healthcare professionals will continue to play valuable roles, we should not increase funding for services with poor outcomes, nor assume that current models of leadership, management, governance and service commissioning are always preferable. Instead, we should prioritise investment in more effective alternatives, and move funding priorities from fragmented biomedical services to integrated, whole-person, and community care. As psychological health issues often have social or environmental causes, psychological health services would most effectively meet our needs if they were able to prioritise prevention and early intervention and be more closely integrated with both physical health services and local authority social and educational services.

We must reform our public mental health campaigns, moving opinion away from biomedical messages to a psychosocial perspective. The general public, the media and mental health professionals require accurate information about the nature, origins and resolution of psychological health issues. We must de-medicalise and de-pathologise public discourse, helping to promote a more constructive and less-stigmatising public relationship to behavioural and emotional difficulties, and encouraging people to take more active steps to protect and improve their psychological health.

We must reform those institutions that uncritically maintain and promote the current unsuccessful approach to psychological health provision. This will involve substantial transfers of power, from individual clinicians to teams, and from professionals to service users. We must ensure that there is proper representation of service users on expert groups and promote a person-centred approach to psychological health care, which emphasises fundamental human rights and personal autonomy.

Finally, because our mental health—our psychological health—and wellbeing are largely dependent on our social circumstances, we must work collectively to create a more humane society: to reduce or eliminate poverty, especially childhood poverty, and to reduce financial and social inequality.

This is indeed a manifesto for change. It might even be revolutionary. But it's also achievable. I am an optimist.

Index

Printed by Printforce, United Kingdom

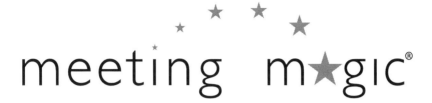

meeting magic®

A practical guide for business managers who want to make their meetings productive.

By Katherine Woods and Ingrid Uden

www.meetingmagic.co.uk

"I have worked with Meeting Magic over a number of years; with Ingrid while I was at Microsoft, and with Katherine since I took over as CEO of Artilium. I highly recommend working with Meeting Magic; their rigorous preparation and innovative facilitation techniques guarantee a successful outcome. Their book contains a wealth of practical advice on making meetings productive."

Robert Marcus, *Chief Executive Officer, Artilium plc*

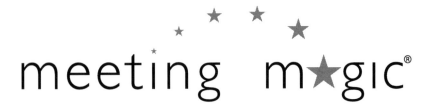

meeting m★gic®

by

Katherine Woods & Ingrid Uden

Copyright © 2007 Meeting Magic Publications

ISBN: 978-0-9557788-0-3

Published by: Meeting Magic Ltd in conjunction with Writersworld Ltd
www.meetingmagic.co.uk

Printed and bound by Antony Rowe Ltd, Eastbourne

WRITERSWORLD
9 Manor Close, Enstone, Oxfordshire OX7 4LU
England
www.writersworld.co.uk

Contents

Chapter

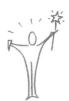

Acknowledgements

We owe a great deal of thanks to lots of people in the writing of this book. Many of our friends and family have offered support and encouragement along the way. In particular, however, we would like to mention the following.

First and foremost we have to thank David Sibbet. David is the President of The Grove Consultants International and one of the founding fathers of Graphic Facilitation. In our early days as facilitators we were fortunate to be trained by David himself and many of the tools and techniques that we now use are those that he and the Grove team developed. The many principles of facilitation that we hold most important, and upon which the advice in this book is based, are explained in greater detail in The Grove's work. More information can be found in the bibliography. The Grove Consultants International is now a strategic partner to Meeting Magic Ltd.

Next we must thank the people who directly helped us to write this book. Lynne Kennedy, Alex Smeed, Lis Long, Stephen Uden and John Handy all gave their time to read drafts of the book and give valuable feedback. Lesley Holden spent hours digitising the hand-drawn illustrations which Steve Yard-Young used in the design of the book layout, and Graham Cook, Sue Croft and Charles Leveroni of Writersworld have helped with everything from cover design to copy editing. Lastly Nigel Temple has given invaluable advice on marketing this book.

Our final thank you, however, is saved for the people without whom none of this would have been possible – our clients. Through sharing with us their stories of meeting nightmares and working with us in their meetings, we have been able to understand what problems people encounter. In turn they have helped us learn how to avoid or overcome these pitfalls. A special thank you to those whose stories we have used to bring the advice to life.

1

Introduction

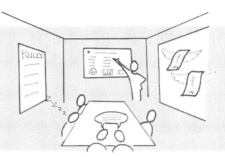

Our guess is that if you work in an organisation where groups of people have to hold meetings to get the work done, you will regularly experience frustration, boredom, irritation and a whole host of other negative emotions at work. You might say this is a lucky guess, based on the fact you are reading this book, but it isn't. Sad to say, it is a known fact that millions of pounds, dollars and euros are wasted every year in the time that managers spend in ineffective meetings. Quite apart from the formal research into the subject, workplaces are rife with jokes alluding to awful meetings, many of the themes being very well explored in the ever popular Dilbert cartoons. Sadder still is that this seems to be accepted, so often, as the natural order of things; something that can't be changed.

Those of you who have ever experienced a well-planned and facilitated meeting will know that in fact, not only can a lot be done about it but that, if you know what you're doing, a meeting can be transformed into a productive and inspiring way to get work done. The trick is to know what you're doing. If you could afford it of course, it would be wonderful to have a professional, independent facilitator to run every meeting you ever called. But in the real world this tends to happen only for the more expensive or critical meetings. For the majority of meetings this just isn't an option and so managers are left trying to contribute to discussions as well as manage the flow of the meeting.

Having stated that something can be done to improve matters, let's also be clear that it isn't as trivial as is sometimes suggested by the 'good meeting practice' brigade. We have been to numerous meeting rooms in many different companies and pinned up on the wall is a dusty, fading notice imploring the occupant to follow a few simple 'good meeting rules'. Of course they fall into disrepute because they don't work and they don't work because they are just too simplistic. Yes, things would be better if everyone was there within the first 5 minutes of the published start time, but when they're not, then what? The faded notice gives no clue. And yes, we'd love it if everyone was respectful and listened to each other. But when they're patently not and voices are getting louder and louder, what should you do? Again, the sad notice remains mute on the subject.

The other end of the spectrum for achieving effective meetings is occupied by the psychologists who have studied and understand the subtleties of human interactions. There is a great depth of information and insight into group processes and interpersonal relationships within a work context and there are many talented people, who understand the implications and apply them to the art of facilitation. But how about those of you, who just want your meetings to run more smoothly? We doubt you have the time or energy to devote to such study. This book has been written for you.

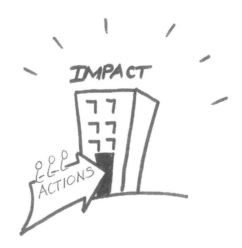

What this book is about, therefore, is getting results from the meetings you call or get asked to manage. Most often it is your meeting, one you've asked people to attend because you need them to help you get some work done. But many of us also find ourselves being asked to run a meeting that we might otherwise be a participant in, just because we're known to be good at that sort of thing. These reasons might confer on you some degree of ownership or leadership for the meeting, but they don't make you a facilitator. So although all the advice in this book is written by two people who have spent many meetings as independent facilitators, it takes the perspective of the hard-pressed manager trying to do a good job. For this reason the language throughout speaks of managers, owners or leaders of meetings and not facilitators.

The Purpose of this Book

We have been facilitating meetings for over 10 years and shared our skills with hundreds of business managers through a variety of different training seminars. Invariably those managers come to the training not because they want to become full time meeting facilitators, but because they want to overcome the problems they have with their meetings, and that is exactly how they tackle it. We might try to structure a training course around lofty principles and models, leading smoothly into methods and practices and finally giving hands-on practice, but time and time again delegates put up their hands and say, "Yes, but last week this happened... how do I cope with that?" Now like any quick fix, it might feel good just to give an answer, but that won't really help because the same situation won't come up exactly the same each time. What you need to understand are the main reasons why a particular problem occurs and then have a range of options for how to cope with those underlying problems. Like any good doctor when presented with a symptom, you first diagnose possible causes and then decide on the best treatment from a range of possible therapies.

This book has been written to appeal to all those managers like those who attend our courses. Each chapter starts with a problem, just like the ones we get presented with. There then follows a review of possible causes for the issue and finishes with lists of ideas for practical things you can do to prevent or resolve the problem. The sections explaining the underlying reasons give enough detail for you to understand the later advice sections, but do not plunge into all the back-up research on a particular topic. For those who are interested in more depth on particular aspects, we refer you to the bibliography at the end of the book.

This book is all about providing practical help. After the diagnosis part of each chapter there follows a section with a list of options written in an instructional way, to make it easy to apply. We use stories and examples to bring our advice to life and in each chapter there is a 'script' for how to tackle a particular interaction. It is not expected that you will be able to follow these scripts, nor any of the suggested ideas, word for word. Meeting facilitation is an art and you will need to find a style of your own through which to express these ideas. What is intended is that you will have many options to try, to play with and to make your own in the many meetings you will be successfully managing into the future.

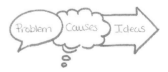

The Style of this Book

This book is intended to be flexible in the way it is read. It could be read from cover to cover, but it also intended to be rewarding if you just read the chapters that suit your needs, or want to browse through the problems and summaries of advice.

Each of the chapters has the same broad structure; to help find your way around we have added some graphic codes in the left hand margins.

 Indicates where a problem is being defined. These are written as questions and have been developed from the questions we get asked by managers in training sessions we run.

 Indicates where the root cause of a problem is being explored. These are the underlying complications that are likely to be causing the problem.

 Indicates options for how problems can be prevented. These are written as instructions for things that can be done in advance of a meeting to prevent the problem arising.

 Indicates options for things you can do in the meeting, if the problem is arising. Again, these are written in an instructional style, to make them easy to apply.

 Finally at the end of each chapter is a summary of the advice for how to prevent the problem that has been explored.

You may notice that some pieces of advice are repeated in different chapters of the book. We have done this to make each chapter useful in its own right, without the need for continually flicking to and fro. For example, contacting the participants of a meeting beforehand can prevent a number of different problems from occurring in a meeting. The small graphics embedded in text symbolise the points being explained and are aimed at helping you find your way around the book if you are dipping in and out.

About the Authors – How this book came to be written

We originally met whilst working at Mars Confectionery. Over the years we worked together in different roles, developing a close working relationship and learning that we had a lot in common ......

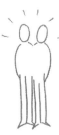

*   Both of us studied Engineering at University, giving us a strong systems thinking to our problem solving.
*   Our backgrounds in Blue chip organisations gave us a breadth of experience in project and people management. We have first-hand experience of leading teams and running business meetings.
*   Through our roles in Communication and Training we gained experience in how to really engage groups, both large and small, to generate business impact.

We both started to learn the art of facilitation whilst at Mars and found ourselves constantly in demand to facilitate key meetings. In 1999 we decided to follow our passion for facilitation on the premise, that other businesses also would benefit from improving their meetings, and Meeting Magic Ltd was born. The business took off immediately and has grown to become the Meeting Magic Network with strategic partners in the USA and Australia.

Over the years we have facilitated a diverse range of meetings. We have worked in the private, public and non-profit sectors with groups ranging from Chief Executive Officers with their leadership teams, to large group consultations. One of the reasons we have enjoyed facilitating so much, is that we have had the chance to experience so many different groups in so many different situations.

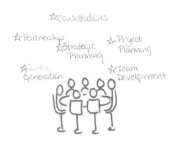

In 2005 Ingrid left Meeting Magic to pursue a career in teaching and we decided to write this book as a way of capturing some of what we had learnt. For two years we wrote the book in our spare time, in between retraining to be a teacher and managing a growing business! Most of the practical examples come from Katherine, as we want to keep them recent.

At the heart of our drive to establish Meeting Magic Ltd and write this book, is a shared desire to show people that there is another way to run meetings. They don't have to be dull and dysfunctional; they can be fun and productive. So we would implore you, read the chapters that sound most familiar to the situations you find yourself in, then go out there and dare to be different:

make your meetings magic!

2

Just talks too much

Q. *It seems so often in meetings that I facilitate, that there are one or more participants who just love the sound of their own voices. They always have an opinion on everything, whether it is an informed one or not, and are without fail the first to answer any open question I put to the group. I like to encourage participation and involvement, but theirs is just too much. When they are talking so much it stops the quieter (more considered or reflective) people from joining in and often I'm sure this must be really irritating. How can I get some balance into my meetings so that everyone gets an equal share of the conversation? I don't want to silence these people altogether but I do need them to be a bit more respectful and make space for the quieter people in the room.*

Problem

A. This meeting leader is right to be concerned about this problem, in particular with respect to the impact it has on others in the room. An important role you can play in achieving a successful meeting is to ensure that all the people there contribute and feel ownership for whatever decisions the group makes. This is very hard to do, if the same one or two people dominate the conversations. There are of course a number of reasons why the phenomenon occurs and we need to consider each of these before we decide what things we can do to correct the balance.

Personal Style

Some people are naturally talkative, where others like to contemplate more before they offer their opinions. This can be because of personal confidence, perhaps related to experience in the subject, but is more often just a question of, for want of getting too technical, personality. Some people will develop their thinking as they are talking, whilst others like to think then talk. Unfortunately these more considered people can find they don't get a word in edgeways, if too many of their talkative colleagues attend the meeting.

In a related way, sometimes there are people attending the meeting who do not speak English as their first language. This can obviously be a barrier to rapid contribution if you have to find your words before you speak. In our experience however, the personality effect is the greater one and if a person is voluble it makes little difference how well they speak the language – they will jump straight into the conversation. Having said that however, we do believe a meeting leader should take into account any possible language barriers using methods discussed in more depth later in the chapter.

Power Play

The reality is, that wherever people gather together, there will be one or more persons who will want to dominate or lead the group. This is true no matter how meek or mild you might think the group would otherwise be; there will be at least one of those shrinking violets who would like to shrink a little less than the others. The people who do this are almost certainly not consciously behaving that way. It is a much more innate human characteristic than that, which you will observe in every group you work with.

This establishing of pecking order will often happen without causing problems for a group. If the people who do want to be more dominant have good interpersonal skills, they will be able to establish themselves high up the social ranking, at the same time as allowing space for the others to contribute. A problem only occurs if there becomes a struggle for the top spot – in which case those slugging it out will ignore the rest of the group in their battle with each other. Or alternatively, the dominant people have very low sensitivity and awareness, and are ignorant of the lack of share of voice others have been allowed, or the frustration that usually mounts as the meeting continues.

Another related cause can be the 'trying to prove something' effect. This is a very natural thing that many people will do when, for example, they are new to a team or have been brought specifically for their knowledge or expertise. In their attempt to demonstrate that they do have value to add to the group, they can sometimes lose sight of the need for others in the group to also contribute.

Finally, of course, within the realms of power play, come the complications of organisational hierarchy between the members of a group, where the boss expects everyone to be quiet and listen because they are subordinate. This whole dimension has a chapter to itself called ***Senior manager knows best*** (chapter 5).

The Experts

Having referred to dominance generally, there is sometimes a genuine imbalance caused by one or more experts being in the room. This can have a couple of knock-on effects. The first is the feeling by the expert, that s/he needs to prove their expertise to the group and will therefore be more dominant as a result.

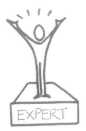

The second effect, in some respects harder to overcome, is when the members of a group hold a great respect for this person and then inhibit themselves from speaking, perhaps in undue reverence.

Whatever the root cause of unequal share of voice, the meeting leader needs to take steps to correct it, if they are to fulfil the objectives of the meeting with everyone's participation and engagement. What follows are specific ideas for things you can do, grouped under Preventions i.e. things to do before the problem occurs, and Interventions i.e. how to handle the situation once you're in it.

Preventions

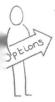

✶ Find out beforehand whether there are **known characters** in the group who are likely to behave this way. If they are well-known by their colleagues for this behaviour, then they are most likely to be the power-play, poor awareness sorts, so getting them to control this behaviour will not be easy. But knowing that they are part of the group is valuable as it enables you to design a meeting style which will minimise their overbearing contributions. (See below for ideas on designing meetings)

✶ At the start of the meeting **establish the ground rules** for how this group will work together. Get the group to agree rules that ensure no one person can over-dominate. For example:-

☆ Make sure everyone has their say (a gentle way to put it)
☆ Equal share of voice (getting a little more definite)
☆ Everyone gets to share one opinion on the topic before anyone is allowed a second say (getting very specific)

Make sure you get agreement to the rules and then explain that your role (probably along with some other things) will be to enforce the rules. Make it clear you will be fair, but ruthless about how you do this.

An example from Ingrid: In a meeting I once facilitated, I had been warned that there were a number of overbearing characters, but that it was really important that everyone had their say. In the introduction I explained to everyone, very calmly, that I would specifically name people who were talking too much and ask them to be quiet until others had had their say on the topic. I emphasised the point a few times that this was really my primary role (on this occasion) and so they could be sure I'd be following through. The effect of this was that I hardly had to use the sanction. Just the possibility of being told, politely, to "shut up because you can't control yourself" was enough to ensure most people did. The worst I had to do in the meeting was ask whether we could "hear from some other voices".

⋆ **Name the problem up front.** It can be a surprisingly successful tactic to tell people, out loud, what the possible problem might be. (See chapter 15 *Naming the elephant* for more on this phenomenon). The effect is often one of relief from those who don't dominate (and wished their colleagues also didn't) and one of guilty acknowledgment from those who do – it is amazing how shy these people can look temporarily. This is a particularly good tactic to use at the same time as making the ground rules. If you name the problem, the group will then undoubtedly propose a rule that addresses the issue, and the brazen statement by you, of the fact that the behaviour is an issue, will do much to help the guilty parties to control themselves, at least for the opening sessions. (For what to do when they forget themselves, see the Interventions section.)

⋆ **Design a process to prevent the problem.** The problem of over-dominance primarily happens when the group is having an open discussion i.e. a conversation that the entire group is party to at the same time. There are many techniques to get people's contributions other than by open discussion. For example:-

　☆　Ask everyone to write their idea on a specific topic onto cards and then put the cards onto a board or poster. This way, all the ideas are there together and (unless specifically marked) carry equal weight. This is an especially good way of getting equal contribution when there is an expert in the room. On topics where everyone's views are valid, everyone will get to contribute equally.

　☆　Pose a question to the group and give everyone (whether they want it or not) thinking time, for example 5 minutes. When the time is up, you can ask everyone to share their thoughts in turn, making it clear that you want to hear everyone's contributions before opening the floor to comments. We have used this technique to very good effect with people speaking English as a second language, where the extra thinking and translating time is especially valuable.

　☆　Split the group into smaller working groups to discuss the topic first. These smaller groups can be anything from pairs to groups of eight. (Groups larger than eight tend not to be effective and for more on this see chapter 10 *Too many people*). How you split the group will depend a lot on how many there are in the room to start with, how many dominant people you're coping with and how much time you have for the groups to report back. Just doing the maths shows, that if you split a group of 20 into 10 pairs, but only allow ten minutes to hear the report back, each pair only has 1 minute, which is not realistic. In these circumstances you might be better splitting into 2 groups of five, or making more time for reporting.

☆ Remember, if you do split the groups to level the playing field, that you do not necessarily want balanced groups (as described in *Too many people*). Here you're trying to give the quieter people an opportunity to have their say, so put the loud folk in a group together. You can rest assured they'll all get their views across, leaving the quieter groups time to share their thoughts and report back in their allocated slot. If you do split the talkative ones between the groups they'll replicate the effects of the large grouping within each small group.

☆ A variation on the above, if you're looking to converge on a single conclusion or decision, is to split the group into pairs. Give them 5 – 10 minutes (or time as appropriate to the size of the decision) to agree on their joint position. It is important they have a single recommendation to take into the next stage. Now get pairs of pairs to form groups of 4 and give them time to discuss their 2 proposals and then agree a single joint position from this group. You go on pairing up groups as many times as necessary until you have just 2 proposals, which can then be discussed with the whole group. As before, try to pair up the voluble characters from the start.

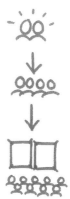

★ *Make space for your experts.* They can tend to push themselves forward, if they feel their knowledge or experience is not being heard. Design a process that has specific times, during which the experience or knowledge is shared and can, if necessary, be questioned to support greater understanding. This can be done in a variety of ways, from a formal presentation slot, to a more open section of the agenda, where you make it clear that the purpose is for the group to get up to speed with the expertise in the room. It might of course be that for different topics, different people become the experts and so you can flag at the start of the agenda, that they'll each have their turn in the spotlight – making them more likely to control themselves at other times.

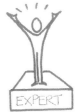

Interventions

★ *Practise public listening.* Often people will keep jumping in because they don't feel they're being listened to or acknowledged – which if they're being over-dominant is probably what is happening. As a meeting leader, you can serve the whole group by actively listening to all contributions and making sure everyone feels heard.

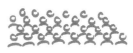

* An invaluable tool to support public listening is to write up what people have said. Record their contributions so that they can SEE they've been heard. The flip chart is the most common tool available for this but is rather limited, if you're trying to record all the ideas being shared in a long meeting. Better to use large white boards (the electronic ones make it easy to capture the information permanently), or our preferred option is to use large sheets of white paper taped onto the wall. We use rolls of paper 1.2m wide that can be rolled out to create a 1.2m deep by 2.5m wide 'page'. This leaves plenty of space to capture the headlines from the discussion and ensure everyone feels listened to. For more on this tool see chapter 13 *Managing information*.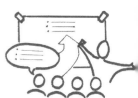

* Creation of large public records of the conversation allows you to use one of the most effective interventions available, namely pointing out that the point the person is making has been heard and recorded. One way this works is as an interruption, "So have I got your point here? (slight pause) Good, can we hear from someone else?" Alternatively if the person is just repeating themselves, you can point to the words you've previously written and say, "Thanks, we have that point, is there anything from someone else?"

* ***Enforce the rules.*** Having got the group to agree to a rule related to equal share of voice – or better still, having primed them to propose such a rule as described above, it is vital that you jump in when you feel the rule is being infringed. Since share of voice can often be seen as subjective (we rarely actually record how long each person in a meeting is speaking – tempting though it might be on occasions), you need to act as a mirror to the group to help them see the behaviour for themselves. It is useful to use an escalating set of interventions, as follows, if the first reminder doesn't fix the problem:-

  ☆ "I feel we haven't heard all the voices in the room yet. Remembering our rule, can we have some other views?"
  ☆ "I'm hearing a lot of the same voices again and again. If we want to keep this rule I'd like some people to make way for the others."
  ☆ "I feel we're not really honouring this rule. Can you (at this point look at the guilty parties) please let some others have their input."
  ☆ "We're really not keeping this rule we set. Can I ask if you're all still committed to having it as a working agreement?" Most groups at this point re-commit to the rule, and do a better job thereafter of keeping it.

* If a number of people are trying to get into the conversation at the same time, make sure you ***acknowledge all*** of them by making eye contact and giving them a quick nod. Then invite them to share their points in turn, asking the quieter people to share their input first. You must make sure, however tempting it is not to, that you get around all the people you've acknowledged, even the louder ones, as cutting them out will only make them exaggerate their overbearing behaviour.

★ If someone if being really disruptive with their behaviour you can always have a **private word** with them during the first available break. We are always polite and unemotional when we do this and would say something along the lines of "You've clearly got a lot to contribute to this meeting and you've made a lot of valuable points already, but we want to make sure we 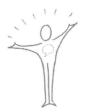 hear from all the people in the room. It is hard for us to hear all the opinions when you have so much to share. What we really need to do is to balance the conversation so we hear from everyone. Is it OK with you if I give you a nod from time to time to remind you to make space for others to contribute?" We've very rarely had anything other than agreement to help from this point on.

★ Invite the **over-talkative contributor closer to the front** or into the centre of attention. Counter-intuitive though this may seem, it does work where the person is merely interrupting as an attention-seeking ploy. We've known this work very effectively, to the extent that the individual has behaved impeccably after being reminded.

★ This chapter focuses on maintaining share of voice in a meeting by managing people who talk a lot. To find out more about how to handle the reverse – please have a look at Chapter 8 *Won't join in.*

Summary

So in summary, our top tips to manage *share of voice* in meetings are:-

★ Identify known talkers in advance and plan ways of handling them.
★ Establish ground rules at the start of the meeting.
★ Name the problem at the start of the meeting.
★ Design processes for equal share of voice.
★ Make space for experts.
★ Practise public listening.
★ Enforce the ground rules.
★ Acknowledge all contributions.
★ Talk to the dominant people in the break.
★ Bring the talkers to the front.

3

Personal conflict

Q. *I sometimes find that no matter how well prepared I am, a meeting just goes off the rails because of a personal conflict between two people in the room. They often dress it up and pretend there isn't a problem, but then they will always disagree with each other and find reasons to contradict what might be very reasonable points of view. It can be very tiresome for others in the room, especially if the arguments are clearly nothing to do with the topic of the meeting and ultimately stop the meeting reaching a satisfactory conclusion. What can I do to stop these personal battles happening in my meetings? I've thought about just telling them not to come, but often we need them there to get the work done.*

Problem

A. Personal disagreements are as old as humanity itself and we're unlikely to be able to change that very easily; this book is offering practical advice, not miracles. You need to have up your sleeve some ideas of how you can at least lessen the impact any conflict might have on the work you're trying to get done. Before we start with what can be done, let's think about some of the main reasons for these conflicts.

Personal Dislike

Some people just don't get on. It isn't one person's fault or the other's; they are just not suited to each other. After all, can you honestly say you have liked everybody you've ever met? Now, by and large, we can choose who we spend time with and so surround ourselves with people we like, but unfortunately within a work context, we don't always have that luxury. People can find themselves forced to work with colleagues who annoy them and, like a small stone in your shoe, the longer you go on, the worse the irritation, until anything they say, including a perfectly innocent comment like, *"Would you like a coffee?"* can sound like a wind up – *"They're having a go at me because I had a coffee five minutes ago and didn't offer them one!"*

Now the good news is that most of us can keep our feelings in check and manage our relationships in a reasonably mature way, but we should be aware, that for some this does require some effort!

History

Although some personal antipathies are written in the stars, many more are manmade. Misunderstandings and upsets happen all the time, mostly as unintended consequences of different people's actions. Sometimes these are addressed, resolved and forgiven, but occasionally they are left to fester and can then build into major

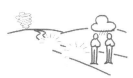

conflict. As time goes on people's memories may change to reinforce their own position with respect to their adversary, whereas the truth will lie somewhere between their two versions of the situation. Some people are better at letting go of such issues than others and a lot depends on the personalities of those involved, which is what most of this chapter is about.

Power Play

From the dawn of time, individuals have sought power over each other – which is why this idea crops up a number of times in this book. For those people who like to be in control or to be in a position of power, there will always be others who are, or who are perceived to be, trying to stop them. This then is the root of another common cause of personal conflict.

Now as the question suggests, the above types of personal conflict are not usually very visible. In the playground we shout names at each other and occasionally resort to physical violence. By the time we're adults, we've learnt to control ourselves (well, most of us have) and so we present a civilised exterior. This however only covers over our real emotions and these can leak out in the way described above. So what can we do to manage this type of situation?

At the heart of all the solutions to managing the conflict are two ideas. The first is to try and find the shared values that individuals might hold. For instance, "Never mind any personal disagreements for now, can we agree that you both really value the success of this project".

The second is to find the common ground in the more pragmatic aspects. This is usually done by taking a broader perspective. "If we can agree that it is in everyone's interests to make sure this project is successful, now let's work through our differences, keeping our agreed goal in mind." So let's look at specific preventions and interventions related to these ideas.

Preventions

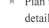

★ If you know that there are people who don't see eye to eye, try and **talk privately with each of them before the meeting.** If you don't know it already, find out if there is any history to the disagreement. We're not suggesting you will be able to magically resolve any long-standing disputes, but to be forewarned is to be forearmed. Once you have an insight into any difficulties you could:-

  ☆ Plan an agenda that steers clear of any hot topics
  ☆ Ask each party, specifically, to keep their dispute from your meeting, assuming it is unrelated.
  ☆ Have a meeting with the two of them before the main meeting, to find out what rules need to be in place to avoid any disruption. This alone might well embarrass them into behaving in your meeting!

★ **Establish some ground rules** as to how this group will work together in the meeting and agree these with everyone at the start of the meeting. Make sure these include some that are pertinent to the issue of personal conflicts. For example:-

  ☆ "All views are welcome, so I'd like to make sure we hear from everyone." (a gentle way to put it)
  ☆ "To encourage different views, I'd like us to ensure no put-downs." (getting a little more definite)
  ☆ "Everyone's views are valid. We can state a different point of view but no one will make negative comments about others' views." (getting very specific)
  ☆ As mentioned in an earlier chapter, explain your role as enforcer of the rules. (Remember, fair but ruthless!)

★ Plan to use **large public displays of information.** This is explained in much more detail in chapter 13 Managing information, but the essence is that you will be able to ensure that everyone can see their contribution has been heard and recognised, as this can defuse emotions. It is also a way for people to SEE that they do agree on things after all – important when they may have stopped listening to each other some time ago!

★ Our final word on preventing conflict is about **knowing the limitations of facilitation.** As facilitative managers there is a tendency to think that we can facilitate our way out of everything. However, there is a level of trust required for facilitation to work and some people just don't want to get on!

   ☆ Check that you have sufficient trust and agreed outcomes to be able to lead the group through a process with high participation, ownership and creativity.

   ☆ Consider involving a negotiator to moderate the group in exploring interests and crafting contracts.

   ☆ If the trust is really low, then you will need to consider involving an external mediator/arbitrator. This area is really outside the scope of this book; we are talking about improving business meetings, not solving the Middle East conflict!

Interventions

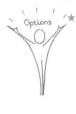

★ Start all your meetings by **clarifying outcomes, agenda, roles and rules** (can be remembered as OARRs). By having these ways of working established at the start of a meeting we can then anchor back to them, to resolve conflicts, later in the meeting. So, for example, if a heated debate is disrupting the flow of a meeting, we can then check back to the outcomes of the meeting and ask whether this discussion needs to be resolved to achieve them. Often when there are historical issues between people they can end up being raised inappropriately, and this kind of intervention can stop them derailing the meeting.

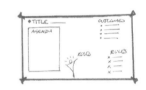

★ **Be clear about what you will not cover.** At the start of the meeting, state very clearly what will and importantly will not be covered by this meeting. This is your opportunity to put out of bounds any topic that might ignite the old conflict – although you'll have needed to do your homework to know what the root of the problem might be.

★ **Practise public listening.** As a meeting leader you can serve the whole group by actively listening to all contributions and making sure everyone feels heard. An invaluable tool to support public listening is to write up what people have said. Record their contributions so that they can SEE they've been heard. The flip chart is the most common tool available for this but is rather limited if you're trying to record all the ideas being shared in a long meeting. It's better to use large white boards (the electronic ones make it easy to capture the information permanently), or

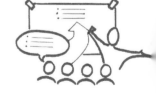

our preferred option is large sheets of white paper taped onto the wall. We use rolls of paper 1.2m wide that can be rolled out to create a 1.2m deep by 2.5m wide 'page'. This leaves plenty of space to capture the headlines from the discussion and ensure everyone feels listened to. For more on this tool see chapter 13 *Managing Information.*

★ A useful technique for getting people to see another's perspective is to get them to literally **sit in each other's chairs.** This can be easily set up by getting people to label their chair with their name (and sometimes the area of expertise or role they represent). You then ask people to move around, to sit in someone else's chair and to consider the situation from this new position. It can be useful to get people to record the insights or key challenges they see as they move from chair to chair. There are usually two productive outcomes from this type of session:
   ☆ The conflicting parties get to see the situation from the other's perspective.
   ☆ People are usually pleasantly surprised by how accurate the insights are, which helps them to feel understood.

★ The previous technique can be modified for larger groups by getting people to write their name at the top of a piece of flipchart. As people walk round the flipcharts they take that person's position and make notes of insights, challenges etc on the flipchart.

★ **Swapping sides.** When people feel that they are not understood, there is a tendency to do more and more talking at the other party, in an attempt to get a point of view across. A more effective means of getting people to listen and understand can be to get the different parties to present the other side's point of view. This approach makes the parties feel heard, when they hear their perspective being presented back, and also makes the different sides understand better, as they need to assimilate the information in order to present it. People often find the reason in an argument when they have to work through it and find a way to communicate it themselves.

An example from Katherine: I was asked to facilitate a meeting between two companies who had been working together for some time and who were encountering problems in their working relationships. When I first got the brief for the meeting there was a draft agenda in place which included two presentations at the start of the meeting, one from each company to the other company about their goals, ways of working, issues etc. I persuaded the client to modify the design so that company 1 was given a wall-chart template to complete about company 2 and vice versa. Each template contained key questions they needed to answer about the other company e.g. business objectives, expectations from the project, culture/ways of working, possible frustrations with the project. Once the two templates were completed they were posted up and the groups swapped over and read their own template (as completed by the other company). Both companies were surprised by how accurate the other company had been and felt understood. The great thing about this technique was that it demonstrated to each party what was known and the focus of the discussion that followed was on what wasn't known. I imagine that if they had prepared presentations to each other the meeting would have started with 'death by PowerPoint' rather than a demonstration of mutual understanding.

★ One of the best tools in managing conflict between two parties is to **take a break and talk with them both privately**. Away from the rest of the group someone is much more likely to open up about what is really going on for them and be open to suggestions about how to move forward.

★ Generally, personal conflicts are most disruptive when a group is in open forum discussion. This format of discussion allows people to hold the limelight and also provides a stage for personal conflicts to play out in front of an audience, whilst the audience falls asleep! By **changing the process** of a conversation in a meeting, we can change the impact that any conflict is having. What we mean by changing the process is that in a group of 12 people you could choose the following process options:

☆ Discussion as a whole group of 12, open forum discussion
☆ Individual thinking time leading into open forum discussion
☆ Paired discussion before sharing in the whole group
☆ Four groups of   3
☆ Three groups of 4
☆ Two groups of   6
☆ Or even combinations e.g. paired discussion, followed by pairs forming groups of 4 to find commonalities in discussion before coming back to the main group.

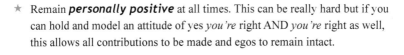

The power comes in switching formats. If what you're doing isn't working, then change to something else.

★ Remain **personally positive** at all times. This can be really hard but if you can hold and model an attitude of yes *you're* right AND *you're* right as well, this allows all contributions to be made and egos to remain intact.

Summary

Our summary of top tips for handling *personal conflicts*:-

★ Clarify outcomes, agenda, rules and roles at the start of the meeting.
★ Practise public listening by recording points visibly.
★ Get the conflicting parties to sit in each other's positions.
★ Take a break in the meeting and talk privately with conflicting parties.
★ Change the process of the discussion.
★ Remain positive at all times!
★ Talk privately with conflicting parties before the meeting.

4

Can't stick to the agenda

Q. *One of the most common problems I face in meetings is people going off track. We either go off track because people reiterate the same points in circular discussions or someone raises a topic and we end up diving down some irrelevant rat run. However much I ask people to keep to the point and emphasise the time constraints, I just can't seem to run the meeting to plan.*

Problem

A. Yes, you and millions of other people running meetings would cite this as the number one reason meetings are unproductive. Ensuring that people get the chance to share their views and explore a topic and still keep to the agenda can be a real challenge.

The tendency is to blame one or two people for rambling or getting side-tracked, but actually keeping on track in a meeting needs to be a shared responsibility.

In this chapter we will look at what makes people stray from the agenda and what we can do to make our meetings run to plan.

Lack of clear outcomes

If people don't have a clear sense of where they are going it is no wonder they can't stick to the path to get them there, and if they all have different views on where they are heading they are likely to take different paths.

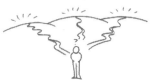

If the group have some sense of where they are going, but not a specific end in mind, they have no sense of what level of depth they need to explore a subject. They can find themselves delving into detail where it may not be needed or going round and round a subject when they actually have enough perspectives to do the work required.

It is inevitable that new subjects get raised in meetings as, when a group of people come together to discuss a topic, they will be likely to have different perspectives. Therefore without a clear outcome it is difficult to determine which subjects need to be covered and which need to be resolved elsewhere. Consequently the group can find themselves exploring a whole topic that actually doesn't need to be covered to achieve the final outcome.
(We talk in detail about lack of clear outcomes in chapter 6 *Unclear outcomes*.)

Group Composition

There is usually a mix of different styles amongst the members of a group. There are task focused people who want to get the job done and see the results, and people/process focused people who are concerned about how the work gets done and how people

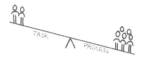

interrelate. In most groups the diversity of both types gives a group balance. However, some groups find themselves particularly strong in some areas and weak in others.

If there is a lack of task focus in the group they are going to find it harder to stick to the agenda. They will probably spend a lot of time talking about how they tackle things without worrying about drawing conclusions.

The subject matter

Subject matter can also cause problems for agendas. Maybe the subject is too complex for a single meeting, or maybe the complexity wasn't understood until everyone came together. Either way, there can be legitimate reasons why another topic that was not

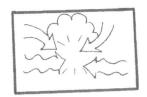

planned for ahead of the meeting, needs to be discussed.

I know we are called Meeting Magic, but even we cannot magic extra time into the day (although there have been many times when we've wished we could). However, there are ways for you to cope with the need to add additional agenda items, and these we will explore in this chapter

Preventions

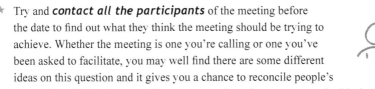

Let's start by looking at ways we can prevent a meeting going off track.

★ Try and **contact all the participants** of the meeting before the date to find out what they think the meeting should be trying to achieve. Whether the meeting is one you're calling or one you've been asked to facilitate, you may well find there are some different ideas on this question and it gives you a chance to reconcile people's expectations before the start. There are a number of ways you can do this depending on time, number of people, who is involved etc. For example:-

☆ Make a 5-10 minute phone call with each participant before the meeting. The call could go something like, "Hello, I am calling you about the meeting we have scheduled on *date*. The purpose of the meeting is *state the purpose of the meeting.* However, I am wondering if you can spare me a few minutes to share your thoughts on what we should be aiming to achieve in the meeting." Having conversations with people in advance enables you to understand the potential issues for a meeting. You may also pick up on things that might send a meeting off track, in a timeframe that allows you to prevent the potential problem.

★ Meetings often go off track because the group are unclear about where they need to get to and how they are going to get there. So designing **Objectives and an Agenda** in advance of a meeting and then communicating this beforehand and at the start prevents a lot of common problems arising. It is also important to be clear about the objectives and agenda for each *individual session* within a meeting e.g. is the outcome to be shared understanding or is a decision to be made?

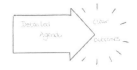

★ Make sure you restate the outcomes and agenda at the start and ideally have them written up and visible throughout the meeting so you can refer back to them.

★ When planning the agenda for a meeting you really need to design the detail of a session to enable accurate time allocation. By this I mean having a **process to manage the conversation** in that part of the meeting, and thinking through the detailed steps at each stage of the process e.g. if you want to share some information and get feedback in a session, you will need to make time to set the session up, then share the information, then allow people to give feedback in an agreed format, then close the session.

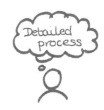

★ ***Beware the meeting agenda without outcomes*** ☠! Clients often come to us with draft agendas that are usually a stream of (unrelated) topics. These are the kinds of meetings that are most likely to go off the rail! The topics on the agenda have no clear outcomes and no structured processes. There is no clear purpose for the meeting, no objectives and therefore no logic in the flow of topics.

An example from Katherine: *I share with you exhibit A, an example of the kind of information I am often sent in advance of an initial briefing session.*

	Global Sales & Marketing Meeting
8:00	Breakfast
8:30	Reviewing last year (Marketing Director)
9:15	Organization, Goals, and Objectives for this year (Marketing Director)
10.00	BREAK
10:15	Product Overview (Marketeer)
11:45	Marketing Plans for this year (Marketeer)
12.45	LUNCH
14:00	Project Update (Project Owner)
14:45	Services & Support Processes (TBD)
15.30	Close (Marketing Director)
15:45	BREAK
16.00	Sales Training (Consultant)
17.30	DRINKS and DINNER

*I have modified the names on this example, to protect the innocent! No, seriously, the reason I share this example with you is because it is **so typical**. I'd bet there are hundreds of meetings going on as you read this, with agendas as ill-defined as this one. Looking at this example, this agenda could be improved by:*

★ *Having a clear and stated purpose. (Clarity about why the meeting is being held and what will happen as a result of this meeting, that otherwise would not happen)*
★ *Clear objectives for the meeting*
★ *Obtaining input from key participants (both people known to be positive and those who are sceptics) about what they want from the meeting. (This agenda had been put together by a couple of senior people who were to lead the meeting without understanding the expectations of the participants coming to the meeting.)*
★ *Clear objectives for the individual sessions on the agenda*
★ *Having a structured process for the sessions. The intention was that the sessions would kick off with a short presentation and then lead into an open forum discussion with 25 people. This kind of process is the most likely to overrun for the following reasons:*
  ☆ *Short presentations need to be well prepared; people tend to ramble more when they are not prepared.*
  ☆ *An open forum discussion without clear outcomes has no end!*
  ☆ *Open forum discussions are the easiest to hijack by dominant people etc*

A sample process – there was a need for clarity about where the organisation was going, so a session was designed as follows.

Outcome: Everyone to understand the new organisation, the business goals for the next year and the Sales and Marketing objectives.

Steps:

1. *Presentation from Marketing Director*
2. *Individual time to think about*
   * *what I liked about what I heard*
   * *what surprised me*
   * *what questions of clarification I have*
3. *Discussions in groups of 5, to produce a maximum of 3 questions*
4. *Group discussion reported back to the main group with questions. Questions collated from all the tables*
5. *Answers to questions by Marketing Director and CEO.*

★ Another practice that can help meetings stay on track is giving people **time to think** about a question before they speak. People often ramble as they think aloud their answer to a question. By giving people even just a couple of minutes to collect their thoughts privately before discussing as a group, you are much more likely to get good quality input. This technique is particularly helpful when people are working in a second language.

★ Sometimes a group of people will have a propensity to run off track because there is a **lack of task focused people** in the group. You can support groups like this by either taking the task focused role yourself (even if it is not your preferred style you will be doing a service to them) or supporting the task focused minority in the group.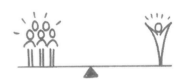

★ Taking time in advance of a meeting to **prepare any information input** to the group can have huge benefit, for example, putting information into templates for ease of digestion in the meeting and preparing posters with information for the walls of the meeting room. This can save time by making the information quick and easy to absorb during the session.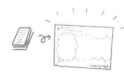

★ **Appropriate use of pre-work** can also help meetings stay on track, although we are always very realistic about what pre-work people will really do in advance of a meeting. We tend to use pre-work to expose people to the meeting content, making good use of 'questions for consideration'. It is always useful, of course, to be prepared for people who have not done the pre-work requested.

Interventions

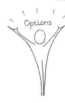

Now let's look at options we can use in a meeting that is likely to veer off track.

★ Make sure you restate the **outcomes and agenda** at the start and ideally have them written up and visible throughout the meeting so you can refer back.

If you have the outcomes and agenda visible throughout the meeting this can help you bring people back on track in a number of ways:

☆ If people start discussing something that sounds as if it is outside the scope of the meeting, you can point to the outcomes and ask, "Do we need to have this conversation in order to achieve these outcomes?" If the answer is no then the group will usually realise the error of their ways and get back to the subject in hand.

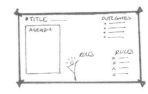

If, however, the group think they need to have the discussion then:-

☆ you can refer back to the agenda to work with the group to reallocate time. For example, "How long do you think we need to cover this?" or "How can we fit this in and still achieve the outcomes?"

☆ you can offer a different process for having the conversation. For example, if the energy is dropping you could split the group up and get them to discuss and come back with their key conclusions.

☆ you could re-jig the agenda in a break and then run through your proposal when you come back.

★ Have a **ground rule** established at the start of a meeting that topics get discussed in their allotted slot on the agenda e.g. "We have a lot to cover today so I am going to propose a ground rule for this meeting that we keep focused in each session on the topic for that session, and don't allow ourselves to get diverted. Can everyone agree to this?"

Then enforce the rule during the meeting. For example, when you hear an 'off topic' discussion arising you can intervene with,

☆ "Do we need to cover this right now?"

☆ Or, getting less subtle, "This sounds like topic X which we have on our agenda at this point (point to visible agenda). Can we come back to discussing topic Y right now?"

☆ Or, getting serious now, "We seem to keep diverting off the subject onto other topics, which means we will overrun if we carry on like this. Do we need to revise this rule, change the agenda or change our finish time?"

★ Share and enforce an 80:20 ground rule. Some group discussions could go on forever but if you get 80% value in 20% of the time then quit while you are ahead. You can share this thinking in the meeting to sense-check the value of continuing the discussion. The kind of intervention we suggest would be, "We could talk about this all day but my sense is that we have covered enough to get the value from the discussion…."

★ ***Recording progress*** can help keep on track as people can see points of discussion being recorded and then move on. If you use wall-chart templates they can assist by not only showing the progress made but also the areas/topics yet to complete. This tends to make the group keep themselves on track. See chapter 13 *Managing information* for more on this.

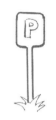

★ If you record progress it allows you to indicate where points have already been made and are now being repeated. You can then push the group to contribute different points rather than repeating what has already been shared.

★ Have a ***car park*** for topics that get raised that will not help achieve the outcomes of the meeting but need to get picked up outside the meeting. Make sure you check that the topic can be parked with the group and that there is a means to pick up the car park topics after the meeting.

> *A warning example from Katherine: I was speaking to a participant of a meeting in preparation for my design work for their meeting. When I asked if he had any issues or concerns about the meeting he vehemently requested that we did not have a car park in the meeting. When I asked him to elaborate he explained that the senior person who had led the meetings in the past had repeatedly used the car park to park difficult issues that he didn't want to address. After each meeting the car park would mysteriously disappear, leaving no record of the hot topics that everyone needed to resolve.*
> *So what this story reminds us to do is:-*
> > *a) use the car park properly – to record topics that are not within the scope of the meeting rather than to avoid conflicts.*
> > *b) have a process for following up on these topics outside the meeting or make sure actions get allocated against the car park items during the meeting.*

★ Having a ***flexible agenda*** can allow for the ebb and flow of meeting discussions. This can be done by starting the meeting with a list of potential topics (either collated in advance or in the meeting or both). The group then prioritise these topics (dot voting works well for this) and build an agenda. If some topics overrun then at least the highest priorities are covered. If sessions take less time, other topics can be added.

★ It can be useful to start a session with an initial brainstorm of possible points for discussion. This brainstorm can be recorded onto a mind map, connecting related points as they build up. The group can then pick out the priorities for discussion.

★ If we know we are likely to need the agenda to flex, we tend to write the agenda items on large (A5) sheets, or use post-its or cards and place them onto a wall chart. This means we can move them around to reflect the changes as the agenda develops.

★ Build plenty of ***breaks*** into the meeting design. This means there is slack in the agenda if sessions overrun. You can also use breaks to have informal discussions about any changes to the agenda that are needed after the break.

Summary

So in summary, our top tips to ensure you *keep your meeting on track* are:-

- ★ Speak to participants in advance of the meeting.
- ★ Clarify the meeting purpose, outcomes and outputs.
- ★ Have clear processes for each stage of the agenda, with detailed timings.
- ★ Clarify the outcomes, agenda, rules and roles at the start of the meeting.
- ★ Have these written up and visible throughout the meeting.
- ★ Use a car park to record topics for discussion outside the meeting.
- ★ Record contributions so people can see they have been heard.
- ★ Keep referring back to the outcomes throughout the meeting.

5

Senior manager knows best

Q. *The hardest thing I have to cope with is senior managers who think they should be involving their people in important decisions but only so long as they produce the "right" answer. I was recently asked to facilitate a group to create solutions to a particular problem and to make sure they got the answer they were meant to. This wasn't too bad if I'd known in advance but I didn't and then all hell broke loose in the meeting when the senior person arrived and got all heavy handed about what people were suggesting. It was only after the meeting that I finally worked out what was going on. I wonder, what techniques are there for getting the group to the same solution that their management want, in a way that doesn't leave everyone feeling manipulated?*

Problem

A. Oh dear! What a horrible mess. And I'm afraid you've asked the wrong question here. To paraphrase, you've asked, "How can I successfully manipulate people so that they feel good about it?" There may be books out there that give you that sort of advice, but this isn't one of them. But don't despair; there is a solution to the problem you present. In fact there is a range of options appropriate to your situation that you can try. As ever, all you need to do is decide why the problem might be happening and then choose your approach.

Personal style

It always feels as if a manager behaving this way is just a complete control freak, and that of course may be the case, but why do they feel that only they have the right answer?

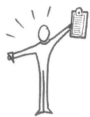

For some it will simply be a desire to be in complete control. They are the 'it might be the wrong decision but at least it is my decision' school of management. Others may not naturally lean in this direction but may be following a lead from above. They've been told to make something happen (and very often a particular something) and so happen it will.

Finally there are those who feel they need to establish their credibility. Insecure managers might not feel confident letting others influence the decisions and so feel they have to ensure the 'right' decision gets made. Now this is all very well; throughout time strong leaders have taken decisions without recourse to a dozen meetings; they decide – they tell – others do. Go back not so long ago and industry the world over ran this way. So why are these same managers now arranging complicated meetings so their staff can come up with the same decisions they've already made?

Too much management training

Over the years more and more books have been written about the importance of a more collaborative style of management. Following the books have come endless hours of training for managers across all levels of organisations. Now all these books and training

have created a belief and expectation that every decision should be collaborative or at least consultative. And this belief exists not only in the people managing but also in those that they are responsible for.

Before going on, we should say that we are 100% committed to the use of collaborative working. After all, this book is essentially about making meetings more productive through ensuring better contribution and collaboration. However, the many hours of management training can sometimes miss two important points.

The first is that collaborative working is *not* always the right answer. There is a spectrum of choices for how to work effectively with a group and whilst collaborative working is excellent for many circumstances it is not always the best choice.

Secondly, and related, is that groups do not always want to be involved in the decision-making. There are times when groups want to be led; they want a manager to make a decision and direct them towards what they want to do. The bottom line, as in so many cases, is to choose the right tool for the job.

So how does this relate to the question above? Most importantly a situation should be handled with honesty. Be honest with the senior manager if a different approach is needed. Get them to share their solutions with the group. If they want the group to buy in then they are more likely to get it by being transparent and letting the group explore the solution. Be honest with the group and credit all participants with intelligence. If they are not going to be involved in the decisions, our experience is that nearly every group we have worked with in this situation is fine, as long as it is made clear from the start. Here are ideas for how to do this effectively.

Preventions

★ Try and **contact all the participants of the meeting** before the date to find out what they think the meeting should be trying to achieve. Whether the meeting is one you're calling or one you've been asked to facilitate, you may well find there are some different ideas on this question and it gives you a chance to reconcile people's expectations before the start. There are a number of ways you can do this depending on time, number of people, who is involved etc. For example;-

☆ A 5-10 minute phone call with each participant before the meeting. The call could go something like, "Hello, I am calling you about the meeting we have scheduled on *date*. The purpose of the meeting is *state the purpose of the meeting*. However, I am wondering if you can spare me a few minutes to share your thoughts on what we should be aiming to achieve in the meeting." Once you have understood their expectations of the meeting you can ask a follow-up question; "With these objectives in mind, is there anything that is likely to get in the way of achieving them in the meeting? Have you any issues or concerns?"

★ As well as understanding the expectations and concerns of participants you will also get an insight into their **expected level of involvement** in decisions. We often find that, when we have these conversations, the team members are asking to hear from their leader, to understand their views. This can be useful to give the leader confidence that it is OK to present something to them and for the leader to know what it is the group want to hear from them.

★ The most important people to contact before the meeting are the most senior people coming, the key stakeholders or decision-makers. With these people it can be useful to have a conversation along the lines of the one described above but also include,

☆ "Are there any 'givens' for this meeting, anything that we need to work with, that cannot be changed?" This will enable you to get really clear about what needs to be achieved in the meeting and what is 'up for grabs' versus givens. The latter is particularly important to clarify when working with senior people as there is no point in spending time in a meeting coming up with plans for things that cannot be changed.

☆ And "How do you propose we make decisions in this meeting? Who will be the decision-maker(s)?" These questions are related to the question above but get more specific about what level of involvement is required in decision-making.

★ There is an excellent model for **understanding different types of decision-making** appropriate to different situations, which was developed by Peter Senge. It identifies that at one end of the spectrum there are times when it is appropriate for an individual to make the decision and then tell those affected, whereas at other times there are benefits to having everyone involved.

The real importance of the model is the understanding that there is not one size fits all. You need to consider the situation and find an approach that works. And if you've chosen appropriately and everyone understands the method adopted, then you will greatly increase your chances of success. When people are given the impression that they are being involved and then find out that the boss wants to tell them the answer, that's when they feel manipulated.... and rightly so!

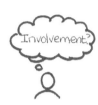

★ It is often **appropriate to use different styles for different sessions** within a meeting e.g. a meeting might start with a leader telling the group her views on their direction. This might be followed by the leader testing top-level plans with the group before the group goes on to create for themselves the tactical action plans.

★ It can be useful to challenge yourself/the meeting owner about **why you want to involve people** and what you will do with their input i.e. what will they do if the group's decision takes them in a very different direction? Another way of thinking about this can be to be clear about the scope for making decisions and making sure this is clarified right at the start of the meeting.

★ Your **choice of style** at any point in a meeting will need to be reflected in your choice of decision-making method. For example, if the purpose of the meeting is to have a shared vision, you could:-

  ☆ create the vision and then tell/sell it to the group – executive decision-making before the meeting

  ☆ create a draft vision and get feedback from the group for you to modify the vision – executive decision-making after the meeting

  ☆ consult with the group about the vision and then develop it yourself– executive decision-making after the meeting

  ☆ get the group to create the vision with you– participatory decision-making during the meeting.

For more on decision-making see chapter 11 *Decisions that stick*.

★ Once you have agreed on the right style for your meeting, it is also important to agree your **role with the senior person** at the meeting. The way you work with them needs to support the style of working you have chosen for the meeting.

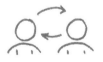

An example of selling a vision: We did some work with a leadership team to develop a long-term vision for their business with the aim of creating a more aligned action in the organisation. Once the leadership team had formed a clear view of what the vision

looked like, they needed to communicate this to the wider organisation. To do this, we facilitated a series of meetings at which the leadership team presented the vision and then facilitated discussions amongst people in the group to clarify their understanding of the vision, before they thought about the implications for their plans.

The interesting twist to this story is that the leadership team intended to sell the vision in the meetings. However, in the first meeting, with their management team, they couldn't help but ask, 'What do you think?' So the first meeting ended up being a test. The key thing to point out here is that they used the feedback from the test to make amendments to the vision, otherwise this could have turned into the kind of manipulated involvement that people detest.

Interventions

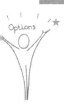

★ Start every meeting by clarifying the **objectives, agenda, roles and rules.** By this we mean, the objectives you aim to achieve by the end of the meeting, the agenda or series of topics you plan to follow through the meeting, the different roles within the meeting and the ground rules that will ensure a successful meeting. As you go through the agenda it can be useful to explain the different styles of the sessions and the proposed decision-making to sense-check this with the group right from the start.

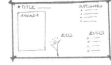

★ If you get into the meeting, however, and find that things aren't quite going to plan then one of the best interventions you can choose is to **take a break.** During this break talk 1:1 with the senior person using the following strategies:-

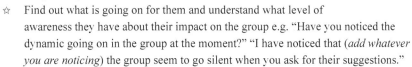

  ☆ Find out what is going on for them and understand what level of awareness they have about their impact on the group e.g. "Have you noticed the dynamic going on in the group at the moment?" "I have noticed that (*add whatever you are noticing*) the group seem to go silent when you ask for their suggestions."

  ☆ Find common ground to build on e.g. "I think they know you have views and want to hear them, as much as you want to hear their views. How about you share your thoughts with the group up-front and then hear what they say? Be clear about the fact that you have views and that you will make the final call, but that you want to understand their views too."

  ☆ Identify the sticking points and try to find solutions to solve them e.g. "I think the group think you have an answer in mind that you have not presented to them. Is that the case?"

  ☆ Look at the values behind their solution e.g. "What is it about involving the group that it important to you?"

  ☆ Look at the bigger picture e.g. "If you have had good experience elsewhere in the business and want to share that here, I am sure the group won't mind hearing that. You can still get their buy-in by letting them explore and modify the approach to suit this particular region."

☆ Challenge the scope of the meeting e.g. "I think we need to work with the vision you have rather than wasting time getting the group to develop a vision. We can then use this meeting to talk about the actions needed to make the vision a reality."

★ Make sure you **do not fall in love with your original meeting design** as you may need to be able to improvise with what happens in the meeting. Don't be afraid to go back into the meeting with a change of plan. That change of plan could be to move further up or down the spectrum of involvement. We have facilitated meetings where the manager has planned to tell the group about something and in the meeting decided to consult. We have also run meetings where we planned to co-create something and the group have agreed they just want the manager to decide.

Summary

So in summary, our top tips on making sure you are *facilitative and not manipulative* in the way you involve people are:-

★ Speak to people before a meeting to find out what level of involvement it expected/wanted.
★ Decide on the appropriate type of decision-making style for the whole meeting and for each session on the agenda.
★ Clarify roles with the senior person coming to the meeting.
★ Start the meeting by clarifying objectives, agenda, roles and rules.
★ If it starts to go pear-shaped, take a break and speak with the senior person 1:1.
★ Be prepared to improvise.

6

Unclear outcomes

Q. *The other week I got a briefing from someone who wanted me to run his meeting. I had some difficulty getting him to be clear on what he wanted from the meeting but in the end thought we had enough of an understanding. When it came to the day of the meeting it all went very wrong. I started the meeting by clearly stating the objectives, only to have him contradict me. Someone else who'd been invited at short notice thought the meeting was about something else completely and before I knew it people were arguing with me about the agenda. Most of the meeting ended up being a discussion about what we wanted a meeting for and hardly any of the original work got done. How can I avoid this in the future? I thought I'd done a good job getting clarity with the meeting owner beforehand, but maybe I'm just not perceptive enough to spot when he isn't clear himself.*

Problem

A. Ah, yes, the classic 'waste of time' meeting. Probably the most common cause of people complaining about meetings being useless is that there is no clear sense of what the meeting is trying to achieve. You are lucky to have had the situation described above, where people actually get to discuss what they think the meeting is about. Most often people sit through what feels like an interminable conversation until they are told they are free to go. They don't know why they went and nothing was achieved. If you take only one piece of advice from this book it is to make sure that for any meeting you attend there is a clear, agreed outcome. This chapter will tell you possible causes of unclear outcomes and how to go about resolving them.

Fogged thinking

While in an ideal world everything falls into nice neat patterns, the day to day reality is that life is messy. How can you get started on this project when it will be so impacted by the impending reorganisation, which in turn is being affected by business performance which in turn will be dramatically affected by the project that you currently have on hold? Ah! Even the clearest thinkers amongst us sometimes have difficulty pulling out the strands of what needs to be tackled, let alone those of us who are less clinical in our thought processes.

It is usually the case that a subject like this will fall into the remit of any given meeting and deciding what should and should not be included can be difficult. It is possible in the case described above that the manager only clarified his thoughts after the discussion with the facilitator.

A big source of fogged thinking can be deciding at what level you need to tackle the issue. That is, do you need a tactical 'quick fix' or are you looking for a more strategic solution? Such is the potential for confusion in this area that we have a whole chapter which deals with it – see chapter 7 *Vision, mission, goals, strategy, tactics...?*

However, just because it is difficult is no excuse not to try and resolve the issue before you have a room full of expectant participants.

Poor communication

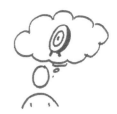

Let's assume the best of people and believe that nobody would arrange a meeting if they didn't have a sense that it would be useful in some way; either to them, to the people attending, to the organisation, or best of all, all three. But a surprisingly common mistake made is in believing that your colleagues are psychic and that since you understand the value of the get-together, so must they. Sadly there are few such gifted people and so without more conventional communication, meetings often proceed without clear outcomes.

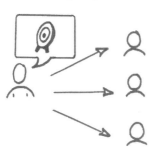

This assumes, of course, that we don't have the problem mentioned above and that there is some clarity in the meeting owner's mind. It is highly possible that what gets communicated doesn't really reflect what will be needed.

Speed of change

Whilst poor communication is something we usually have a degree of control over, the speed of change that many organisations experience is often something that we have little control of. In large organisations in particular, something significant can 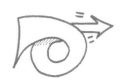 have changed between the meeting being planned and the time it finally goes ahead. Or a meeting owner might make careful arrangements based on one set of assumptions, only to have a more recently informed attendee at the meeting challenge them all. In either case this can be a frustrating situation and if not managed carefully can lead to conflict of the sort described. The bottom line is that everyone attending the meeting needs to have a common understanding of the meeting outcomes. The rest of this chapter deals with how to ensure you achieve this and what options you have if you find yourself adrift.

Preventions

★ ***Clear the fogged thinking.*** If you (or the meeting owner in the case where you've been asked to facilitate for someone else) have a case of fogged thinking, try to structure your thoughts towards a decision using any of the following as appropriate:

☆ Write down all the issues that need to be resolved. Use a large piece of paper and scatter them all over it – don't just make a list. When you can see them all on the same page together, look for groups of issues that are related or similar. Take a new page and rewrite these groups or 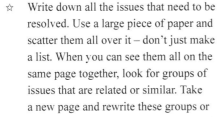 clusters (just a generic title or word will do for each group). Now look for where these groups of issues might impact on each other i.e. we can't address this topic until we have resolution in this area. Draw between the groups to show these inter-relationships. Now stand back and look at your map of the issues. From this you should be able to determine what your meeting should try and tackle and in what order.

☆ Think really big. What are your goals? What ideally are you trying to achieve, not just in a single meeting but overall? Where are you trying to get to? Once you have some picture of future perfection, think about what steps you need to take to achieve the end goal. What needs to happen first? What follows on? Can this all be tackled in one meeting and if not, what scope will you set for the planned session?

☆ What processes or procedures are already in existence in your organisation? Can you use these or part of these to support the work you need to do? Will this help to untangle your ideas for what needs to be done?

Make sure you get real clarity about the level at which you want to, or need to, work. For more advice about this consult chapter 7 *Vision, mission, goals, strategy, tactic...?*

* Try and **contact all the participants** of the meeting before
the date to find out what they think the meeting should be trying
to achieve. Whether the meeting is one you're calling or one
you've been asked to facilitate, you may well find there are
some different ideas on this question and it gives you a chance to
reconcile people's expectations before the start. There are a number of ways you can do
this depending on time, number of people, who is involved etc. For example:-

  ☆ A 5-10 minute phone call with each participant before the meeting. The call could
  go something like, "Hello, I am calling you about the meeting we have scheduled
  on *date*. The purpose of the meeting is *state the purpose of the meeting*. However,
  I wondering if you can spare me a few minutes to share your thoughts on what we
  should be aiming to achieve in the meeting."

  ☆ E-mail everyone with a set of questions. For example, you could send something
  like,
  "Thank you for committing to come to the meeting on date. The purpose of the
  meeting is, *state the purpose of the meeting*. I would appreciate your input into the
  design of the meeting, so please can you spare a moment to consider the following
  questions and send me your replies by date.

    ☆ What would you like us to achieve in the meeting? What specific objectives
    do we need to achieve?
    ☆ Do you have any issues or concerns about the meeting?
    ☆ Do you have any ideas for the meeting?
    ☆ Is there anything else it would be useful for me to know before the meeting?

  ☆ Contact everyone with a clear proposal for the meeting outcomes and ask for
  feedback.
  ☆ If there are lots of participants, making the above ideas too cumbersome to carry out,
  you can target any of the approaches at a few influential or representative people.

Bearing in mind the speed of change issue, however, don't canvass views too early.
Some people (although not all by any means!) like to plan promptly and have everything
wrapped up well ahead of the meeting date. If you do want to get ahead of the game, do
this by all means, but in this case you should do a quick check-in with participants much
closer to the date, to ensure no major changes need to be taken account of.

* Once you've collected the various views about the meeting you must take into account
any differences you find. At the very least you should be clear in your communication
what the meeting is and is not going to tackle. But don't just dismiss any ideas that do not
accord with your own. Be open-minded and consider how you can help meet the needs
of the other participants. After all, you presumably have invited them to the meeting
because you need them to support you in your work, so helping them with what they
need only makes sense.

* If there are very divergent views you might need to dig deeper. Question some more on
what lies beneath these different views. You might find there is a common root cause
around which you can structure some shared work.

★ If you have been asked to facilitate the meeting for someone else, like our contributor above, plan to spend some time with them before the meeting to **play back what the meeting outcomes will be.** If you've followed the earlier advice these may be subtly different from what they thought they wanted so be prepared to spend time making sure they understand any changes and why these are necessary.

★ Having done all this preparation work you MUST now **communicate the outcomes** clearly with all meeting participants. If appropriate, send these out by e-mail or in paper form, ahead of the date itself. In any case always start the meeting by re-stating the outcomes. This might feel like overkill but it really is worth it. Say everyone does know and agrees with them, the worst case in repeating them is that everyone nods as you talk through them and you move on; time expended 30 seconds. Worst case if you do not talk them through is that there is still some lingering misunderstanding or disagreement. So you start the meeting and rapidly get bogged down with people challenging what the meeting is discussing: back to square one. And what do you do if you quickly talk through the outcomes and someone challenges them? Read on to the next section for ideas on this.

One final word of caution. When running the vast majority of meetings we'd urge you to take the above advice. Consult with the participants and ensure they are on board with the purpose of the meeting before you start. However, for one type of meeting, namely creative or idea generation meetings, it is best to avoid too much of this involvement up front. This topic is covered in much more depth in chapter 16 *Out of the box,* so best look there if you regularly run these sorts of meetings.

Interventions

The following ideas are things you can do if the meeting is unravelling because of unclear outcomes. But before you decide to trigger any of the following strategies you need to know, that the problem is indeed that of unclear goals. If you're lucky someone will directly challenge the purpose of the meeting, but luck isn't something to rely on, so some symptoms that also point to unclear goals are:

☆ people challenging the agenda, wanting to talk about different things.
☆ people putting lots of seemingly unrelated items onto AOB.
☆ people wanting clarification of the scope of the meeting.

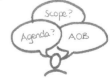

If the meeting is starting to unravel in any of the above ways then the following interventions can be used to get you back on track.

★ If someone hasn't already said it, **state directly** that there appear to be different ideas about the meeting outcomes. It may be that you do in fact have agreed outcomes but that some participants have just forgotten. By openly putting it to the group that people are not working towards common outcomes, everyone has the opportunity to realign.

- ★ Clearly **restate the outcomes** to which you think you have agreement. Challenge, gently, any work or lines of discussion that are not in support of achieving these outcomes. You can use approaches such as:-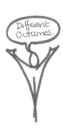
  - ☆ "We have these outcomes for the meeting and if we want to be productive we need to stay focused on them."
  - ☆ "Is the current line of discussion related to the outcomes?" [proceed accordingly, depending on the answer]
  - ☆ "This is an interesting line of discussion but it doesn't directly lead us towards our outcomes. Can we make a note of it and come back to it later if we have time?"

- ★ If there is no common understanding on what the meeting is about, you need to stop the discussions you are trying to have, temporarily, and **get some agreement on the outcomes.** You can use some of the same approaches used in the Preventions section. In summary:-
  - ☆ Go around the group and get everyone to state their ideal outcomes for the meeting. If there are power issues within the group, such that people might not get to share their views equally, use some of the ideas in chapter 2 *Just talks too much*. Once you have a list of everyone's ideals you can find the common ground and agree what the meeting will or will not cover.
  - ☆ If people are having trouble articulating their thoughts in terms of outcomes, collect issues that they feel need addressing. Sort them and order them as described earlier in the chapter and then get agreement about how to proceed.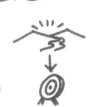
  - ☆ Get people to describe the end goal as they see it. Try to develop a shared view about the bigger picture and then work down to what this particular meeting should work on.
  - ☆ Refer back to existing procedures or processes in use within the organisation. Ask for everyone's views on where the meeting fits within this and then look for common ground to move you forward.

- ★ Sometimes the goals appear quite clear but people disagree about the specifics of what needs to be discussed and in what order. In this case you can use a **flexible agenda** approach to get the meeting moving again. To make this work, collect the ideas for what needs to be discussed i.e. the agenda items. Write them onto separate piece of paper and tape them to the wall or whiteboard so that everyone can see them. Ask people to state how much time should be spent on each item and write these onto the papers. Then determine if there is a particular order the items need to go in. You can now start to rearrange the papers on the wall so that they are in the flow of the meeting. You can look at how much time each item will take and start to plan in short breaks or lunch as necessary. By the end, you should have an agenda that everyone has created and is therefore happy to abide by. If more time is needed than has been planned for, the participants can choose to drop an item, change the time spent on each topic or plan to reschedule.

An example from Katherine: I was once asked to facilitate a one day meeting for a manager and his team. The broad purpose of the meeting was to get the team working effectively together. When I got the brief from the client the outcomes seemed a little woolly, but I wasn't unduly concerned as I planned to speak with all the meeting participants beforehand. However, when I consolidated all the information from my pre-meeting phone calls there were no clear themes in the objectives and everyone seemed to have different views about what was broken in the team and therefore what needed fixing. The approach I chose to take was to set the meeting up with a process to agree the meeting outcomes as a group. This was intended to get the group sharing their views about the team and self-diagnose what needed to be achieved in the meeting. The process I used was to post up four, large, blank pieces of paper on the wall (2m high x 1.25m wide) with the headings

☆ *The facts/data about our current situation*

☆ *Ideas/solutions to our current situation*

☆ *Problems/concerns regarding this team*

☆ *Other/miscellaneous*

I let the group of 8 form pairs, with each pair starting at one of the pieces of paper. They spent time writing their comments under that heading, then moved onto another piece of paper where they read the comments up there and added to them. When everyone had written on all the boards, we reviewed all the comments together to CLARIFY (not solve) the points written up.

In different pairs, they then started to agree on the outcomes for the meeting. Each pair then joined another pair to consolidate their outcomes and finally the whole group came together to agree the meeting outcomes. We then took a break during which I developed an agenda to achieve the outcomes, which I proposed to the group on their return. This process took about 2 ½ hours at the start of the meeting, but it meant that the group had complete ownership of the meeting and they had already started to work in a constructive manner through the process of creating their agenda.

Summary

So in summary, our top tips to ensure you have *clear outcomes* for your meetings are:-

★ Try our techniques for clarifying fogged thinking.
★ Contact participants in advance to find out their desired outcomes.
★ Communicate the outcomes
  ☆ in advance and
  ☆ at the start of the meeting.
★ State when you hear different outcomes in the group.
★ Clarify where there is agreement.
★ Take time out of the meeting to agree outcomes.
★ Use a flexible agenda to clarify the specifics.

7

Vision, mission, goals,
strategy, tactics....?

Q. *Help! Every group I work with seems to have a different idea of what constitutes a vision or a mission, let alone the confusion around goals, strategy and tactics. Worst still, sometimes a group becomes paralysed because there are such different views about what they all mean. Last week we had a meeting where a simple task of brainstorming some strategies got completely stuck. We argued for 30 minutes on whether the first contribution was a strategy or not and the meeting barely recovered from there. Can you give me some simple guidance about how to avoid this confusion?*

A. We feel particularly for this contributor. How many meetings have we facilitated where this issue has raised its head! The frustration can become tangible as people increasingly talk at cross-purposes or feel that they are just not understood. But why is this situation such a hard one?

Different language

Many organisations these days are multicultural, either because they operate across different countries or because people increasingly choose to live and work in places other than their country of birth.

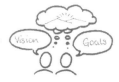

This is great in terms of bringing together the best ideas from the widest range of perspectives, but can, and often does, give rise to some confusion. Whilst the language skills of our multilingual colleagues often leave us, as native English speakers, in awe, it is easy to forget that the subtleties of precise meaning become even more complex across languages. Being open about these challenges, and having a discussion about what we mean by the words we use, is the only way to unpick the difficulties

Different strengths

The pleasure (and pain) of working with groups is that we are all different. Some of us have great talents for thinking the big ideas whereas others think through all those bothersome details that ensure a plan won't come unstuck at the first hurdle. It is vital that all these strengths

are present within a group if we want real success, but sometimes these contradictory strands of thinking can cause conflict.

One place the problem can surface is when groups are trying to agree missions, goals and tactics. These terms can take on very different meanings depending on the level at which you normally do your thinking. For example, if you are a real detail person then the goals become specific, often short term, tactical achievements; you'd be ready to leap into action once you'd agreed them. On the other hand, a colleague whose mind is always on the next grand idea would regard the goals as large strategic elements, each requiring further levels of thought and planning before you could action them, let alone achieve them. Neither approach is right or wrong. Again it is simply a matter of defining and agreeing the approach.

Different strengths

We are all fashion victims to one extent or another. Businesses and organisations are no less prone to following the trends in management thinking. This can sometimes give rise to a sudden urge for groups to 'synergise resources' or some other such latest buzz idea.

Often the work and processes are the same or very similar to those that have been used for decades, but if new terms are introduced for old ideas it isn't long before different interpretations are creeping in and before you know it, there is confusion and disagreement about what the group is trying to do.

Whatever the underlying reasons for confusion, the approaches to prevent or move the problems forward are the same and come down to clarification of meaning. Specific ideas for how to do this follow.

Preventions

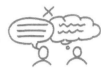

Here are some things you can do in advance of a meeting to prevent terminology problems...

* The key to making sure terminology doesn't become an issue in the meeting is to clarify what the participants mean by the terminology they are using, so **don't assume...**

* Terminology can be clarified before the meeting by **asking people exactly what they mean** in advance. Approaches to getting clarity may include asking for examples, asking how 'it' will be used.

* By having some **standard definitions** to work from, people can choose what most closely represents their need. Some organisations have their own definitions so it's worth checking whether these exist. Here are some examples we have found useful. They are not intended to be the 'right' definitions, just a starter to enable the clarification discussions.

  * ☆ VISION: a compelling image of a desired future state; where we imagine we could get to in the very long term.
  * ☆ MISSION or PURPOSE STATEMENT: a statement of what the organisation is here to do; a team or company's reason for being.
  * ☆ GOALS: results the team/company expects to achieve in a particular timeframe, usually medium/long term.
  * ☆ OBJECTIVES: results the team /company expects to achieve in a particular timeframe, usually short term. Objectives can be formed in the SMART format (Specific, Measureable, Achievable, Realistic, Timebound); sometimes with the addition of ARSE (Aligned, Relevant, Stretching, Enthusiastic)!!!!
  * ☆ STRATEGY: how to achieve the goals (not at a tactical level). Typically strategy statements are structured – achieve X (goal) through Y (strategy).
  * ☆ VALUES/PRINCIPLES: the fundamental code that governs how we do things. Things that you/the team hold to be true, that guide the way you work or interact with others.
  * ☆ TACTICS: the detailed actions that make up the plan for how to achieve the goals.

* Once you have agreed on the terminology it is useful to **communicate** this to all the participants. We would usually do this when clarifying the outcomes and agenda in an invitation e.g. 'for the purpose of our discussions in this meeting, strategy means....'

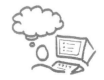

* **Metaphor** can help bring theoretical definitions to life, so rather than trying to get clarity about vision and tactical actions for a project, it may be easier to talk about 'what the cathedral will look like when it's built' (vision) and 'what the stone masons and carpenters need to do' (tactics).

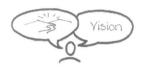

* Having said that and without wishing to contradict all the above, it actually doesn't really matter! One man's strategy is another man's tactic but as long as the group in the meeting have a **common language to work with** then it really doesn't matter. It only becomes an issue if there needs to be common language across different groups within an organisation.

Interventions

Options you can use in a meeting to get a common language to work with are....

* Make sure you **always clarify what is meant.** If someone suggests 'we need to agree on the goals and action plans for x', make sure you clarify what is meant by goals and what level of detail is required in the action plans.

* By **providing definitions** for a group you can help them unlock what it is they mean. So it can be useful to keep some 'standard definitions' up your sleeve, to use on occasions when the group are getting stuck on terminology.

* **Listen for differences**. One of the causes of decisions getting undone after meetings can be that subtle differences are not being picked up in the meeting. By listening for the language and definitions within the group you can help them to see where they agree and where they disagree.

* When you need to **get clarification of terminology** this does not mean that you, the facilitator/meeting leader needs to answer the question. You can **use the group** to get the clarity needed. We always look for a 'saviour' in most groups, someone who will see what is going on and see what's needed. So when the group has said they want to brainstorm a list of strategies and the list ends up as a mish mash of tactics, values, strategies... it can often be your 'saviour' who will spot that the list is not consistent and needs to be sorted. Interestingly, your saviour may not be who you expect. We once facilitated a meeting in which the most strategic thinker was the most junior person.

* One of the reasons groups get hung up on terminology can be difficulty with process. Theoretically it makes sense to work on strategy and then cascade down to tactics. However, it is our experience that people can often find this a difficult way to work. Brainstorming tactics, then clustering to identify strategies can unlock groups.

Example from Katherine: *I was facilitating a meeting once where the group needed clarity on what we meant by strategy. I started by offering the definition above, but this was not really what they were after. In the end we resorted to consulting a dictionary. The reason this approach worked for this group was that the definition was not owned by any one individual in the group; it was independent. The group agreed to work with the dictionary definitions they found and it enabled them to progress with the work they needed to do.*

Summary

Our top tips for making sure you have a *common language* for a group to work with are:-

* Do not assume you know what people mean.
* Ask people what they mean before and during the meeting.
* Communicate terminology before a meeting.
* Have some standard definitions to help the group, but don't get wedded to them yourself.
* Work with the group to get clarity on terminology in the meeting.
* Metaphors can help bring theoretical definitions to life.

8

Won't join in

Q. *Some groups seem to be really difficult to get any contribution from. If you're lucky there will at least be one or two people with something to say but from time to time you get groups where no one joins in. It can be like pulling teeth getting the conversation going. What can I do to shake up a group like this and get the meeting going?*

Problem

A. Painful isn't it, when no one will speak. You find yourself starting by asking lots of open questions and as the silence rolls on you fill the space with easy yes/no questions, desperate for someone to help you out. The problem is you've no idea what everyone is thinking and whether, what you're getting them to agree to, is actually what they think. Worse still, you're wondering why they are like this and what you could do to get them to contribute.

Just before we explore reasons why people may not want to speak up, a note of caution. People do need thinking time. Sometimes participants will not be able to jump straight in with an answer and you need to ride the silence until they are ready to contribute. Don't immediately assume that no one will speak just because there is a pause for thought. When you are leading a meeting, a 20 second pause can feel like 20 minutes, but if you fill all the silences then the participants can't speak. However, if you've tried several questions, and you've given people time to respond but there is still silence, then the ideas in this chapter may be just what you need.

Fear

A simple answer in many cases for people not speaking up is fear. They may be intimidated because they don't know each other and don't want to look foolish. They may feel in awe because they are part of a very large group (see chapter 10 *Too many people* for working with big numbers of participants) so that speaking up is almost like public speaking. Then again it could be that the culture of the organisation doesn't reward, or worse still punishes people, who speak their mind against the prevailing mood.

Whatever the reason for people being nervous, you won't overcome their reluctance by simply repeating the question and waiting.

Lack of engagement

The majority of people like to be engaged in what they are doing. They have an interest in the success of their work and their actions are driven by a desire to see this success. Unfortunately some organisations, by their actions, don't encourage participation and engagement. Over a time people learn not to bother and enthusiasm turns to apathy. The more times people see their contribution not making a difference, the less likely they are to be bothered next time.

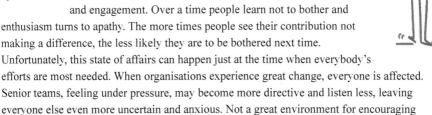

Unfortunately, this state of affairs can happen just at the time when everybody's efforts are most needed. When organisations experience great change, everyone is affected. Senior teams, feeling under pressure, may become more directive and listen less, leaving everyone else even more uncertain and anxious. Not a great environment for encouraging people to speak up.

Complex subject

Not every day, but sometimes, we come across meetings where the content of the discussion is really mind-boggling. Some things are just hard to understand and think about, often because different aspects are inter-related and so unpicking where to begin is challenging. Many of us need time to think before we can contribute in situations like this. At the very least we need a bit of

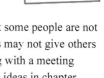

guidance about how to tackle the subject. The potential danger here is that some people are not so inhibited and will jump into a discussion, no matter how complex. This may not give others a chance to gather their thoughts and before you know it you're struggling with a meeting dominated by a few individuals. For more on that particular issue read the ideas in chapter 2 *Just talks too much.* In the meantime the rest of this chapter gives you useful strategies for dealing with the challenge of no one contributing.

Preventions

Here are some options for preparing to get the contribution you want.

* Try and **contact all the participants** of the meeting before the date to find out what they think the meeting should be trying to achieve and any potential issues. Even if you just get to speak with a few people coming to the meeting, you are likely to get an insight into any big issues this way. There are a number of ways you can do this depending on time, number of people, who is involved etc.
For example:-

  ☆ Make a 5-10 minute **phone call** with each participant before the meeting. The call could go something like, "Hello, I am calling you about the meeting we have scheduled on date. The purpose of the meeting is state the purpose of the meeting. However, I am wondering if you can spare me a few minutes to share your thoughts on what we should be aiming to achieve in the meeting." Once you have understood their expectations you can ask a follow-up question, "With these objectives in mind, is there anything that is likely to get in the way of achieving them in the meeting? Any issues or concerns you have?"

  ☆ **E-mail** everyone with a set of questions. For example you could send something like,
  "Thank you for committing to come to the meeting on date. The purpose of the meeting is state purpose of the meeting. I would appreciate your input into the design of the meeting, so please can you spare a moment to consider the following questions and send me your replies by date.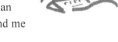

    ☆ What would you like is to achieve in the meeting? What specific objectives do we need to achieve?

    ☆ Do you have any issues or concerns about the meeting?

    ☆ Do you have any ideas for the meeting?

    ☆ Is there anything else it would be useful for me to know before the meeting?

By identifying low contribution as an issue before a meeting, it is possible to prevent it getting in the way of achieving the outcomes.

* **Design contribution into the agenda.** One of the best ways to ensure contribution in meetings is to design processes that ensure you get it. Often meetings have agenda points identified but no process within each agenda item. This means all discussion happens as open forum, which is most open to patterns of contribution arising such as some people over contributing whilst others under contribute. Here are some of the process options that encourage equal contribution in meetings.

  ☆ Giving people time to think before contributing allows them to collect their thoughts. This not only gives people more confidence in their contributions but often saves time as it prevents rambling!

☆ Using techniques in which people contribute on post-its or cards and then share. Again these processes allow thinking time as people write their points up, and there is the added benefit of contributions visually carrying equal weight if you choose to post them up in the debrief. Some tips for making these types of processes work well are:-

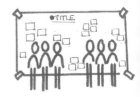

Tips for using cards or post-its

☆ Make sure your instructions are clear about what exactly you are asking people to write down. Ideally have a question written up for people to refer to, one point per card etc.

☆ Think about how much contribution you want/can manage. If you allow someone 5 minutes to write their thoughts onto cards they can produce a lot in the time, so prioritise before sharing, asking people to only add new points in the debrief.

☆ Think about the debrief process you are going to use. If people share their points one at a time this can mean the last person has little to add. An option we find quite useful is to ask for a point, find out if anyone has anything similar to add, allow the group to discuss this point and then move on to a different point.

☆ Make sure you have enough space to see and manage the cards and post-its as they come up.

☆ Think about how you plan to use the final display. If you need a record of all the points, a simple solution is to photograph the chart. However, you need to plan for this by allowing the right size of cards and pens and instructing people to write their points clearly.

☆ You can buy cards and post-its for these kinds of processes from Neuland. www.pinpoint-facilitation.com

☆ Using *large wall-chart templates* also encourages contribution for a number of reasons and gives a clear focus for the group discussion. The structure of the chart should clarify what contribution is required and the white space intuitively signals the need for contribution. These templates can be used in different sizes for different group formats e.g.

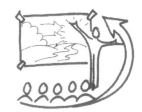

☆ Wall-sized charts for facilitating whole group discussion (approx 3m wide x 1.25m high)

☆ Table top (A1/A2) for small group discussion

☆ A3/A4 templates for paired discussion or for individual contribution

☆ For more information on this subject see chapter 13 *Managing information*. By breaking the group up you also encourage contribution, as the smaller the group the harder it is for people not to contribute. Options include paired discussions, table discussions (8 or less per table), small group discussions etc.

* ***Good joining instructions*** for a meeting can assist contribution in meetings in a number of ways:-

    ☆ By clarifying the purpose and outcomes people can see what they are committing to and understand the content of the meeting.

    ☆ Joining instructions can also set the tone and style of a meeting in advance and therefore ensure people come with the expectation that their contribution will be required.

    ☆ We are always very realistic about how much pre-work people will do in advance of a meeting. However, just asking people to consider some questions prior to the event can be a useful way of getting people into the meeting content in advance and ensuring good quality contribution in the meeting.

* ***Check your behaviour***. If you want contribution in your meeting and communicate this in advance of a meeting, you must be sure that your behaviour in the meeting encourages contribution and that the actions that follow up the meeting support this too. This is partly about the style you use to lead your meetings; is it open, friendly, encouraging? And also about being clear where you do and where you don't want contribution and how that contribution is to be used. Chapter 5 *Senior manager knows best* talks about this in more depth.

* Watch out for:

    ☆ People getting shouted down when they do contribute – "I hear what you say but…"

    ☆ Car parks being used to sideline issues and then not followed up – "I don't think that topic is relevant to this meeting, I think we should park it."

    ☆ Actions not followed up after meetings – "We agreed that at the last meeting but I don't think anyone did anything about it."

    ☆ Contributions not being used – "We've been asked about this before but nothing seems to happen as a result."

* When holding a meeting to tackle a complex subject you need to ***break the task down into manageable chunks of conversation.***
    Thinking through the journey that the group needs to go through is all part of good process design for the meeting and sometimes you need to go slow to go fast. For example, asking a group to go straight into purpose/role clarification discussions can be hard work. By providing a framework to lead into this type of conclusion can really help e.g. get the group to discuss the work they have been engaged in; get them to add areas they think they should be working on; pull out themes and then conclude with purpose/role clarification.

    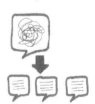

* ***Sharing context.*** Linked to the above point is the whole area of setting context to lead into decision-making. Getting people to share context gets them talking and exchanging information and often leads to better quality decisions.

An example from Katherine: I was asked to facilitate a meeting for a group of six regional managers with the purpose of developing a plan for the overall business. From my conversations with the participants before the meeting I knew that there was not a great deal of mutual trust and respect in the group. Rather than launching straight into the planning process, I made time on the agenda for sharing context first. I combined the context sharing with personal introductions by giving each manager an A2 chart with some general questions about their region and a couple of questions about themselves i.e. What is the size of your region? Who are your biggest customers? Who are your competitors? What are the challenges you currently face? How long have you been in this role? Where did you come from into this role? Each participant had 20 minutes to complete their template before sharing the headlines with the group. The whole session took about 90 minutes but meant there was much better mutual understanding about where each of them was coming from as they went into making decisions about their business plan.

★ Once a **group size** gets to about 18-20 people the group dynamics change, making it harder for people to contribute in the whole group. Techniques for working with larger groups can be found in chapter 10 *Too many people.*

★ If you know that there are likely to be low contributors in your group then it is important to **be realistic** about how you work with them. Don't assume that by using all the tools and techniques in this chapter you will instantly get high levels of contribution! You will need to build up to the level of contribution you need.

Interventions

Some options for dealing with low contribution in meetings:

★ **Setting the tone for a meeting at the start** is very important. Using an open and collaborative style right from the start invites contribution. When we know that contribution is likely to be a challenge we name problems up front e.g.
  ☆ Acknowledging the different styles in the room and inviting everyone to contribute.
  ☆ Acknowledging where there have been problems in the past e.g. actions not followed up, car parks getting lost.
  ☆ Expressing that differing views are OK and you are open to people challenging.

★ The other tool we find useful at the start of meetings, is to do some kind of **check-in** with people to find out how they are and what they want from the meeting. This gives a chance for people to express expectations, concerns, distractions etc and gives the meeting leader a sense of where the group is at. There are vast quantities of resources for creative introduction session some of which can be found in chapter 16 *Out of the box.*

★ If a group are **going through change** it is important to accept that people will be in different places. There is a model, sometimes known as the Four Room Apartment, that describes our reactions to change in four phases; denial, resistance, exploration, acceptance. This model is useful in the context of contribution as it explains why we can sometimes hear very different contributions from people who are in the same situation, for example:-

☆ **Denial** – "I know everyone is talking about X but I've seen these things come and go and it won't actually happen."

☆ **Resistance** – "I can see why they need to do this in Department X but I don't need to do it, I'm alright."

☆ **Exploration** – "So what would it mean to me if we started working in this way?"

☆ **Acceptance** – "I didn't like the sound of it initially but actually it's been an improvement."

There are no rules for how long a person is going to spend in any one phase but if we are aware that people may be in different phases then we can promote conversations that allow exploration from different perspectives, to help people move through the change process.

✳ What we are about to say now may sound as if we are contradicting everything previously said: that it is also important to **let people contribute in a way they feel most comfortable.**

An example from Ingrid and Katherine: We once facilitated a meeting in which we used many techniques to invite contribution, yet there were two people who barely said a word when we were in open forum discussion. However, whenever we checked in with these people, in breaks etc, they were completely happy with the way the conversation was progressing. Their views were being incorporated in the paired and small group work and they had nothing to add once we came together as a whole group.

✳ Related to the above point is the need to **appreciate people's different styles** and how that relates to the contributions they make e.g. some people have a tendency to be more 'towards' focused, whilst others are more 'away from' focused; some people are more future focused and others relate to the past; some people focus on the task to be done whilst others think about the people concerned and how it will be done.

An example from Katherine: In my early days as a facilitator I remember facilitating a meeting for a leader who didn't want any discussions about the past in his meeting; he just wanted to talk about the future. This was set as a rule at the start of the meeting but inevitably ended up getting broken.

As facilitative meeting leaders, we need to embrace the differences that exist in the groups we work with. Our challenge is to find ways for these different styles to contribute and be harnessed to give better quality decisions. I have worked with this leader since that meeting and, having persuaded him to let me facilitate a meeting that allowed the past-focused people to be heard alongside the future-focused participants, he can see the benefits.

Summary

Our top tips for *getting participation* from the whole group in a meeting are:-

★ Contact participants in advance to identify potential contribution issues.
★ Design processes into the agenda that ensure contribution.
★ Break complex tasks into manageable chunks.
★ Allow time on the agenda for sharing context before making decisions.
★ Provide good joining instructions and tell people where you want their contributions.
★ Set a collaborative tone at the start of the meeting.
★ Accept that people will be in different places as a group goes through change.
★ Appreciate different styles e.g. towards/away; future/past; task/process.

9

I feel like a spare part

Q. *It really annoys me when I've spent so much time preparing for a meeting and planning the agenda that some people in a group then seem to think they know best and refuse to do the tasks I propose. It just seems so rude of them and when I tell them why what I'm suggesting is best, they often don't seem to listen and instead, just insist they prefer their way. I wouldn't mind so much, but the group often seems to take their side, leaving me feeling rather redundant. What can I do to stop this sort of rebellion in my meetings?*

Problem

A. Oh, what a difficult situation. Difficult because as a facilitator in this situation, you're being given some very immediate feedback about how useful you are being to the group at that moment. But don't despair, that doesn't mean you're necessarily doing a bad job. It could be, not what you're suggesting so much, as how you propose the work. And it could, in fact, be a very positive thing; a symptom of how well you've run the meeting or group until that point.

Job done

In the early stages of getting a group to work together, they need a lot of support; they need leading through the processes to get the discussions flowing and make the work happen. Whilst this stage is vital as a kick-start, it can leave teams very dependent on the facilitator or process leader and with no real sense of

ownership for what they achieve. There is a danger that if there isn't someone around to organise them and tell them what to do, then nothing happens (no doubt that sounds familiar to many of you!)

If groups are to be really successful they need to become independent and so, as work progresses, the meeting leader needs to take more of a backseat or supporting role. When you're preparing for a meeting or workshop you should plan for gradual transfer; a shifting in the balance of leadership, and ultimately, ownership. There are ideas in the rest of this chapter, which explain how to make this transition smoothly. If you do your job really well in the early stages of a meeting, a group can take you by surprise and grab the initiative from you. Although a little disconcerting when it happens, a good facilitator will welcome the group taking charge, provided they have first checked that this friendly takeover is for the right reasons as opposed to one of the following:

Unclear instructions

When you ask anyone to do something they need to know *why* they're doing it and exactly *what* they have to do. This is true for an instruction to an individual but even more so when you start communicating to a group of people. We need to examine the *why* and the *what* separately, so let's begin with the *why*.

Not many people are happy to do things if they don't know why they should. (And do you really want to work with people who are happy just to *do*?). And the *why* operates at two levels. There is the question **why bother at all?** By this we mean what is this piece of work all about? Where does it fit into the big picture? This is a vital question to answer and if you don't have a good reason you should challenge yourself about the need to do that work.

The other *why* is the one that meeting leaders often come unstuck with. Picture the scene. You've read this book cover to cover (except for this chapter) and have developed some really interesting ways to get the meeting to be effective, to get the work done and done in a way that makes the decisions stick. Then armed with all these great ideas you bounce in on an unsuspecting group at the office and suggest they start writing their top three issues onto post-it notes, which you'll put on a chart on the wall. They've never seen this approach before and haven't read the book and being a little stuck in their ways they decide they don't fancy that. But they're too polite to mock you directly (after all that's what they're thinking) so they suggest a different thing instead and there you are – the spare part facilitator. So what went wrong? You didn't explain why it would be a good idea to write ideas on post-its. You didn't take the time to remind them of the interminable circular discussions and the groans of despair at the coffee machine that always follow the usual session of this group. You didn't explain **why this process.** You'll be delighted to know that this chapter gives you ideas for how to do this effectively too.

So that just leaves the **what.** This seems the most obvious but because of that, it is easily overlooked. If you have a designed a great, involving method for getting the work done, you MUST take the time to explain to everyone EXACTLY what they have to do. Probably more than not knowing why, a group will rebel when they don't understand the instructions. People are too embarrassed to say they don't understand, so instead, they suggest a different task – one they understand and can explain, even if it isn't going to be as effective for achieving the aims of the meeting. The first step in getting this right is being clear in your own mind what it is you're asking people to do. After that it is a simple question of how to communicate clearly. There are more ideas for how to do this later in the chapter.

Unhelpful help

Having examined two possible causes for this type of problem in your meetings, we need to consider a final prospect. You need to challenge yourself that maybe the group have a point; that you are providing unhelpful help.

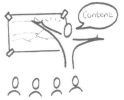

As independent facilitators we often have people share with us their stories of bad facilitation experiences. Amongst the best (or worst, depending how you look at it) is the facilitator who decided during the early part of the meeting, what the 'right answer' was for the group. This was despite the fact that he was independent of the business, had not worked with this group or with this type of project before, and in fact knew nothing of the industry sector either. Having come to his decision he then facilitated the group to agree with him, or at least he tried to. Every proposal he made led the group to the 'right answer' and as this became increasingly clear the group began to rebel. It started with one or two voices and ultimately became a unified group. Now a unified group is in general a good thing and so you might consider this facilitator performed a tremendous service by providing everyone with a common enemy to unite against. We'd like to suggest that unless you have an armour-plated ego that doesn't mind being universally hated, that you try and find more constructive ways of being helpful.

So what exactly is it that counts as unhelpful help? One of the things it is useful to separate out when designing and running meetings is the difference between the process and content of a meeting. The process is the way in which a conversation is held, the content is the subject matter or topic being discussed. To use a metaphor, it's like cooking; the ingredients are the content and the whisking, folding, chopping, baking are all processes! As illustrated above, getting involved in the **content** of the discussion is usually unhelpful. If you want to have a really effective meeting, you need to carefully guide the **process.** Mixing up your contributions between the two will leave the group confused and potentially frustrated as it can appear very manipulative. Now, we know that some of you reading this will be in meetings, where you have a part in the discussion, as well as trying to bring some effective working through facilitating the process. Don't despair. Despite all we've just said, this can be done. The crucial thing is not to confuse the two roles, either in your own mind or in the minds of the other participants. It does take some careful planning, but it can be done and more suggestions for how are provided in this chapter.

In previous chapters we have used the format of Preventions and Interventions to give lists of options you can use to address the problem being explored. In this chapter all the options are interventions, so we have provided them in a different structure.

Be there for the group

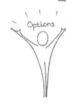

If you believe the group has the answer to the question being raised in the meeting and you genuinely want to involve them in decisions then your role is to provide the most effective conversation format for the group to unlock the answer for themselves. (For more about how you want to involve the group in decision-making refer to chapter 5 *Senior manager knows best* and chapter 11 *Decisions that stick*). This means behaving in a way that supports the group....

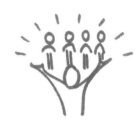

★ **Do not evaluate individual comments** from the group either verbally or non-verbally e.g. by not writing a comment down.

★ **Ask others in the group for a response** e.g. "What does everyone else think about this?" "Are there others that share this view?" "What other different views are there?"

★ **Be open to being persuaded.** One of the best bits of advice I got in my early days as a facilitator was *don't fall in love with your design.* It's sometimes hard to do when you have put days of work into preparing for a meeting, but if you genuinely want to support the group you may need to change plan mid-meeting.

★ **Hold no opinion.** It is the group's discussion and you are there to facilitate the process not the content.

★ **Design your meeting process to ensure equal/joint input**
   ☆ Contribute on post-its
   ☆ Allow thinking time before asking for contributions
   ☆ Add your comments last if you need to add to the content but beware of the 'summarise and then pounce' attack!
   ☆ For more ideas see chapter 2 *Talks too much*

★ *Find ways to contribute your opinion that do not manipulate the group*
- ☆ Contribute on post-its. This means your views sit alongside others' equally.
- ☆ Contribute using templates i.e. charts with the key questions on that get answered during the meeting. You can either complete your own template or fill one in with a syndicate group.
- ☆ Send a discussion document before the meeting so the group know your position in advance.

★ *Support the lone voice.* Maybe the group can talk them round but don't let them get browbeaten. I have seen the lone point of view, when supported, enable a group to come up with a far more robust solution. (You need to bear in mind the decision-making process you have chosen for your meeting, see chapter 11 *Decisions that stick*).

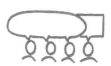

An example from Katherine: I read the theory about supporting the lone voice a long time before I really 'got it' through experiencing the benefits in a meeting I facilitated. I was working with a group of senior managers in a two-day strategy workshop. At one point in the meeting we were about to make a critical decision when one person did not agree. I made space for this person to make his point before the rest of the group descended on him, trying to browbeat him into agreeing. (I have never found browbeating a great way to get commitment!) I suggested a break and took the chance to speak with the individual who had a different view. He did have a very different perspective on the decision and felt he wasn't being understood so, when we came back from the break, I suggested a change of process.
  1. *First I asked him to restate his view.*
  2. *I allowed the group a few minutes to ask questions (for clarification only).*
  3. *The group had to collectively list the positive aspects of his idea before identifying the issues they had.*
This process forced the group to listen differently to his view and the ensuing discussion lead the group to a completely new decision that was far more robust than the original decision that had so nearly been agreed on.

★ *Respect everyone.* Don't get drawn into negative group dynamics. Everyone in the meeting should be heard and involved.

★ *Be explicit* when you are using an idea that comes from the group.

Be clear

Here are some options for ensuring the participants in your meeting are clear about why they are there, why you are using this process and what they are being asked to do.

★ Start every meeting by sharing a bit of context about why the meeting has been called and clarifying the purpose of the meeting. This helps people to understand why they are there. For example, "Thank you all for coming to this meeting. The reason I have called us all together is...... What I hope to achieve is....."

* Then go on to clarify the **objectives** for the meeting, the **agenda**, the **roles** within the group and the ground **rules**. This enables clarity about the specifics of what needs to be achieved and what you will be doing together. We strongly recommend you write this up and keep it up during the meeting, to refer back to.

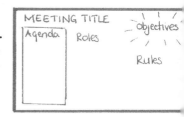

* **Stories and metaphors** can be useful to elaborate difficult concepts. For example,
  * if you are at the start of a project or working with a new team and taking time to discuss goals and direction, then using the metaphor of a journey can help explain why it is important to be clear about the end destination.
  * if you are going to talk about different roles in a group then the metaphor of a football team could explain the need for different roles and clarity about who is doing what.

* **Show the whole journey.** It can be difficult for people to take part in a discussion if they don't know where it's heading. One of the tools that can help with this is using large wall charts with the headings for the discussion. This shows the group the framework for the whole discussion before starting to tackle one aspect. (For more on this see chapter 13 *Managing information*)

* Have a flipchart with the **purpose and steps** for each agenda item and give really clear instructions when you ask the group to do something. Use the flipchart to start the session off and keep it there to refer to at the start of the session and then throughout the whole session.
  * Make sure the steps go into detail e.g. the exact timings, the numbers of post-its per person, how you will debrief the discussion etc.

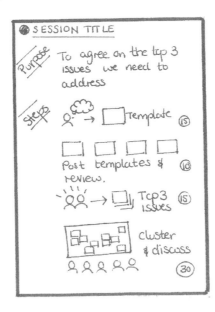

* Answer the questions before they are asked.

* Give examples to illustrate what you are asking the group to contribute.

* Provide frameworks to clarify understanding. Whilst business models for the sake of intellectual debate are not useful for a group, providing a framework to help facilitate a discussion can be very helpful.

  Katherine's example: *I was facilitating a meeting for a new manufacturing head and his management team. We had spent some time exploring the history of the group, and the new leader had shared his goals for the future and we were stuck in a discussion about all the problems preventing the group from achieving the goals. After taking a break, we introduced the Stephen Covey model of Sphere of control, Sphere of influence, Sphere of concern. We used this model to sort through the issues. Most of the actions identified were to resolve things within the group's control and a small number of actions were identified for the new head to take away and try to influence.*

When to lead & when to follow

Choosing to manage your meetings in the way we propose in this book is about choosing a facilitative style of leadership. Any leader needs to know when to do the leadership thing and when to support the group's work.

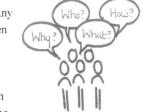

* You need to lead a group into decision-making, so usually the start of any meeting or process requires the most leadership. In practical terms, what this means is making sure people have the answers to some key questions before being ready to commit to a decision.
  * "Why are we here?" "What is the purpose of this work?" "How does this fit in to the big picture?"
  * "Who are we working with?" "How do I fit in with them?"
  * "What are we aiming to achieve?" "What's my role in it?"
  * "How are we going to do it?'"

* The things you need to clarify before you start making implementation decisions include:-
  * The context and purpose of the work you are doing.
  * Taking time to ensure everyone knows who is there and their role in the work.
  * Ensuring that the goals of the work are clarified.
  * Setting out your ways of working for any ongoing work.

* Once a group gets into implementation you need to accept that your role will be in following/supporting their work.

★ When a group are working well together sit back and enjoy it; your job is done ☺! The kinds of things that you can usefully do at this stage are,
   ☆ recording/documenting
   ☆ making notes on process for learning reviews
   ☆ helping with process design where appropriate
   ☆ NOT intervening unnecessarily!!!

Summary

Our top tips for ensuring you do not *feel like a spare part* in a meeting are:-

★ Be honest with yourself about whether you want the group involved in the work. If you do, then behave in a way that supports their involvement.
★ Clarify the objectives, agenda, roles and ground rules before and at the start of your meeting.
★ Clarify the purpose and steps of each agenda item at the start of the session.
★ Design your meeting to allow time to lead into decisions.
★ If the group is working well, don't feel the need to intervene.

10

Too many people

Q. *Is there a "right" number of people to have in a meeting? I find I can manage about 15 people, as long as they're not too argumentative, and still keep control. Once the numbers get much bigger I find it too difficult to focus sufficiently on what someone is saying at the same time as trying to watch out for other contributions or possible disagreements. What often happens is that bit by bit people in large meetings switch off as they find it hard to get their say. I recently ran a meeting where we thought about 18 people would come and in the end 35 arrived. At first I was pleased because obviously everyone was very interested in the subject, but the meeting was a disaster because people felt frustrated that they couldn't contribute as much as they wanted. I was run ragged trying to manage everyone and make sure I captured everyone's ideas on the flipchart. In the end we muddled through but it wasn't very satisfactory.*

Problem

A. Well, congratulations that so many people wanted to come to your meeting; you must be doing something right. But we do sympathise trying to manage as many participants as that, using methods designed for smaller numbers. In fact your question doesn't have a straight answer. Despite what many people will tell you there is no 'right' number. You need rather to think about it as the having the right meeting planned for the people who need or want to contribute. The ideas that follow should allow you to have successful meetings no matter how many get involved.

Getting the Right People

If meetings are going to be effective, and particularly if any decisions are going to be made and followed through (more on this in chapter 11 *Decisions that stick*), you need to have the right people in the room. If the right number is five then you have yourself a fairly easy meeting to manage but if the number is 500 you'll have to plan a little differently. Conventional wisdom often advises that meaningful discussions can't take place once you have more than about 20 people in a room, but they can and must if the decision requires input or participation of greater numbers.

The reasons for this are very apparent if you think about it for any length of time. Imagine a project that impacts all the divisions and departments of an organisation. And worse than that, it's a pan-European organisation with inevitable differences from country to country, and this project will impact all of them. How can you possibly get all the information from across this complex system so as to be able to make good quality decisions? And how can you ensure you have the buy-in from all the diverse areas of this organisation? Of course, these will remain challenging questions no matter how you organise your meetings, but you certainly don't help yourself if your first action is to exclude lots of people from the discussions because you artificially restrict your numbers. When it comes to meetings it isn't a choice between quality and quantity; sometimes you only get quality if you go for quantity.

Right people, wrong process

So you've invited all the people you need to your meeting and whatever that number is, returning to the original question, you now have the *right* number. A better question to ask at this point is *What is the right process to use?* The reason our contributor had so many problems was that the plan for the meeting wasn't appropriate. Managing large numbers, even many hundreds, is possible but you do need to use very different methods. This chapter will give you the tools you need.

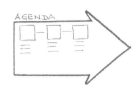

Preventions

Here are some things you can do in advance to ensure you have the right people and process for your meeting.

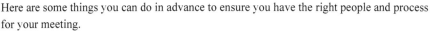

★ **Decide who needs to be in the meeting.** If you have called the meeting then you will have an initial view of who the key people are. It is then advisable to have brief discussions with some of the key people to find out their views. There are a number of ways you can do this depending on time, number of people, who is involved etc. For example, you could:-

☆ Make a 5-10 minute phone call with each participant before the meeting. The call could go something like, "Hello, I am calling you about the meeting we have scheduled on *date. The purpose of the meeting is state the purpose of the meeting.* However, I am wondering if you can spare me a few minutes to share your thoughts on what we should be aiming to achieve in the meeting….. Given these objectives, who do you think needs to be in the meeting?"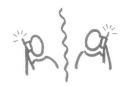

☆ E-mail everyone with a set of questions. For example, you could send something like,
'Thank you for committing to come to the meeting on *date.* The purpose of the meeting *is state purpose of the meeting.* I would appreciate your input into the design of the meeting, so please can you spare a moment to consider the following questions and send me your replies by *date.*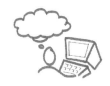

  ☆ What would you like us to achieve in the meeting? What specific objectives do we need to achieve?

  ☆ Do you have any issues or concerns about the meeting?

  ☆ Who do you think should be at the meeting?'

★ The key to getting the right people in a meeting is to be really **clear about the roles** of the people participating. While it is important not to stifle good decision-making by limiting the numbers, it is also important to make sure the meeting isn't full of voyeurs!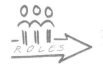

★ If some key **people cannot make it** to a meeting it is worth considering whether you can **get their input in advance** of the meeting and then incorporate their views without them being there. This can be particularly effectively done through the use of partially-completed wall charts, populated with the views of those people not able to attend. The big question with using this type of approach is whether they will have/need ownership of the decision made in their absence.

★ Once you have decided on who needs to be at the meeting, it is important to make sure you have **enough space.** For large groups this means there is enough space for the group to be seated in a 'cabaret' layout with space to move between the tables. 'Cabaret' means the group is arranged around circular tables, ideally in groups of no more than 8.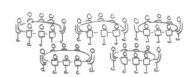

★ Once you know who needs to come to the meeting you can get on with the meeting design. Having a robust meeting design is even more critical with large groups as it is more difficult to improvise.

Large-meeting techniques

There are some common techniques that make for good meeting design when you are working with large numbers of participants.

★ One of the key principles to large group design is enabling *share of voice*. If you imagine yourself in a situation where there are large numbers of people and then ask yourself how you feel about contributing in these situations you are likely to feel emotions like, 'I don't want to speak up in front of all these people'; 'There's no point, I am just one person'. So, in designing meetings for large groups we need to **allow people to be heard** and **make it easy for them to contribute.**

★ Techniques that facilitate this are:-

☆ Designing the discussions to be held in **small groups** (usually at tables) and then connecting back to the main group. It also helps to allow **personal reflection** time in the small group discussions, as this helps people collect their thoughts before contributing. This is why the 'cabaret' style layout works so well with large groups.

☆ Cabaret layout allows for a style of working whereby the depth of discussion happens at tables. This is facilitated by setting up the discussion to the whole room and then allowing small groups to hold discussions at their tables. To aid this process it is useful to have a session brief on every table, stating the purpose and steps of the session. A great way for groups to manage their discussions is to provide them with a tabletop chart (usually A2 or A1 size), divided into sections with questions to fill in. (See more about this in chapter 13 *Managing information*)

☆ The other aspect of working in table groups is to establish some **ways of working** at the tables from the start of the meeting. We usually recommend that table groups share the jobs to be done in discussions and ideally rotate these roles throughout a meeting.

☆ Facilitator – to lead the discussion

☆ Recorder/Reporter – to make notes and report back for the group, if required

☆ Timekeeper – to keep the discussion to time

☆ When the groups have completed a discussion it is important to connect back to the whole group. This can be done in various ways:

☆ Presentation from each table or a selection of tables.

☆ Posters or completed tabletop charts hung round the room. Then everyone invited to walk around the room to review the outputs. (See more on templates in chapter 13 *Managing information*).

☆ Asking for key points from each table and looking for different points to be added each time until there are no new points.

★ Graffiti walls are a great tool for larger meetings. They are literally a wall of blank paper for people to write comments on. Conversations can develop over time and this allows people to express views and have side conversations publicly.

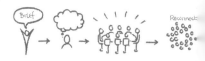

★ Mind maps are a way of connecting information about a topic by putting the topic at the centre of the page then creating themed branches off the topic to form a diagram of interconnected branches around a central topic. Large-group mind mapping is a way of capturing lots of different views 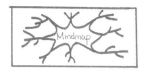 quickly in a way that allows people to see the linkages between them. This tool usually requires someone to facilitate the discussion and someone to record. It starts with an explanation of the central topic/theme for discussion. When the group starts to contribute they say whether their point is a new branch on the mind map or they name the branch their point is related to. It is important to have a competent recorder so that you can keep the pace up in a session like this. I have witnessed these sessions run very slowly and low energy when the recorder can't keep up. One way round this is to use two recorders, each taking alternate points.

★ When designing meetings for larger groups **'don't do for the group what they can do for themselves'.** For example, handing out a document in a meeting of 12 people you could pass a copy to each person. Now imagine the same task with 200 people – handing out becomes impracticable. So, the benefit of thinking in this way is twofold.
　　☆　It is not practicable to do everything for everyone in a large group
　　☆　It encourages shared responsibility for the work being done, rather than the usual lemming mentality that can occur in large meetings.

★ The practical solution to encouraging the group to support itself in a meeting is to **provide resource tables** with materials available for a table representative to collect.

★ One of the great benefits of having a large group can be the diversity of perspectives you get in the meeting and the wealth of experience. However, you only get the real benefit from this if the table groups are mixed and change throughout the meeting. Sometimes work needs to be done within functional groups, in which case sitting them all at one table can be beneficial. The key is to **think about the impact of the seating arrangements** as part of the design in the preparation.

★ Once a meeting size becomes more than about 30 people the tendency is to go for meetings that are 'death by PowerPoint' i.e. loads of presentations and one-way information. These types of meetings rarely have any long-term impact; at best they create a bit of a buzz on the day. By **minimising the amount of presentation** you maximise the amount of working discussion that gets done in a meeting and make the most of the brainpower in the room. We try to apply this principle in both large and small group meetings!

An example from Katherine: I recently had a conversation with a client that went like this…
CLIENT: "I have decided to call a meeting of all the people who work in X. We are going through lots of change at the moment and it's causing a few problems. There are lots of

rumours flying around about what might be happening, most of which are unfounded, and people are not working well together as there is a lot of mistrust. I thought we could spend a day together, give everyone a better sense of where we are heading and clear the air."

ME: "Sounds like a good idea. Do you have any plans for the agenda?"

CLIENT: "Yes, I have got a presentation about the overall business direction. I've also asked each of my Divisional Heads to prepare a presentation about their functions. I thought we could have a few questions and answers and then I have invited an external consultant to come along at the end of the day to do something motivating with them."

This example shows a common mistake made in meetings. The reason people need to come together in meetings is to have conversations, not to be presented at. Conversations are even more important if there is conflict in the group. A well-run meeting will have well-structured conversations to achieve the overall objectives, whatever the size of group.

★ The other critical point to define before any meeting, but particularly one with larger numbers of participants, is the **decision- making process**. In the absence of any defined decision- making process, people in a group tend to think they are being asked about something, so they make the decision, which assumes consensus decision-making, the most time-consuming process.

For example, if the outcome of the meeting is to understand the vision for the future, what position are you in?

1. You have a vision that needs explaining to get common understanding.

2. You have a vision that you need to get buy-in to.

3. You have a proposal and want to get ideas to improve it.

4. You don't have anything yet and want to collect ideas as input to your proposal.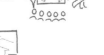

5. You don't have anything yet and want everyone coming to the meeting to jointly create the vision.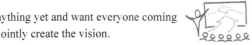

For each outcome of a meeting it is useful to really think through which style of decision-making is appropriate.

★ The final thing to consider as part of the design of your meeting is the **onward communication.** What needs to be communicated, and to whom, after the meeting? By thinking about this in advance it is possible to design it as part of the meeting. There are also options for sending out templates from the meeting with spaces for additional contributions afterwards, but only use this approach if you plan to take action on the comments!

Interventions

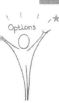

Options

* If you find yourself in a meeting and start to realise the **right people aren't there,** the key thing is **not to ignore the problem.** Any decisions or agreements that get made without the right people in the room are likely to get overturned anyway, so it really is a waste of time just ploughing on. The tactics I have used are:-
    * ☆ Front the issue with the group if they seem to be ignoring the problem *'Do we have the right people in the room to make these decisions?'*
    * ☆ If the answer is 'no' then it can be useful to ask, "How can we get the right people involved?" and "What actions can we take to convene a meeting where the right people will enable effective working?"

* If you find yourself with **more people than expected,** one of the first strategies we would suggest is to thank everyone for coming (and congratulate yourself on your meeting magnetism!)

* By clarifying the meeting purpose and outcomes at the start you can **sense-check that everyone is there for the same reason** and not for something else.

* We would recommend being transparent with the group about your surprise and be explicit about what you will need to do, something like this...
    "Thank you all for coming to our meeting today. I am surprised and pleased to see how many people are keen to get involved in this matter. I have to confess that I did not anticipate getting such a response to my invitation and my agenda was for a smaller group. My proposal is that we aim to have the same conversations in the same order but I will need to improvise the process to make it productive with a larger group. We will need to start the meeting as one group, to get everyone on the same page, so it may feel like the start of the meeting is a bit hard work. However, once we get going I will make opportunities to split into groups to allow depth of discussion."

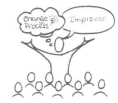

* Find ways to **break the group up into smaller groups** to have the conversations (see more about this earlier in this chapter), for example,
    * ☆ Working in pairs
    * ☆ Small group working (up to 8 per group)
    * ☆ Divide the task into working parties
    * ☆ Work in parallel streams

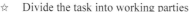

* **Only sort out in the meeting what you really need to**
    * ☆ Find areas of common agreement early.
    * ☆ Focus the time you have together on resolving areas of difference.
    * ☆ Put things to the vote early.
    See more about decision-making in chapter 11 *Decisions that stick*

* Assuming you do have the right people in the room and you have designed the meeting to work effectively with a large group, then you are a long way down the road to success. However, there are some useful tips for facilitating large groups.

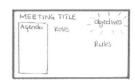

  ☆ When you open the meeting, make sure you talk about the *objectives* you want to achieve in the meeting, the *agenda* for how you plan to achieve the objectives and the *roles* and ground *rules* expected in the meeting.

  ☆ *Give clear instructions.* When you set up a group task there are some key tips to getting this right by being clear about why and what you are asking (see more about this in chapter 9 *I feel like a spare part*).

  ☆ The key thing with a large group, though, is to give it your best and then let them get on with it. Don't ask for questions of clarification as you will either get stunned silence or anarchy!

Summary

Our top tips for ensuring you have the *right number of people* in your meetings are:-

* The most important aspect of having a productive meeting is having the right people there, regardless of how many.
* If you need a large group (more than about 18 people) to get the work done, then design the meeting using large-group techniques.
* If you realise key people are missing at the start of a meeting, decide whether the meeting is worth continuing with.
* If you know in advance that key people cannot come to the meeting, consider ways to obtain their input and include it without them present.
* If more people than expected turn up to your meeting, modify your design to use large-group techniques.

11

Decisions that stick

Q. *How do you get a group to make a decision that sticks? So often when I follow up on a meeting I find that the agreements that we all thought we had made have come unstuck and that people aren't doing their actions or have started a rear-guard action to reverse the work of the meeting. What is the point of everyone voting in a meeting to agree something if they then change their mind?*

Problem

A. What a very common situation. And what a frustrating one for everyone involved. If this happens too often the decision-making in meetings doesn't stand a chance at all as everyone then has an expectation that it will mean nothing. Of course decisions only stick if everybody involved is onboard with the decision. Onboard doesn't mean you have to have 100% agreement. In fact consensus is very hard to achieve; what you need is a decision that once it is made, everyone will abide by. So let's start by exploring what goes on when people have to agree, before looking at strategies for making it happen.

What stops people agreeing?

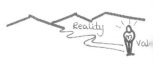

If we were all clones with identical life experiences we'd find we never disagreed with each other, but what a dull existence that would be. Life is full of interesting, different people and if we occasionally find people with whom we disagree then that is a price worth paying.

So what is it exactly that causes the disagreements? There are two dimensions that cause us to come to different judgements. The first is that we have different realities. Through our education and life experience we all have our own view of what is real; of what we know to be true if you prefer. It isn't necessarily that one person is right when another is wrong. Think of it more as no one has the whole picture. We all only see the bits that have been shown to us along the way. Depending on which bit of the picture we've seen, we may well form very different ideas about the world to those of our neighbour and this can become a cause for conflict. Second, and in many ways harder, is that we might have different values. We may all have the same view on the facts of a situation but if we value different things, we can easily come to different decisions about what is the right thing to do. This is particularly tricky, as the only way to reach agreement is to find common ground on those basic beliefs.

The basics

Clearly a good decision can only be made if there has been a thorough exploration of the information relating to the decision as well as, in some cases, the values by which the decision will be judged. This means the people with the information need to be included in the process and if this means a large number of people have to get involved, then so be it. See chapter 10 *Too many people* for more on this. If values are to be explored then it isn't just a case of handing out a few facts and figures. There may well be the need for some lengthy discussions around and behind the topic before you can move to decision time.

Decision types

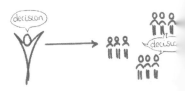

There is increasingly a feeling that people who are affected by decisions should be involved in decisions. But involvement doesn't have to mean they make the decision. There is an excellent model for understanding different types of decision-making appropriate to different situations, which was developed by Peter Senge. It identifies that at one end of the spectrum there are times when it is appropriate for an individual to make the decision and then tell those affected, whereas at other times there are benefits to having everyone involved.

The real importance of the model is the understanding that there is not one size fits all. You need to consider the situation and find an approach that works. And if you've chosen appropriately and everyone understands the method adopted, you will greatly increase your chances of success.

Decision-making methods

Quite apart from which overall approach you need to employ, there is also the choice of method to gain the final agreement. Again, different choices will work better or worse depending on the dynamics and relationships within the group. At one end of the scale, hierarchical decision-making can work well, where the group respect their leader and trust him or her to make a good final decision.

At the other end of the scale consensus decisions give everyone an equal voice and no agreement is reached until everyone is happy. In the middle of these two are the most popular methods of rule-based decision-making. Any type of voting system would fall into this category and these can work very well, as long as everyone is agreed on the rules!

Sometimes a meeting won't do

In some situations you need to face the truth, that a meeting, even a well-facilitated one, is not the panacea for all problems. There are sometimes situations where agreement is not possible through a polite, if robust exchange of ideas. These are the times when mediation or arbitration is necessary. This requires a whole different set of skills and this book will not attempt to stray into that area, other than to flag that some situations do need other skills and you should make sure you use the right tools for the job.

With all of this in mind when you want to have a meeting to make decisions that stick, it is important to consider two main aspects:
     1. making sure you get all the information and
     2. designing the process for making the decision itself.
In this chapter we will be looking at options in these two areas.

Getting all the information

    ★ Whatever the meeting you are leading it will involve people, so it is important to make sure the meeting is designed to handle the group dynamics. In practical terms, what this means is making sure people have the **answers to some key questions before being ready to commit** to a decision.

☆ 'Why are we here?' 'What is the purpose of this work?' 'How does this fit in to the big picture?'

☆ 'Who are we working with?' 'How do I fit in with them?'

☆ 'What are we aiming to achieve?' 'What's my role in it?'

☆ 'How are we going to do it?'

All too often meetings are convened where groups form solutions for how things need to be done – action plans – but without the answers to the preceding questions being clear. These are the kind of action plans that rarely get implemented as there is usually a lack of commitment behind them. By ensuring your meetings take time to share the information that answers all the questions, you will be much more likely to make decisions with commitment to them.

★ Good decisions are **informed decisions** so it is also important to enable information to be shared to give people the context and perspectives for making quality decisions. This means allowing time in the agenda for information-sharing and data-gathering processes. Time spent at the front end of a meeting sharing information usually saves time later on in decision-making because people understand the different perspectives and feel their perspectives are understood.

It is important to flag up that sharing information is usually most effective when done **through discussion rather then presentations.** Discussions allow people to ask for the information they need and acknowledges the information they already know, rather than *assuming* what they need and planning long presentations.

★ We take a view that different perspectives are what help to make better quality decisions. If this is true then taking time to **explore these different perspectives** is valuable. To do this we broadly need to explore:-

☆ People's actual experience, which can be past experience of similar situations or current experience of the wider context that is impacting on their view.

☆ People's values, which are the principles that guide people in the way they make decisions. Exploring values can allow groups to find common, shared ideas that enable them to reach decisions more easily, especially if their realities are very different.

★ **Decisions sometimes need to be made iteratively.** You may be familiar with this style in making individual decisions, where you can start to form a view and then revisit the decision, coming at it from a different perspective. The same can be true for groups; they sometimes need to revisit decisions. This can be done

☆ in separate meetings

☆ after some reflection time e.g. on the second morning of a two day meeting, after a lunch break

☆ in different formats e.g. splitting the group into pairs or small groups to discuss the topic, share headlines from the small groups as a whole group then re-form different sub-groups for discussion… this can be repeated several times.

* Contrary to the above view there can also be times when it is best to leave a decision **partially complete,** such as when the principal decision has been made and the detail is not yet agreed. These decisions can be useful when either the detail is not important for the next stage of the process or the detail can be refined outside the meeting.

* Agreeing the **criteria for any decisions** to be made can unlock groups. For example, if someone is looking to resolve a problem by finding the ideas/solutions that are going to be the easiest to implement, he is going to choose a very different path from the person who is looking for the most innovative, long-term solutions. Having an up-front discussion about these different criteria is much more productive than arguing about the course of action to be taken.
Few decisions are simple enough to have one criterion, so having some kind of ranking/ sense of priority of the different criteria involved can be useful.

* Agreeing any 'givens' up-front can prevent a lot of wasted time in meetings. By setting out **things that cannot be changed,** a group can understand what needs to be decided and what does not.

* **Creativity meetings** usually have three phases with different decision-making at each phase.
    1. Idea generation – in which you are actively trying to prevent decisions from being made. This is a data-gathering phase.

    2. Idea selection – in which the most promising ideas are selected. Decision-making at this stage can be done using any or several of the following methods:
        a. an expert decision-maker
        b. a small group of experts making the decision
        c. a group poll
        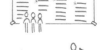

    3. Idea development – in which phase decisions are usually made by experts or by the person who owns the problem.

When looking to generate creative decisions, there are specific techniques that can assist with creativity; these can be found in chapter 16 *Out of the box.*

* The one aspect of getting all the data that seems to be forgotten most frequently is the **value of reviewing the past.** By getting a group to share its history you can learn a lot from the successes and mistakes of the past, as well as about the personal histories of individuals in the room. The other advantage of allowing time for this kind of conversation is that it acknowledges all the past experience in the room, so if you know you are going to have people who keep saying, 'but we tried that before and it didn't work', then using this technique can tease out exactly what was tried before and why it didn't work, before looking to the future and what needs to be done. We often use large sheets of paper on the wall to create timelines with groups in support of this kind of conversation.

An example from Katherine and Ingrid: In a meeting for a group that had been formed through acquisition, we proposed a session at the start of the agenda in which the history of the group was explored. In the weeks running up to the meeting this session became known as the 'History Bit' in discussions with the client. Not having experienced our facilitation before he had no experience of this kind of thing and clearly did not see the value. Despite attempts to delete the 'History Bit' from the agenda we protected it and ran the session. It proved to be one of the most valuable sessions of the day...
It allowed older members of the team to feel valued.
It enabled newer people to understand the legacy.
It developed a shared understanding of where they came from and why the current difference existed.

Processes for decision-making

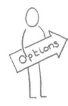

It is absolutely key to have process for decision-making when you are working with a group and that process needs to be made clear up-front, usually in the rules of the meeting. Once a decision has been agreed it is important to distil it by being clear about who will deliver what and when. This clarity can be improved by writing it down publicly (for more on *Managing information* see chapter 13).

This section outlines a number of different decision-making options; the art of running an effective meeting is in choosing the right option for the group/situation you are in. It is useful **to consider using more than one decision-making process to make a decision** e.g. you may decide on a dot vote, then remove the least favourite options and have a discussion about the remaining options on the table. The other thing to consider when making decisions in groups is making the process iterative i.e. giving people the chance to explore options, then start to form a decision, then continue the discussion before making the final decision.

* *Hierarchical*
  ☆ The most senior person in the meeting makes the decision.
  ☆ The most senior person makes the decision outside the meeting.
  ☆ The person with the most expertise makes the decision.

* *Consensus*
  ☆ Through discussion i.e. talk about the subject until the group forms a consensus.
  ☆ Negotiation i.e. each party discusses and modifies options until an option that meets everyone's needs is agreed on.
  ☆ Dialogic. This type of decision-making is about gaining an understanding of the principles behind different perspectives/options. Once a group can agree to one or more common principles, the solutions that everyone can agree with tend to come quickly.
  ☆ The important thing to remember is that consensus decision-making takes time! It's also important to consider what you will do if you can't get the whole group to agree.

* **Rule Based**
  ☆ **Dot voting** – often done using sticky dots or ticks of the pen. Each person gets a number of votes that they can place against their favourite options. This allows the group to see the weight of interest for each option.

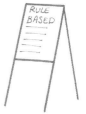

To make dot voting work well you need to give everyone the right number of sticky dots to ensure you will have clear 'winners' in the decision. A useful rule of thumb for this is to count up the number of options/ideas that you are choosing from, divide it by 3 and then round up. E.g. if you have 19 options to choose from you would give each person
$$19/3 = 6.3 => 7 \text{ votes.}$$
It is also important to ask people **not** to put several votes from one individual against one option. This rule of thumb works well up to 10 dots. People usually struggle to place more than 10 votes so that tends to be the maximum we hand out, even when there are hundreds of options to choose from.

A couple of variations about how you dot vote are:-
1. Give people their dots and get them all to come up together and vote.
2. Ask people to consider their choices and write them down before placing their dots.

  ☆ **Criteria based** – where a set of criteria are used to evaluate a number of options. The criteria can be agreed in advance and given to the group or determined by the group in the meeting, but it is better not to have too many; we usually aim for up to 6.
  There are then options about how you use the criteria to evaluate the options. This can be done intuitively by the participants.
  1. Tell everyone the criteria
  2. Ensure everyone understands them
  3. Let everyone place their votes

Alternatively, criteria can be used in a scoring mechanism whereby each option is given a numerical score against each of the criteria. The option(s) with the highest scores are then selected. For example 0= lowest and 3= highest against criteria shown in the grid below

Criteria ⇩	Option 1	Option 2	Option 3	Option 4
Cost				
Impact				
Time to implement				
Total score				

The 'watch out' I would give to this approach is that the scores can be surprising and it is useful to allow the group time to discuss the findings when the 'scores on the doors' have been calculated.

Similar to the above approach is the use of a ranking mechanism e.g. A, B, C for each option against the criteria. The decision is made by looking at the options with the most promising rankings e.g. the most As across all the criteria.

☆ **Higher/lower** – we tend to use this approach visually with groups. You can write the different options onto cards or A5 post-its and then post them up on the wall. You then go through each card placing it higher or lower on the wall, depending on how promising it seems. Another option around this method is to get the group to come up to the wall and move the cards around themselves in silence. When the cards are all static you let the group discuss the placing of the cards to sense-check the prioritisation.

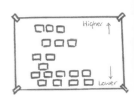

☆ **Show of hands** – often used in meetings to make majority-based decisions. The interesting thing about this option is there is clear visibility of each person's individual decision. This can lead to peer pressure, with people raising their hands when they see who else is!

☆ Another variation is to get everyone to do **'fist to five'** – where a hand raised as a fist = 0 and a hand raised with all 5 fingers = 100% agreed. Each person is asked to make their hand formation on their lap before being asked to raise their hands.

☆ **Majority/minority voting** – Most of us are familiar with majority voting, where the options with the most votes get selected. Minority decision-making is when the option with the least votes gets selected i.e. when you are looking to eliminate the least favourite option.

☆ **Eliminating the least favourite** – by removing the options that are least favoured, the group can then focus on discussing the most promising options. Determining the least favourite can be done using any of the options above.

☆ **Electronic keypads** – it is possible to hire electronic keypad systems to use in meetings, usually for large groups. These work on the basis of offering the group options labelled as A, B, C or D and then everyone individually selects by pushing the appropriate button on their handheld device to give an overall vote.

☆ **Shareware** – is the next level of technology available beyond the keypads, where individuals or small groups work from laptops running specialist software to support group conversations e.g. WebIQ, Group Systems. This type of approach allows large amounts of information to be exchanged and processed quickly and allows large groups to do more iterations of debate than most low tech approaches can facilitate.

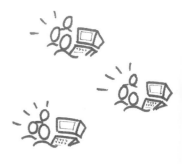

Summary

To summarise, our top tips for making *decisions that stick* are:-

* Make sure you consider the group dynamics and lead a group into decision-making.
* Allow time for sharing context and perspectives including historical information to enable informed decisions.
* Consider.....
  ☆ Iterative decision-making
  ☆ Partial decisions
  ☆ Using more than one decision-making technique
* Decision-making methods are....
  ☆ Hierarchical or
  ☆ Consensus or
  ☆ Rule Based

12

Keeping everyone energised

Q. *I find that during some meetings the energy really flags. As a result I'm a big fan of energisers. I have my favourites to use after lunch or during the slow, low-energy slots mid-morning or afternoon. They can be really effective for getting a group going but sometimes I find they don't really do the job very well. Some people just don't join in properly and the group can still be just as lethargic afterwards as they were before. In some cases it seems to make it harder to get the work done, not better. How can I avoid this problem and ensure my groups are always lively and respond well to energisers?*

Problem

A. You're so right to have the energy of the group in mind when planning or managing your meeting. However, you've asked slightly the wrong question. A better question would be. 'How can I ensure the energy levels of my groups are always right for the work we need to do?' Your question implies that high energy is always good but some pieces of work require quiet reflection or focused concentration. It could be that your difficulties are due to the energiser not matching the work you're doing. Let's start by thinking about the reasons the group energy might not feel right.

Time of day

It is natural that people's energy varies through the day. We all have times when we feel more awake and when we find it easier to concentrate. This varies for different people but by and large we are more alert at the start of the day and we dip later in the morning as blood sugar runs low. We can often feel a little sleepy after lunch but revive later in the afternoon once our digestive system has had a chance to work. How well we all ride these changes depends on many factors, but certainly the length of time we're expecting to work and when we plan our breaks can have a big impact.

Wrong process / wrong style

Quite apart from the natural rhythm of the day, people's energy levels can be greatly affected by what they are being asked to do. You know how it is, you may be feeling a bit tired and lethargic but if someone suggests an exciting or interesting trip out then more

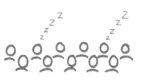

than likely you'll suddenly perk up and be set to go. And it isn't just what we're being asked to do, but also *how*. The application of this to meetings is two-fold. Firstly, too much of the same thing gets boring and saps energy. Using the same approach over and over will stifle a meeting and the worst culprit for this is endless presentations. However, don't think it isn't true for other processes. One reason our contributor may be having difficulty with icebreakers is using the same type over and over. Secondly, you need to try and match the type of work to the right time of day. Generally people are more alert at the start of the day so use this time for absorbing information rather than trying to slog through it after lunch. You can exacerbate energy problems by doing the wrong work at the wrong time.

Finally, related to this idea of the wrong type of work is the style the facilitator uses. If you manage your meetings by always pushing the group, they'll quickly tire. Conversely, if you always pose big open questions, leaving them to fill the gaps, the group will again run out of steam pretty quickly. You need to get a balance of these 'push' and 'pull' styles to best manage the energy of the group.

Lack of commitment

One big danger with using icebreakers is that you may use them like sticking plasters and fail to notice that something more serious is wrong for the group. Often it is tempting to see low energy as a need for a coffee break, or a need to get up and jump about for a while. But low energy can also be a symptom of people in the group being in conflict. Not everyone displays their disagreement

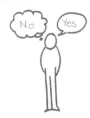

by ranting and raving. Some simply withdraw and become observers of what is going on – they may be looking for opportunities to sabotage at a later date.

While you don't want to jump to this conclusion every time your group has an energy dip, you should keep it in mind. And certainly if a long coffee break and a change in process haven't made a difference, you should certainly start exploring whether there are any hidden disagreements that need to be aired. When preparing your meeting it is useful to consider the energy of the group as part of the design for your meeting. Here are some things you can plan to do.

Planning the energy of your meeting

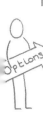

★ *Minimise, or ideally eliminate, presentations.* There are all kinds of statistics quoted about how long people really pay attention in presentations; suffice to say it is not very long. We all know this and yet so many meetings are 'death by PowerPoint'. So, challenge yourself about presentations

☆ Is a presentation really the best means to share information?

☆ Do people already know it? Many presentations waste time giving information that people already have.

☆ Set time limits for presentations. But beware…. if we had a pound for the number of times we've heard someone say, 'I'll only need 10 minutes', and 30 to 45 minutes later they are still up there presenting, we'd be very rich! If someone is to present for 10 minutes, they should only have 1 or 2 slides….. and this does not mean each slide has 30 bullet points! The other 'beware' about setting time limits is, people just try to talk faster!

☆ Could you use large wall charts to share information? These can be prepared in advance or you can produce charts with blank spaces for people to complete information during the meeting. (for more on this see chapter 13 *Managing information*).

☆ Information produced on wall charts can be reviewed by inviting people to walk around the room and read the charts.

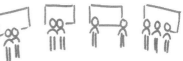

★ *Keep presentations to the morning* when people tend to more alert.

★ Make sure the sessions *before and after lunch keep the group active.* Sessions like small-group activities, paired walks, standing brainstorms, all help keep the group energy.

★ *Plan the ups and the downs of energy in the meeting.* For example there is no point in expecting a group to be high energy if they are doing some in-depth analysis. Just prepare for this kind of intense-thinking energy and allow a break afterwards.

★ *Your energy* can keep the energy of the group going. So even when you are feeling low energy, try to keep your pace and tone lively if you want to keep the group energised.

★ Allow **plenty of breaks** during a meeting but be realistic about time; a 5 minute break always ends up being 10!

★ If you have smokers or caffeine addicts in the group make sure you allow time in breaks for them to get their fix ☺ They do need it and won't work very well without it, whether you approve or not.

★ Give people an **opportunity to talk.** If the people in the meeting see each other infrequently then allow time in the agenda for them to catch up. We always allow long lunch breaks (1½ hrs) in our internal meetings as we so rarely get the chance to catch up without there being a specific piece of work to discuss.

★ **Change the format** the group is working in from session to session.
By different formats we mean
  ☆ Whole group discussion
  ☆ Small group discussion (different sizes of groups)
  ☆ Pairs
  ☆ Individual thinking time

★ **Use processes that encourage movement** during the meeting such as standing up and sticking post-its on a board, walking around to review charts etc.

★ Make sure you have an **environment that keeps energy in the meeting.** We won't bore you with our war stories about awful venues we have worked in, but our worst experience of a venue's impact on group energy was one where the two day meeting finished half a day early because everyone had headaches!

★ So, ensure the following aspects of your meeting environment work for you;
  ☆ Natural light in the room
  ☆ Comfortable temperature
  ☆ You may choose to arrange your room with zones, to create different working environments for the different sections of the meeting.

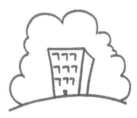

  ☆ Sufficient food and drink. Make sure you have the right quality of food and drink to keep people's bodies and brains healthy in the meeting. Plenty of water, fresh fruit and nuts available as snacks and a light, healthy lunch are best for the brain, but experience shows that people really like bacon sandwiches, chocolate bars, biscuits, crisps and sweets!
  ☆ Toys to play with. It has been shown that having something to fiddle with can help many people concentrate in meetings. So, better to provide suitable toys than find someone irritatingly flicking the top of their pen throughout a discussion. Look for toys like juggling thuds, stress balls or tangles, not toys like puzzles, which detract people's attention from the meeting.

An example from Ingrid: I was facilitating a creativity session in a London Hotel and had requested a large spacious room with natural light. When I got to the venue I found we had a room on the third floor... of the basement... with no natural light... that was usually used as a dining room so had very dim lighting! So I had the challenge of compensating for the awful environment by using other methods. Throughout the meeting I kept people standing and moving around. I mixed the groups and used different formats. We had regular breaks and big posters with sunshines drawn on them and I bounced about like a lunatic for the entire 3 hours of the meeting!

Interventions

If you get into your meeting and find that the energy in the group is an issue, here are some things you can do

★ **Change something!** We would offer this as a principle if any aspect of your meeting isn't going well, like the old saying, 'if you keep doing what you've always done, you'll keep getting what you've always got!'

☆ Front it out and find out why. Say something like, "Is it me, or does everyone seem a bit low energy right now?" Usually this is enough to get a sense of the group feeling and some people will offer reasons why.

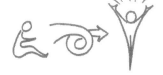

☆ Once you have established that everyone is a bit low energy you can offer some suggestions. "OK, we are all feeling a bit tired, so let's…

☆ take a break"

☆ change the way we are working. Let's get into pairs for this next discussion." You could also choose to work in small groups or allow some individual reflection time.

☆ look at this subject from a different perspective."

☆ check whether this discussion is helping us to achieve the outcomes for today, or if it is best handled elsewhere." But BEWARE of people using this as a means to avoid conflict.

★ If you *take a break* you can try to work out why the energy is low

☆ either by asking around the group

☆ or by changing something and then observing the impact.

★ **Be prepared to name the conflict** i.e. re-open the discussion in a way that allows people to express concerns or differences of opinion.

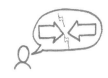

★ Create space for discussion and listen for people's objections.

★ *Finish early.* If everyone is exhausted, there's really no point in pushing the group to the planned finish time.

★ *Finish late.* By offering more time you can change the energy by allowing people the space to discuss things properly.

★ *Use energisers.* Try to make these relevant to the meeting content and always make sure they are appropriate for the group. You *don't have to* use explicit energisers to do a good job of managing energy. I frequently run meetings where I manage the energy throughout the meeting using methods described above. It is worth remembering that some people hate energisers, so be sure of your audience if you use these.

Energisers

There are lots of great resources to give you ideas for energisers (see bibliography). In this section we outline four categories of energisers and give you a few ideas of each.

★ **Raising physical energy**

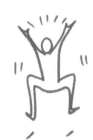

★ Orange race – split group into 2 teams and line up in rows. Give front person an orange/ball to pass over their shoulder and through the next person's legs until the orange gets to the back. The back person runs to the front with the orange and restarts the process. The winning team is the first to get back to its original configuration.

★ Shake hands – give everyone 2 minutes to walk round the rooms and shake hands with people. You can find out how many hand-shakes people have done at the end.

★ Team formations – get people in small groups and then give them a configuration to get into e.g. 2 hands on the floor, two in the air and 4 feet on the ground. The groups have to organise themselves into a formation that achieves this. BEWARE if physical contact is inappropriate for the group.

★ Sitting circle – get into a circle, with everyone's shoulder into the middle and all facing the same way. Get everyone to sit down slowly until everyone is sitting on someone's knee.

★ Tangle – in a circle with everyone facing inwards, get people to hold hands in pairs. Get the spare hands into the middle and everyone grabs someone's hand. The group then needs to untangle and usually end up in 1 or 2 circles.

★ **Morning starters**

★ Walk through the previous day – get everyone to walk around the room reviewing the charts produced on the previous day.

★ Reflections – give everyone a chance to share their overnight reflections on the previous day's work.

* Stretching exercises

* Go for a walk alone or a paired walk to discuss reflections on the previous work.

* How are you? Getting people into the meeting by asking 'How are you?' with the intention of genuinely listening to how people are and allowing people to share whatever is on their mind at the moment.

★ *Focusing Attention*
  Anything that engages both sides of the brain helps with this.

* Hands to knees – standing with hands outstretched, get people to raise their knees one at a time in front of them and touch opposite hands to knees.

* Hands to feet – standing with hands outstretched, get people to raise their feet one at a time behind them and touch opposite hands to feet.

* Patting heads and rubbing tummies, and the reverse.

* Figure of 8 – stand up and hold one arm outstretched in front of the face. Then form a fist with this hand and raise the thumb. Move the thumb in a sideways figure of 8 whilst keeping focused on the thumb throughout the movement. Make the figure of 8 bigger until you cannot see it without moving the head.

* Stamp, clap click – get the group into pairs. Get them to count to 3 alternately. Then replace the 1 with a stamp and repeat. Then replace the 1 with a stamp and the 2 with a clap. Finally replace all 3 with stamp, clap click.

★ *Getting creative*
  Anything that gets people being playful can help with creativity. See more on getting *Out of the box* in chapter 16.

* Hand out rubber bands/paper clips and ask everyone to brainstorm different things they could do with them.

* Get people into pairs or threes and start to tell a story. BUT they are only allowed to tell one sentence of the story at a time before passing onto another person.

* Get the group to design a poem, song, sketch or mime about the subject they are going to be talking about.

* In pairs tell jokes/funny stories.

Summary

To summarise, our top tips for *managing energy* in meetings are,

★ Minimise (or eliminate) presentations. Keep them to the start of the meeting.
★ Think about energy as you plan your agenda – allow plenty of breaks. Keep people active around lunchtime. Give variety of format.
★ Make sure you have the right environment.
★ If energy starts to plummet in a meeting, do not ignore it, do something!
★ Use energisers appropriately for the particular group you are working with.

13

Managing information

Q. *I've had a lot of experience running meetings and I'm pretty successful with managing all the people dynamics that arise. The problem I have is how to manage all the information. I always keep a couple of flip charts handy to record actions as they come up and to park issues that we can't discuss at that particular point, but I sometimes feel this isn't enough. Sometimes a group is discussing a very complex subject and people get lost with different understandings of what has been said. Or in a long meeting, over several days, we end up with so many different ideas on different bits of flip chart paper that the group start to forget what we've discussed. What can I do to keep a better track of all the information?*

A. Congratulations that you successfully manage the people in a meeting. And how perceptive to realise that taming the information is just as much a challenge. Meetings are all about information exchange. If we didn't need to share or jointly create data and ideas there would be no need for getting people together at all. Getting this aspect of a meeting right can therefore make a huge difference to the success, or otherwise, of any forum.

Holistic thinking

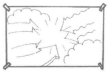

Why is information management so hard? Well, at the heart of the problem is the fact that information can only be shared sequentially. One person speaks and others listen (if it's going well) and then the next person adds to the information pool and so on. Unfortunately, to make sense of the information and craft it into something we need, we have to be able to see all the information at the same time. Now whilst some of us have good memories, even the best of us find it hard to hold all the strands of a complex subject in our heads at the same time.

This inability to hold lots of ideas in our heads is not something we should be ashamed of. We have two factors working against us. The first is our brain's basic memory capacity. We can hold approximately seven things in our head at a time. This is why most of us remember long telephone numbers not as 11 different numbers but chunked into groups of 2 or 3 numbers. So for instance, instead of remembering 0, 7, 8, 7, 9, 8, 1, 3, 2, 8, 9 it is easier to learn 0787, 981, 32, 89.

The second thing many of us find difficult is visualising large, complex pictures or maps. So much information is presented to us in sequential, logical lists we're just not used to trying to piece it all together in our heads. We're fine if we can see it written down on paper or screen; it is the challenge of creating the picture in our minds that we find so hard.

The eyes have it

If you could get a print-out of the different inputs the brain is receiving you'd realise that by far the dominant sense is your sight. Yes, we make sense of the world around with touch and hearing as well as smell and taste but a lot of what the brain uses comes from what we see. When we ask our brains to gather information only by listening we rather handicap ourselves – particularly if we ask it to do this for a whole day or longer. It becomes even more of an issue when we add the fact that the brain just can't concentrate 100% of the time. We do have small periods of down time and if something is said during one of our 'out' moments then we've lost it. Visual inputs have the potential to be there and stay there awhile, giving ourselves a much better chance of catching up when we come 'back on line'.

The Flipchart

The problem with the flipchart is exactly that; you write on them, then flip them. If we are to address the issues mentioned above we need to use anything we write down as a way to reinforce the ability of people to absorb the information and do something with it. Having lots of unmanageable lists on separate pages may do little to support the work being done. This chapter describes the basics of how to use a technique called Graphic Facilitation to make the information useful within meetings.

Graphic Facilitation overview

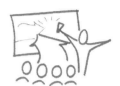

* Graphic Facilitation simply means that information that is shared in the meeting is captured, real time, in large displays (approx 1.25m x 3m) on the wall, often in a graphical fashion.
And why does it work so well? Because:

* When people's contributions are recorded onto a large display they can literally SEE that they have been heard. This encourages participation.

* All the information is visible together so it is much easier to understand how different aspects inter-relate. The group can SEE the whole system that they are discussing.

* When the record of the meeting is created in the room, in front of everyone, the agreements that are made are much more likely to stick! When everyone can SEE what they are agreeing to, it gives people an opportunity to speak up if there are still issues to resolve.

* Having a large display in the meeting really focuses the attention of a group and gives a focal point for discussion.

* It plays to the fact that people obtain the majority of their information through visual means.

Preventions

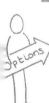

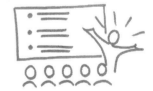

* **PowerPoint** – there are lots of jokes about 'death by PowerPoint' and they come from its overuse or poor use of in meetings. However, if managed carefully PowerPoint can be a useful means to present information, particularly to large groups. Some watch-outs from our experience are:-
    * ☆ **Not too much!** – both within a presentation and within the meeting. Someone should not be using 20 slides for a 10 minute presentation. And within a meeting you don't want endless hours of PowerPoint presentations if you want the participants engaged and awake!
    * ☆ **Don't repeat what people already know** – many presentations give endless amounts of context that the group largely knows, so when the speaker finally gets to the point the audience have lost the will to live. I remember sitting through a half hour presentation in which the presenter took 27 minutes giving contextual information about the current market and climate for his department. By the time he reached the crux of the presentation, the goals for the forthcoming year, he'd run out of time.

* **Booklets/handouts** – these can be helpful for presenting information to a group as they are useful for people to make their own notes on and also allow people to have the information to hand in subsequent discussions. We sometimes give information in handout format where we want people to discuss it in smaller groups and come back with questions.

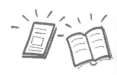

* **Templates** – templates can be used to capture information before or during meetings. They can be produced in various sizes from A4 through to large wall charts (1.25m deep and 3m wide). Whatever the size of the template it is usually divided into a number of sections, each section having a title or a question explaining the type of information in the section. Graphics/shapes can also be used to divide the template in to sections, which can make it easier to use. Templates are useful for presenting key points and also for providing a common framework so readers can access the information easily. Below is an example of a template.

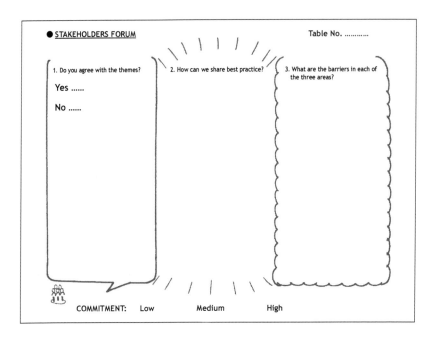

* Before a meeting – a template can be circulated to presenters. The completed templates can be sent out before the meeting or templates can be completed in the meeting to share information.

An example from Katherine: '*I was asked to facilitate a sales meeting with representatives from different regions around the world coming together. When I first talked to the client about his plans for the meeting he explained that everyone was going to prepare a presentation about their region and they would start the meeting with these presentations. I worked out that these presentations were going to take about 5 hrs of a 2 day meeting! Instead of this I designed the following approach.*

I found out that the key pieces of information people were interested in were the size of each market, the main customers in the market, the competitors in the market and the key challenges they were facing. We asked people to think about these aspects of their markets in preparation for the meeting but not to prepare a presentation.

At the point in the meeting where we needed to share context about the different markets I handed out A3 graphic templates to regional representatives. They completed the templates in about 15-20 minutes, posted them up on the wall and then reviewed the templates from the other regions. Once everyone had reviewed all the templates, which took about 20 minutes, I then facilitated a discussion amongst the group about any questions that people had. This took about 30 minutes. By the end of the session everyone understood the salient points about each region, everyone knew who was who and some interesting debates had been started about some of the common issues.'

☆ Templates sent out in advance of a meeting can be used to prepare a single, consolidated presentation for use in the meeting. For example, if you are getting a group together for a learning review of a project, it can be useful to send templates to all the participants to get them to highlight the events, highs, lows and learning before the meeting. This information can then be consolidated beforehand for presentation in the meeting.

★ **Posters** can be used to present information that may not be necessary for the core discussions but provides background or subliminal information. For example a welcome poster with the name, date of the meeting and the names of participants.

★ **Sharing information in a market place** set up is a great way of people getting what they need rather than listening to endless presentations and filtering out what they don't need. In a market place people set up stands/market stalls with information for people to look at. At its simplest level a market place could just be people with flipcharts/wall charts/posters with information on. However, marketplaces also lend themselves to demonstrations and even audience participation.

An example: *We once ran a market place with a prize for the most creative stall. The variety and creative energy put into each group's information sharing was tremendous. We enjoyed sketches, songs and demonstrations!*

★ The real crux of presenting information in any format is to **be clear about the purpose** i.e. what do you want the group to do as a result of this information? If you want the group to understand a new piece of legislation whose implications they need to understand but can't change, then the method needs to be fundamentally different to presenting information with a view to changing attitudes.

Participants recording

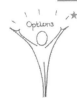

Graphic templates provide a great means for participants to record key points of discussion in a meeting. Templates can be produced in all sizes to suit different needs e.g. A4/A4 for individual recording, table-top templates for small-group recording, wall-sized charts for larger group work. The great thing about templates is that a well designed template will be intuitive for the group to use. It is still important, however, to give clear instructions for use e.g. record key points, make sure writing is clear, how completed templates will be used.

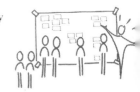

Participants write onto post-its or cards. This is particularly useful when needing to draw comparisons by clustering the post-its i.e. grouping them, with similar points together. To make this type of approach work, you need to think about how you will handle the cards and therefore how to handle the quantity of cards. Some tips for making this type of technique work are:-

☆ Making sure you are explicit about one point per post-it, sticking to key words.

☆ Making A5 post-its and using large felt pens – this means they will be legible when posted up onto a board or the wall.

☆ Managing the quantity of input written onto the post-its; this can be done by
  ☆ limiting the time
  ☆ asking people for a specific number of post-its
  ☆ asking people to prioritise their post-its

☆ Managing the debrief of post-its can be done by:-
  ☆ One person debriefing at a time – beware of the first people covering all the points and also be mindful of energy when using this style.
  ☆ One person giving a point and then people with similar points adding theirs, so you cluster as you go – make sure you have plenty of space to differentiate between different clusters.
  ☆ One person giving a point and you move on to looking for a new/different point. This approach avoids duplication but you lose the sense of how many people had the point.
  ☆ Everyone silently putting up all the post-its and sorting them into clusters based on what they read. The discussion starts once the post-its are clustered.
  ☆ .... and there are probably more.
  ☆ But we would warn you against making assumptions about the words people have written on their post-its and doing the clustering for the group. Check back with them, saying things like, "What was meant here?" "Can someone clarify this point?" "Are these points the same or different?"

Make collages. Many of you may not have done collage work since you were at school but they are a very powerful way for groups and individuals to communicate complex concepts/feelings/emotions without needing great drawing skills. We usually provide a selection of business-specific journals and general magazines/colour supplements for people to cut up and paste onto a collage. Flipchart sized collages usually work well for small groups of about five.

★ We often used collage techniques when developing visions with groups. Sometimes people worry about whether people will get into making collages but our experience is that everyone gets into it and the results are much more than could have been expressed in words alone.

★ Collages are also a great way of communicating complex feelings/emotions so we have used them in sessions where there is conflict in the group. Getting each member of a group to create a collage of what it feels like to be part of the team can lead to a much richer discussion that starting with words alone.

★ **Enter data into a projected spreadsheet.** The key here is the *projection*, which makes the information much clearer to everyone than an individual with a laptop entering data in the meeting. When the information is clear and visible then everyone can engage with it.

★ **Create a book as the output for a meeting**. This usually works best if you provide a format for the book at the start of the meeting so participants have a structure to work with.

> **An example:** *We ran a meeting once where the aim was to identify problems in a project and then how to solve them. At the start of the meeting we had two letter trays, one letter tray was full of blank A4 pro formas, the other was empty except for a front and back cover to the book we were going to produce. When we got to the part of the meeting where problems had been identified and prioritised, small groups of people took a problem to work on and completed a pro forma with information about how to resolve each problem if it occurred. When they finished tackling one problem they moved onto another, until the list of problems was gone and the book letter tray was full of completed pro formas. There was powerful symbolism in the project leader walking away with a completed book at the end of the meeting.*

★ **Use graffiti walls/actions/car parks.** These are all examples of where a large blank piece of paper can be put up at the start of a meeting for people to contribute to as the meeting progresses. Graffiti walls are great for capturing ideas/thoughts throughout a meeting and can lead to some interesting streams of discussion if left up during a meeting that spans several days. Beware of car parks being used to park contentious issues that need to be faced up to by a group that is avoiding conflict.

★ **Set up power time / café style.** This type of participant recording involves setting up a meeting around a table or tables covered with paper. In the centre of the table is a question written on the paper. Individuals then write their response to the questions around the paper and then move round adding comments to other people's contributions as they go. This is done without the group talking and can produce a great deal of information really quickly.

Facilitator recording – the art of public listening

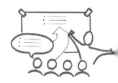

In many schools we are taught the art of public speaking, but rarely are we taught the art of public listening. By being able to record a meeting effectively a facilitator can do a great service to the discussions by helping to acknowledge and clarify contributions, prevent misunderstandings and help people see what's going on.

★ Most information in meetings is recorded in a *list format.* This is partly because the list is a very useful tool for capturing the flow of a discussion but also partly due to a lack of conscious thinking about how best to record the information to help the group make connections.

★ When you need to compare pieces of information, try *clustering.* This can be done either by recording information directly into clusters of common information or by producing the pieces of information on separate post-its/cards and then moving them to form clusters. This usually works best when you use large (A5) post-its and large felt pens, with one point per post-it, so that the group can see what is being written up. By writing onto post-its you have the flexibility to move the information around during or after the discussion.

★ If you need to build combinations of information then using a *grid* is the most useful format. For example, if you want to assess product ideas against criteria, using a grid like the one below would be best.

Products ⇨	Idea 1	Idea 2	Idea 3	Idea 4
Criteria A				
Criteria B				
Criteria C				
Criteria D				

Diagrams such as process maps and mind maps can help show the connections between pieces of information.

★ Mandalas are charts produced around a central theme. Intuitively pictures drawn in this way give a sense of wholeness. If you are working with a group where this is a message you want to convey, managing the display around a central theme can help. For example we have created team targets in meetings, which look like a target with the central mission or vision in the middle, the team goals in the next ring, then individual objectives in the next layer out.

★ If you are confident at *drawing* things pictorially in front of the group, drawings can be a great way of giving meaning. However, if you are not confident about working like this then great effect can be had by creating collages. This can be done by you working with the group as they cut out images to form an overall picture of what is being described.

★ ***The power of metaphor.*** The use of metaphor and imagery can be extremely powerful in helping groups see what's going on in a meeting. One of the most common metaphors used in meetings is the metaphor of a journey, which can be used to help a group explore where they have come from, where they are going and the challenges/milestones on the route.

Metaphors for use in meetings can be developed ahead of the meeting, in the preparation and thinking about how to set the meeting up. They can also evolve in meetings and these can be some of the most transformational as they come from the group and have strong shared ownership.

Once a metaphor has been developed for a meeting it is useful to support its use through imagery in the charts used in the meeting. For example, graphic templates developed around a metaphorical theme for a meeting can help manage the flow of the agenda.

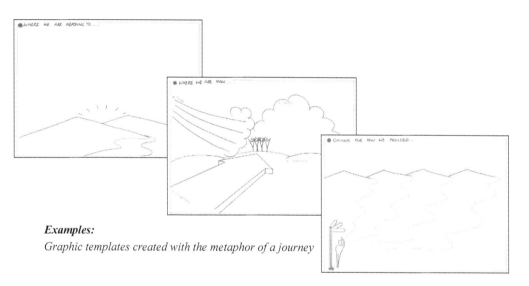

Examples:
Graphic templates created with the metaphor of a journey

★ ***Graphic templates.*** Graphic templates can be used by a facilitator as well as the participants in meetings. Usually the large wall-sized charts are the appropriate size for this use (1.25m x 3m). There are some tips to using templates effectively with groups...

☆ Take time at the start to explain the objective and the overall format of the template. Even though templates are pretty intuitive, it's best not to make assumptions.

☆ Templates give the group the structure for the discussion but it is important to be flexible i.e. move between sections as the conversation moves on; add new sections if necessary; delete sections that are not relevant.

★ ***Blank sheet of paper.*** An experienced graphic facilitator can work from a blank sheet of paper, drawing up the format and adding the content as they go. This is very powerful for the group, seeing their work created before then, but takes years of practice to be able to do. If you are facilitating a meeting where this style of information management would be valuable, there are professional graphic recorders who will work with facilitators to add this level of graphics to a meeting.

Tips for recording

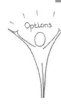

If you want to make your notes clear and easy to read, here are our top tips...

- ★ Have a title to your chart, usually top left and in capitals.
- ★ Usually three dark colours on one chart are enough. Keep light colours, like yellow, orange, red for highlighting.
- ★ We tend to use black for the outline of a chart, the margin, drawings and shapes, keeping other dark colours for the text.
- ★ Use CAPITALS and large lettering for points you want to HIGHLIGHT.
- ★ Keep to lower case for the main text as this is easier to read.
- ★ Have a margin on your chart as it gives you space to improvise.
- ★ Have a format and overall structure to your chart.
- ★ Listen, listen, listen... to the exact words people use and record them faithfully. There's nothing worse than a recorder interpreting contributions incorrectly.
- ★ Leave spaces for bits you miss and come back to fill them in.

Follow-up documentation

Having the right outputs produced after a meeting can do a lot to support the ongoing follow-up of actions afterwards. Some options for output formats are...

- ★ **A book.** A hard or soft copy book with key points from the meeting. See example Participants recording earlier in this chapter.
- ★ **Digital images** of the charts produced in a meeting. The use of large graphic displays can record the events, actions and agreements in real time in a meeting. These can then be digitally photographed, cleaned up and dropped into a file to provide a record of the meeting.
- ★ **Graphic recording.** Graphic recorders can record a meeting graphically, capturing the key points of discussion throughout onto a storyboard. These charts can then be reproduced using digital photography, as described above.
- ★ **Electronic templates** can be created to replicate templates used in the meeting. The outputs from the meeting discussions can then be entered into this format.

Summary

Our top tips for *information management* in meetings are:-

- ★ Plan how you will manage the information before, during and after a meeting. Remember that information is the currency of meetings!
- ★ Think about the different ways you could handle the information.
- ★ Minimise the use of PowerPoint.
- ★ Maximise the use of large displays, templates and wall charts.
- ★ Use the group to help with recording in the meeting.
- ★ There is more to life than just lists ☺!

14

People not there

Q. *My problem is knowing how to deal with people who aren't there for all the meeting. Sometimes people just arrive late, sometimes they pop out to attend to more urgent things and sometimes they leave before the end. The problem is that this can be very disruptive for the group because when they arrive back, and the group has made progress without them, they can then re-open all the discussion again as they may not agree with the decisions taken. Worst of all can be the people who leave before the end, especially if lots of people do this. The participants just seem to leave in dribs and drabs until there seems no point in going on. By this time it is impossible to agree any actions because the people who'd do the work have left already. How do I cope with this type of behaviour in my meetings?*

Problem

A. Yes, we all recognise this particularly frustrating problem that can plague meetings. Your question suggests you're prepared to put up with the behaviour but want to minimise its impact and this might be a reasonably realistic approach for which you'll find ideas in this chapter. But before giving up completely it is worth also thinking about what causes people to arrive late, leave early or plan clashing commitments. By understanding this you open a new set of possibilities to prevent the problem altogether.

Do you need a meeting?

So many meetings happen out of habit or because we feel we should have one. But maybe people are simply voting with their feet when they come and go from a meeting. It is well worth going back to basics and asking, what exactly do we need to get together to discuss, agree or decide. And having thought that through, who actually needs to be there. If you don't do this you may find you have some of the problems described.

Different priorities

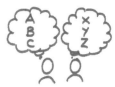

If people don't all have the same sense of the importance of the discussion it won't be long before there is conflict of one sort or another. It can be very frustrating for participants who have a big stake in a discussion to see others treat the subject much more casually by arriving late or leaving early. But it is far from unusual for different parts of an organisation to have different priorities and while they do (or should) all share a broader agreed set of priorities (something to do with the success of the organisation, you might hope) it can be helpful if everyone can see how the individual pieces fit together.

Quite apart from business priorities, people's personal priorities should never be underestimated. If people are asked to travel away from home to attend a meeting you will without doubt bring in to play all the possibility of personal interests conflicting with work. Who wouldn't rather catch a slightly earlier flight home on a Friday than risk the late flight being delayed and keeping them away from their families those extra few hours? Being aware of these dimensions and planning around them can make a big difference to the success of the meeting.

Company culture

Finally, the culture or norms that groups are exposed to makes a lot of difference to their behaviour. If people are always walking in and out of their meetings then it will be what they expect and so what they do. It might be that they have ways that they work around it already, but in most cases it is simply a perpetuating bad habit which is not effectively compensated for. If this is the case then it may well be time to start changing the culture.

An example from Katherine: I once worked with a large food manufacturing firm that had grown rapidly through acquisition. One of the norms that had become established throughout the business was late attendance / non attendance at meetings. It was agreed amongst senior managers that these behaviours were symptomatic of deep cultural problems that were being addressed and that tackling attendance at meetings in isolation from these bigger problems would be fruitless.

Preventions

* ***Adjust the time*** of the meeting to suit the needs of the participants, so that you get the right people there.

* ***Rearrange the date*** of the meeting if necessary, as meeting without the right people is a waste of time anyway.

* ***Check venue and travel arrangements*** to make sure logistical issues don't get in the way. For example, if you have people flying in from different countries it is useful to choose a venue that is close to an airport with regular flights to and from the countries people will be flying from.

* Getting ***travel booked centrally*** means you can work with your travel agent/administrator to ensure people arrive before the start of the meeting and leave after the close.

* ***Plan a shorter meeting.*** This may at least get you started by enabling everyone to meet and get some shared understanding of the meeting topic. If you can gain momentum and commitment in a short meeting, people may be more ready to make time for a follow-up meeting.

* ***Get a senior person to send out the invitation.*** With so many demands on most managers' time these days it can be hard to prioritise what needs to be done. However, if a meeting is clearly being sponsored by someone senior it is more likely to be a priority with participants.

* ***Make it clear what decisions will be made in the meeting*** and that, if they are not there, they cannot be part of the decision- making. It may sound harsh but sometimes this is the most appropriate form of action.

* In preparation for a meeting it is useful to ***call the key people*** who need to be there. The framework we use for these pre-meeting interviews is to understand participant expectations and also any issues or concerns. If you have a concern about attendance at the meeting it can be useful to check how much time each person can give to it and how much time they think is needed to achieve their expectations.

  A 5-10 minute phone call with each participant before the meeting could go something like, "Hello, I am calling you about the meeting we have scheduled on *date*. The purpose of the meeting is *state the purpose of the meeting*. However, I am wondering if you can spare me a few minutes to share your thoughts on what we should be aiming to achieve in the meeting." Once you have understood their expectations of the meeting you can ask a follow up question. "With these objectives in mind, is there anything that is likely to get in the way of achieving them in the meeting? Any issues or concerns you have?" If they don't mention time/attendance as an issue you can raise it with them. "The meeting is being held at *venue* from *start time* to *finish time*. Can you make this?"

★ Make sure all pre-meeting communication is clear and correct. Before any meeting we will always circulate
  ☆ the outcomes for the meeting
  ☆ an overview of the agenda for the meeting, with start and finish times
  ☆ any pre-work for the meeting – we are always very realistic about what people will do beforehand, but it can be useful to give them some things to think about before they arrive.
  ☆ the maps/directions they need to get there – these must be accurate a) so your participants get there on time and b) so they arrive in the best possible mood, not frustrated from having got lost!

Interventions

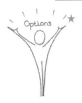

★ Honour your commitment by starting on time. There's nothing worse than busting a gut to get somewhere on time to find that they start late! If there is a genuine issue that makes it wise to start late then check with those that are there that this decision is OK with them.
  ☆ For example, "I know we were scheduled to start at 9am but I understand we have a significant number of people stuck on a train, who will be here by 9:15am. I suggest we wait for them, is this OK?"

★ At the start of the meeting make sure you remind people of the finish time and ask people if this fits with their travel arrangements. Also ask at regular intervals throughout the meeting when people need to leave. At the start of a meeting people are very focused on the work ahead of them and travel plans are usually not in the front of their mind, so gentle reminders throughout the meeting give people other opportunities to check.

★ Ask people in private about their travel plans. They may be more likely to confess that they have planned to leave early!

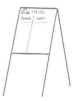

★ Put up a taxi booking sheet for the end of the meeting. That way they have a vested interest in checking the exact time they need to leave.

★ If it transpires that the meeting needs to finish early to accommodate travel plans, you may need to have a discussion with the group about what will NOT get done as a result.

⋆ Plan to finish when people go. It's awful when a meeting fizzles to a close, with people leaving in dribs and drabs through the final hours. Much better to end when most people need to leave and plan to get the additional work done another way.

⋆ If you don't have all the right people at the meeting you may need to change the decision-making process for the meeting. For example, the outcome from the meeting may have been to make a decision about something, but you actually only make a recommendation.

⋆ Sometimes you may need to change the natural flow of an agenda to accommodate the availability of key people in the meeting. While this can lead to a slightly disjointed agenda, it is better to have the right people around for the discussions they need to be part of.

Summary

Our summary of tops tip for *managing attendance* in meetings is:-

⋆ Call participants before the meeting to check their expectations, issues and availability.
⋆ Understand your participants' availability and plan the meeting accordingly.
⋆ Get a senior person to sponsor the meeting and send the invitation.
⋆ Ensure the information in the invitation is accurate.
⋆ State the decisions that will get made in the invitation.
⋆ Honour time commitments throughout the meeting i.e. start on time and start back after breaks on time.
⋆ Sense-check the finish time throughout the meeting.
⋆ Finish the meeting when people need to go.

15

Naming the elephant

Q. *At a meeting I ran last week the most senior person there was very uncomfortable from the start and really didn't seem to be contributing in the way she normally does. At a break I confronted her and she confided in me that she knew there was to be a major reorganisation which would impact the group and whilst she didn't feel she could share this information, it was stopping her being fully able to take part in the meeting. We struggled on with the rest of the day but the team knew something was wrong and bit by bit they changed their behaviour, some becoming quieter and others rather challenging and disruptive. It was terrible knowing the problem but not being able to do anything about it. I've been in similar situations before but have never had such a difficult time of it. What advice can you give about how to handle such things in the future?*

A. Yes, it is a difficult position to be in when you have been given information in confidence but you believe it would be best if that information was shared, particularly in a situation like this where other people sense that something is wrong. And that is the real crux of this problem. If something is afoot then people will often pick it up. They may not notice anything more than a feeling of unease but they will sense something.

You see, for all our sophistication of language, human beings still possess all that innate animal instinct for reading those slight changes in body language, facial expression and who knows what else which contribute such a large part of our communication. Bottom line, whether we tell people or not, they'll know. We all know what it is like having an elephant in the room that no one mentions; we hope that if we ignore it it'll go away.

But what prevents people from just sharing all the information? Why can't we be 100% open and honest?

Political

Often in organisations politics is cited as a reason why people cannot or will not share information. Often decisions take a while to be made. An idea is formed but it takes some time before things are properly worked through and implemented. During this rumination phase it is often felt preferable to keep the information from a broader audience. And this may not be from any sinister motive. Often it is felt to be better not to worry people with things that might never happen. This could backfire, however, as people start speculating worse possibilities in the absence of concrete information.

Holding onto information can, of course, also be a power play. There is a well-known expression that 'information is power' and many hold this principle dear. We've covered power play in chapter 2 *Just talks too much* and there are ideas both in that chapter as well as here for how to manage the situation if this is the case.

Personal

What may be hardest to tackle is where people have personal reasons for keeping things confidential. We all have different approaches to how open we like to be about ourselves and different circumstances will lead us to greater or lesser levels of disclosure. If there are personal dimensions to someone's decision to remain quiet on a subject you have little choice but to respect this.

Fear

Finally we touch upon one of the great motivators for all sorts of human behaviour: fear. We often worry more before an event than we need to. The anticipation of all the things that could go wrong crowd into our minds and squeeze out a more rational evaluation of what might really happen. Very often we think of all the negatives and subsequent bad outcomes without notching up any of the possible good or even neutral options.

We do this as an insurance policy. If we've thought through all the bad things it helps to prepare us should these things happen. Of course, what starts out as a useful strategy often goes into overdrive and we lose our sense of perspective.

The problem for us in this situation is that because we fear what might happen if we share information, we decide to keep everything to ourselves. In fact the more likely outcome from sharing information is either neutral or positive. As managers we need to find ways to encourage people to overcome their caution and trust that other people will often react more favourably if they are kept informed.

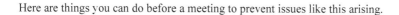

Preventions

Here are things you can do before a meeting to prevent issues like this arising.

* Try and **contact all the participants** of the meeting before the date to find out about their expectations and any issues or concerns they may have. Whether the meeting is one you're calling or one you've been asked to facilitate, you will find people are more likely to be open about issues on a one-to-one basis and it gives you a chance to reconcile these problems before the start. There are a number of ways you can do this depending on time, number of people, who is involved etc. For example you could:-

  ☆ Phone each participant for a 5 – 10 minutes conversation to ask them what they want to see achieved and any concerns about the meeting.

  ☆ E-mail everyone with a set of questions about the meeting, including concerns/ issues/barriers.

  However, if you do identify some issues through these pre-meeting conversations, be aware that they may 'evaporate'. This can occur because your conversations catalyse people to resolving things.

* **Encourage openness** in advance of the meeting. This can be done in the way you have dialogues with participants and the communication that is sent out to them in advance.

* **Plan what can be shared.** A leader can turn this type of situation into an opportunity to generate a great deal of trust within a group if they can disclose some of what's going on. For example, they can share that a reorganisation is going to happen, without disclosing details. In the meetings we have facilitated where people have done this, not only has it had a positive effect on the group, but confidences have been kept when they have been asked for.

* If you know the meeting is going to involve **tackling difficult issues,** make the space for these conversations.

  Katherine's example: I was facilitating a three day meeting for a group of senior executives and at the end of the first day I had concerns that there were some unmentionables in the group that were not being discussed. I didn't want to push the group too much initially, so on the second morning I opened the meeting and then offered the chance for overnight reflections on the work the group had done the previous day. To start with, the group offered reflections that were pretty 'safe', and then someone said, 'I don't think we are being open and honest, I know I am not,' which lead to more contributions along these lines. The discussion went on with people talking about what they hadn't been sharing, and why, which lead into the leader sharing his expectations of the group members and the group fronting their concerns. Two hours into the day we took a break from what had been a pretty fierce but very productive conversation.

* If, in your preparation, you uncover an issue that is going to blow the meeting out of the water, better to postpone the meeting than to continue regardless!

Interventions

If, despite you best efforts, you find an issue like this arising in your meeting, here are some ideas for things you can do.

* Take a **break**. By taking a break you give yourself time to
   1. think about how to handle the situation
   2. talk with key people
   3. prepare something different for the group to do

* **Talk to the person withholding information.** Rather than ask them how they think it's going, it can be quicker and more productive to state, without evaluating, what you are observing in the group, and to ask their view on it. For example, "I have noticed that when we mention the events of 2007 (the elephant), no one makes eye contact with me and it is very hard to get participation. Do you have any idea why this is?"
   ☆ It could be that you are wrongly interpreting the behaviour.
   ☆ Once they are made aware of the symptoms they might be able to shed some light on the problem.
   ☆ If the problem is them, this is the first step to addressing it!

* In a situation like the one described at the start of the chapter, **encourage them to be as open as they can.** Even if they just admit to the group that they know some changes are afoot but don't know what, this is better than a poorly executed cover-up.

* Create space in the agenda to talk with the group without a sense of time pressure. It is important to have the discussion.

* Another option is that **you name the elephant;** share with the group what's going on and see what response you get.

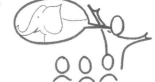

* By **exaggerating the consequences** you can push the group to resolving how they can work productively. For example, "If this meeting carries on at a superficial level the decisions that get made are unlikely to be robust and will be likely to get unstuck after the meeting."

* **Give people permission to leave.** Better this than carry on with a time-wasting exercise.

Summary

Our top tips for getting *open and honest* conversations in meetings are:-

* Contact all the participants before the meeting to understand their expectations and concerns.
* Talk with people who want to withhold information and encourage them to be open and share as much as they can, both before and during the meeting.
* Have the courage to tackle difficult issues.
* Push the group to talk about their issues through
  * naming the elephant yourself
  * exaggerating the consequences of not resolving issues.

16

Out of the box

Q. *What can I do to get people to think more creatively? We seem to be so locked into our thinking. At a meeting last week we spent 4 hours coming up with half a dozen solutions that, quite frankly, I could have jotted down before we started. It seems that if we do get any vaguely different ideas other people just give you all the reasons why they won't work. We did try a new brainstorming technique a while ago but somehow, although we had lots of fun and came up with loads of ideas, none of the ideas have really taken hold. What I want to know is how to get out-of-the-box thinking in my meetings so that we get good ideas that we can put into practice.*

Problem

A. Ah, the holy grail of so many organisations; a truly new idea. How elusive they are! But then, if it was easy to come up with fantastic new ideas any time we wanted, maybe we wouldn't prize them so much. But why is it so hard? Is it just that most people are not creative? We think not. It isn't so much our ability to be creative but, as the above suggests, all the barriers we put in place either before or after we come up with the ideas. Let's examine the root causes of the problem.

Organisational inertia

Cause

Sometimes organisations say they want great new ideas when in fact they rather like business as usual. When an organisation has been very successful for a long time, it can often be hard to believe that change is really necessary.

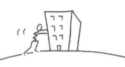

There might be just too much vested interest in business as usual, so subtle ways are found to sabotage new ideas. Favourite sabotage methods are

1. 'We tried that *x* years ago and it didn't work then.'
2. 'That might work in other places but it wouldn't work here.'
3. Delaying the decision to 'think about it'.

Individual barriers

Cause

We are all naturally quite creative but, in general, life does not train or encourage us to use these skills. Throughout our education there is generally a *right answer* that we're trying to learn and in our work it is often compliance to the systems and procedures that is valued above a more maverick approach. And the less we use

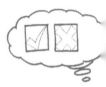

our natural creativity the more we persuade ourselves we cannot do it. In fact we start feeling uncomfortable with solutions to problems that stray too much from the day to day. But this is all just learnt behaviour and if we can learn one way to think then we can learn another.

Problems vs opportunity

Cause

It is an old and much worn joke to refer to business problems as opportunities and this section is not about the semantics of that old chestnut. However, we can all too easily get locked into thinking about problems and trying to solve them, instead of the potentially more

productive arena of thinking about our opportunities. Again, we stress, there is little value in just renaming the one for the other. Instead, by thinking what opportunities we have from the position we are in and exploring how we can exploit them, we might find, when we look again, that many of the problems have diminished if not evaporated altogether.

Overall meeting design

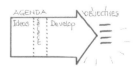

★ In preparation for a creativity meeting it is important to consider **how creative you want to be.**

☆ Do you want to be generating really wild, blue sky ideas or

☆ Do you just want to make sure you consider all the ideas currently out there, before making a decision?

☆ Being honest with yourself about the level of creativity you really require can save a lot of wasted time in the meeting.

★ **Be clear on the objective,** the end point you want to get to. Do you want to stop when you have hundreds of ideas or do you want a solution that you can implement?

★ Having decided on the level of creativity required, you can then start to think about the **appropriate methods** for the meeting. Some examples are:-

☆ Consider using problem-solving techniques – these involve clearly scoping out the problem, identifying solutions, selecting the solutions that look most promising and developing them into actionable plans.

☆ For creative idea generation there are many creativity techniques. Most of them work on the principle of getting people to be playful in their thinking and to use stimulus to get people to look for ideas in different ways.

☆ Opportunity searching is a method of generating ideas based on looking for the opportunities in a situation by viewing it from different perspectives.

★ **Plan three separate phases to being creative:**

☆ Idea generation; generating ideas with the level of creativity desired

☆ Idea selection; identifying the most promising ideas for development

☆ Idea development; working on the ideas to transform them into solutions.

★ **Consider using different people for different phases.** For example, you may choose to invite naïve participants to assist at the idea generation phase and then experts to assist with idea development.

★ **Don't expect too much in too short a time.** If you want to get to tangible, actionable solutions you need to allow 1/3 meeting time for idea generation and 2/3 meeting time for idea development.

The rest of this chapter contains specific ideas for how you could run each of these phases for a creativity meeting.

Before the meeting

★ This is one of the few types of meetings where we would not recommend speaking to all the participants in advance.

The aim is to keep the meeting spontaneous.

★ It is useful to send out **pre-meeting communication** that clarifies the overall purpose of the meeting and the logistical information for people to make travel arrangements.

★ Intriguing and creative pre-work can also help get people to the meeting in the right mindset.

An example from Ingrid: I once ran a creativity meeting to look for opportunities to save money in the pipeline of a manufacturing company. In advance of the meeting we sent an invitation to the participants that included a quote, 'Creative thinking may simply mean the realization that there is no particular virtue in doing things the way they have always been done.' With this quote in mind we asked the participants to do at least one thing differently from their usual routine on the morning of the meeting. Some people put their watches on different hands, or had a different cereal for breakfast. One brave person came with her underwear outside her clothes! But the point of the exercise was to start to get people, before the meeting, into a mindset of doing things differently.

Idea generation

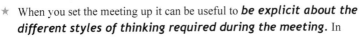

In this phase of the meeting you are aiming to get all the ideas you can from the group.

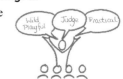

* ✷ When you set the meeting up it can be useful to **be explicit about the different styles of thinking required during the meeting.** In this initial phase of idea generation you are looking for people to say whatever ideas come into their head, without fear of being evaluated, so creating a fun, playful atmosphere is the best way to get started.

* ✷ When setting up an idea generation session it is important not to over-specify the situation. You need to give the group enough context to be able to generate ideas without getting locked into ways of thinking. A useful framework that comes from the Synectics problem-solving methodology is to answer the following questions when introducing the situation:-
  * ☆ Why we are doing this
  * ☆ Brief background
  * ☆ What we've tried already
  * ☆ Our power to act
  * ☆ My dream solution
  * ☆ Desired outcome from today

* ✷ **Warm the group up** to being playful and going with the flow before getting into generating ideas. Any fun games can be used. Here are some ideas...
  * ☆ Get into groups of 3; start with one person saying, 'Hello, please can you tell me why you have a geranium in your ear'. The person they are speaking to has to make up a reply, for example, "I was passing a lovely hanging basket and noticed this geranium matched my top, so I couldn't resist picking it and sticking it in my ear." Then ask the third person something equally ridiculous. This game rarely goes more that 1 round without lots of laughter.
  * ☆ In pairs or threes, tell a story one sentence at a time. Each person has to take a turn and work with it.

★ Use a bit of amusing video footage that sets up the meeting well and also gets the group laughing. Research has shown that being in a *humorous frame of mind* makes people think more creatively.

★ You are probably familiar with the concept of having two hemispheres to our brains, the left brain for logic and language and the right brain for artistic activity. It is thought that we are at our most creative when we *use both sides of our brain,* so getting the group to do exercises that cross both sides of the brain can help everyone physiologically to prepare for being creative. Here are some examples.

☆ Stamp, clap click – get the group into pairs. Get them to count to 3 alternately. Replace the 1 with a stamp and repeat. Then replace the 1 with a stamp and the 2 with a clap. Finally replace all 3 with stamp, clap click.

☆ Patting heads and rubbing tummies.

☆ Touching left hand to right foot and the reverse.

★ Creative puzzles can help to get the participants *looking at things differently.*

☆ Cards with hidden words on.

☆ Brainstorming weird and wonderful uses for ordinary objects e.g. paperclips, elastic bands

☆ Show the group pictures that can look like something different depending on which way you look at it. For example, the black and white picture which shows a candlestick if you look at the white space or two faces in silhouette if you look at the black.

★ When you start brainstorming ideas it is useful to remind people that there is *no evaluation* allowed at this stage in the process.

☆ For example, "In this first phase of our meeting we want to get as many ideas as possible. Later we will be selecting the most promising ones. So, in this phase it is important not to evaluate the ideas that get suggested. Let's just make sure we understand them and accurately record them."

☆ If people can't help themselves, it can be useful to remind them of this rule, "Let's not evaluate the ideas now, we will be doing that later. Let's think of more ideas first."

☆ If the group really persist in evaluating then you might want to initiate a penalty system. "To prevent ourselves from evaluating and critiquing the ideas, I am going to suggest a fine to anyone who evaluates an idea between now and the end of this session."

★ During the idea-generation brainstorm it can be useful to offer *provocations to stimulate people's thinking…..*

☆ In really creative sessions encourage participants to think of illegal, immoral or impossible ideas.

☆ Using metaphor to explore the situation differently e.g. "This situation has been referred to as fire fighting. If we were the fire brigade, what would we be doing to resolve this situation?"

☆ Taking other perspectives e.g. "How would Mickey Mouse approach this problem?"

☆ Use verbal stimulus by looking up random words in a dictionary and finding ways to relate them to ideas e.g. "How could you use a tractor (random word from dictionary) to solve this problem?"

★ Create physical stimulus by getting participants to find objects around the room to relate to ideas.
★ Use pictorial stimulus by using children's playing cards.

★ It can also be useful to let people **brainstorm individually** as well as in small groups or in the whole group.

Selection of ideas

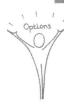

In this stage of the meeting we are looking for a few promising ideas to be selected for further development. It is important the selector(s) still keeps an open mind and doesn't just select ideas that look feasible. The idea development phase can take really blue sky ideas and turn them into something actionable.

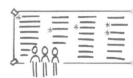

★ It is important to **be clear about how** idea selection will be done before you get into the meeting and state the process in the ground rules at the start.

★ Ideas can be selected by
  ☆ Everyone in the group
  ☆ A problem owner
  ☆ A small group (maybe experts or key stakeholders)

★ The selection process **can be done in a series of cuts** e.g. the group vote on the ideas they like the look of then the problem owner selects from this short list.

★ Voting is one way of **getting group decisions.** For more ideas see chapter 11 *Decisions that stick.*

★ At this stage you **can afford to be bold** and select ideas for development that have potential and intrigue as they are not at final idea stage yet.

★ It can also be useful to think about which **ideas people feel passionate about,** rather than thinking too logically about them.

Idea generation

This final stage of a creativity meeting is about turning the intriguing ideas that have been selected into concrete ideas with detailed actions. Some ideas to help are:-

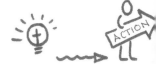

★ Plan to take longer in the idea development than the idea generation. A useful rule of thumb is to use 1/3 of your time for idea generation and **2/3 of your time for idea development.**

★ This is the point in a creativity meeting where a different type of creative skill is required and **expert knowledge** can be of great assistance here. It may be useful to invite experts to join the meeting at this stage to help figure out how to make the great ideas a reality.

★ **Create a chart for final ideas.** Examples of the categories you may have on a chart are:-

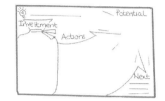

☆ What is the potential of this idea?
☆ What investment is required?
☆ How would you broadly go about implementing the idea?
☆ What are the immediate next steps?

★ For more on graphic templates see chapter 13 *Managing information.*

★ It can be useful to **subdivide** the work at this stage. Either,
☆ give the relevant jobs to the relevant experts or
☆ let people work on the ideas they are passionate about pursuing or
☆ run an open-space style workshop that has a champion for each idea and people coming in and out with different expertise.

★ **Be prepared to get creative again** e.g. if an idea is great but illegal, look for creative ways to turn it into something legal.

Summary

Our top tips for getting *creative outputs* that you can act upon are:-

★ Make sure you invite a combination of naïve and expert participants to the meeting.
★ Set the meeting up by,
☆ clarifying the objectives and agenda
☆ explaining the different thinking styles
☆ clarifying who will make the selection and how
☆ giving a brief overview of the situation and problem

★ Idea generation:
☆ Get people relaxed and playful
☆ Use provocations to stimulate thinking
☆ No evaluation allowed!

★ Selection: Have a clear selection process
★ Idea development:
☆ Use expert participants
☆ Allow 2/3 of your time for this
☆ Create charts to give a framework for it
☆ Subdivide the work.

Bibliography

'Best Practices for Facilitation' by David Sibbet

'Graphic Facilitation' by David Sibbet

'Group Graphics – Visual Tools for Working Together' by David Sibbet

'Principles of Facilitation' by David Sibbet

'The Fifth Discipline' by Peter Senge

'The Fifth Discipline Fieldbook' by Peter Senge

'The Dance of Change' by Peter Senge

'Brain Based Learning' by Eric Jensen

'Future Search' by Marvin Weisbord and Sandra Janoff

'How to make meetings work' by Michael Doyle and David Strauss

'Facilitator's Guide to Participatory Decision Making' by Sam Kaner

'Visual Language' by Robert Horn

'201 Icebreakers' by Edie West

'Coaching for Performance' by John Whitmore

'The Facilitator's Fieldbook' by Tom Justice and David Jamieson

'The Magic of Metaphor' by Nick Owen

'Open Space Technology, A Users Guide' by Harrison Owen

'Expanding our Now' by Harrison Owen

'The Handbook of Large Group Methods' by Barbara Bunker & Billie Alban

'The skilled facilitator' by Roger Schwartz

'Practical Facilitation' by Christine Hogan

'Serious Creativity' by Edward de Bono

'Opportunities' by Edward de Bono

'A Whack on the side of the Head' by Roger von Oech

'A Kick in the Seat of the Pants' by Roger von Oech

'Creative Whack Pack' by Roger von Oech

'What If – How to Start a Creative Revolution at Work' by Dave Allan, Matt Kingdon, Kris Murrin, Daz Rudkin

'Imagine' by Synectics

'The Power of Appreciative Inquiry' by Diana Whitney and Amanda Trosten-Bloom

'The Mindmap Book' by Tony Buzan